D1126346

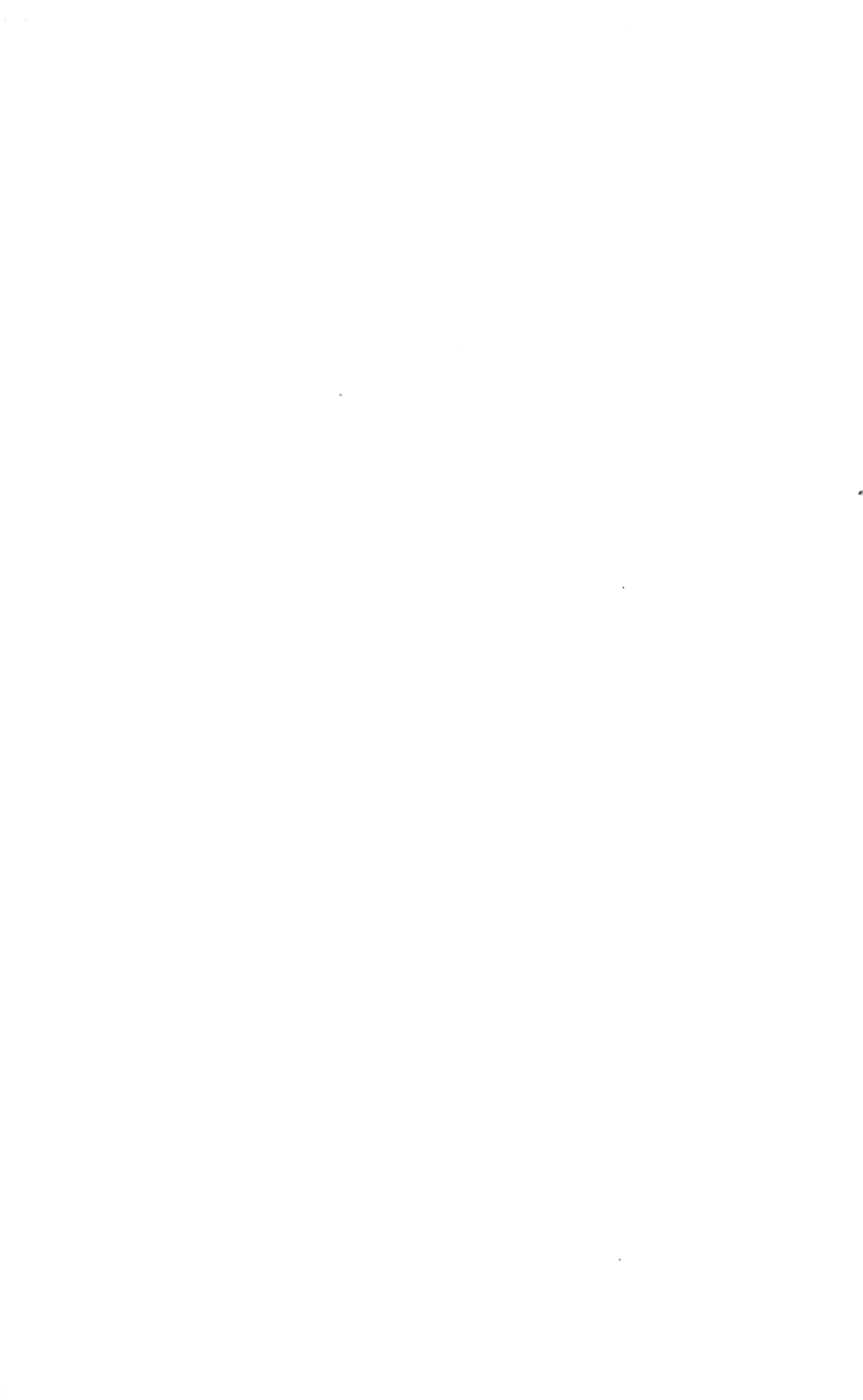

A Public Health Perspective of Women's Mental Health

Bruce Lubotsky Levin • Marion Ann Becker
Editors

A Public Health Perspective of Women's Mental Health

Foreword by Rosalynn Carter

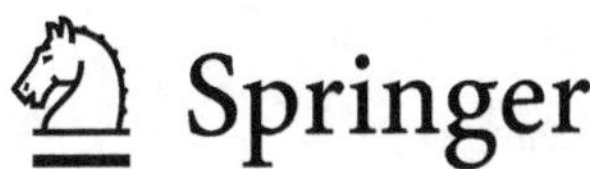

Editors
Bruce Lubotsky Levin
University of South Florida
Florida Mental Health Institute
Dept. Child & Family Studies
13301 Bruce B. Downs Blvd.
Tampa, FL 33612
USA

Marion Ann Becker
University of South Florida
Dept. Mental Health Law & Policy
13301 Bruce B. Downs Blvd.
Tampa, FL 33612
USA

ISBN: 978-1-4419-1525-2 e-ISBN: 978-1-4419-1526-9
DOI 10.1007/978-1-4419-1526-9
Springer New York Dordrecht Heidelberg London

Library of Congress Control Number: 2010921911

© Springer Science+Business Media, LLC 2010
All rights reserved. This work may not be translated or copied in whole or in part without the written permission of the publisher (Springer Science+Business Media, LLC, 233 Spring Street, New York, NY 10013, USA), except for brief excerpts in connection with reviews or scholarly analysis. Use in connection with any form of information storage and retrieval, electronic adaptation, computer software, or by similar or dissimilar methodology now known or hereafter developed is forbidden.
The use in this publication of trade names, trademarks, service marks, and similar terms, even if they are not identified as such, is not to be taken as an expression of opinion as to whether or not they are subject to proprietary rights.

Printed on acid-free paper

Springer is part of Springer Science+Business Media (www.springer.com)

Foreword

From the richest metropolis to the poorest village, mental illnesses take a devastating toll on women the world over. Mental disorders are some of the most complex, misunderstood, and stigmatized public health problems. According to the U.S. Surgeon General, mental disorders are among the leading causes of disability in America and worldwide. For example, major depression ranks second among causes of the global burden of disease and is the leading cause of disability for both women and men in the USA. Epidemiological studies reveal that approximately one-half of American women will experience a mental disorder sometime in their lives. Furthermore, these disorders are a major cause of morbidity and mortality in women.

Mental disorders weigh so heavily because they significantly disrupt daily life and negatively affect resilience to other stressors, coping strategies, and the ability to participate in work, family, and social responsibilities. These disorders can be linked to poverty and to environments and behaviors that compromise women's safety and security. The growing level of poverty among women in the USA suggests that mental disorders are likely to be an ongoing major public health problem for the foreseeable future.

While there have been recent advances in the consumer and advocacy movements as well as in psychopharmacologic and neurologic research, efforts at mental health system reform have not been adequate. Discrimination; disparities in access, quality, and outcomes of care; and unmet needs for the effective treatment of mental disorders in women remain significant challenges in our society.

A Public Health Perspective of Women's Mental Health offers a comprehensive assessment of women's mental health services. Unlike other books which tend to be more narrowly focused on clinical and treatment issues, this text synthesizes an extensive body of literature regarding epidemiology, treatment, and delivery of mental health services for women. It also presents the social context of mental disorders and the implications these issues have on women's mental health policy and services delivery.

Each chapter is written by nationally known researchers, academicians, practitioners, and advocates in the fields of women's health, mental health, and substance abuse services. The text captures both the breadth and depth of the critical issues facing women with mental and substance use disorders. *A Public Health Perspective of Women's Mental Health* is essential reading for students in a variety of academic disciplines, including public health, social work, psychology, psychiatry, education, and nursing. In addition, health and mental health practitioners will find this book an indispensable reference for teaching and clinical practice.

Rosalynn Carter
The Carter Center
Atlanta, Georgia

Preface

Introduction

A Public Health Perspective of Women's Mental Health examines major issues in the organization, financing, and provision of women's mental health services. It also presents an overview of the epidemiology of mental disorders across the lifespan of women, an in-depth discussion of selected mental and substance use disorders that particularly affect women, and includes an examination of emerging issues in women's mental health.

The idea for this text originated during the preparation of a special issue of the *Journal of Behavioral Health Services & Research (JBHS&R* Volume 32, Number 2, 2005) focusing on *The Impact of Co-Occurring Disorders and Violence on Women.* Prior to the publication of this special issue of the *JBHS&R*, virtually all published texts examined women's mental health services from a clinical and/or biomedical perspective. In addition, it became apparent to one of the editors (MB) while teaching a graduate level women's mental health course at the University of South Florida College of Public Health that despite the increased attention in the past decade to women's mental health issues, no text in the medical or behavioral health literature could be identified which offered an extensive examination of women's mental health from a public health perspective. This text attempts to respond to this gap in the literature by providing the current state of knowledge on women's mental health and examining the need for mental health services and the effect of mental disorders upon women's daily lives.

This text was developed with three objectives in mind: (1) to highlight mental health and substance use disorders of particular concern to women, (2) to emphasize services delivery and services research issues in women's mental health, and (3) to provide a discussion of these critical issues from a (multidisciplinary) public health perspective. In order to accomplish these goals, an editorial decision was made to include a diverse set of chapters, ranging from theory-driven chapters to more traditional quantitative and empirically based chapters. The result is an exceptional volume that we hope accomplishes all three objectives.

This text is particularly timely given the substantial changes in financing and services delivery of health and mental health services at the national and state levels.

In addition, this text attempts to fill the void of materials examining women's mental health services in a variety of environments, including jails and prisons, the workplace, and rural areas of America.

Nationally recognized experts in the fields of women's mental health, services research, practice, and policy were invited to prepare chapters specifically for this initiative. The chapter contributors include individuals from various areas of expertise, including public health, social work, psychiatry, public administration, sociology, clinical and social psychology, health behavior/health education, substance abuse, and education.

This text was designed for a variety of audiences, including (1) undergraduate students in the social and behavioral sciences, (2) graduate students in public health, community health and mental health, women's studies, social work, psychiatric and community health nursing, community and medical psychology, medical sociology, medical anthropology, community and social psychiatry, and other graduate and postdoctoral students in the allied behavioral health sciences, (3) professionals currently employed in mental health and substance abuse programs in various healthcare organizations, including health maintenance organizations, women's health centers, hospitals, substance abuse clinics, and community mental health centers, and (4) consumers, policymakers, advocates, and professionals involved in the fields of mental health and substance abuse services within local, state, and federal government.

Organization of the Text

The chapters in this text are organized into three basic components: Part I. *Overview and Epidemiology of Mental Disorders in Women* (Chaps. 1–5), Part II. *Selected Disorders* (Chaps. 6–10), and Part III. *Services Delivery and Emerging Research* (Chaps. 11–20).

In Chap. 1, Becker and Levin provide an introduction to the text and a look at the meaning of a public health approach to women's mental health services. Chapter 2 (Warner and Bott), Chap. 3 (Alexander and McMahon), and Chap. 4 (Kenna, Ghezel, and Rasgon) focus on the epidemiology and treatment of mental disorders in children and adolescents, adults, and older women, with an emphasis on gender differences, risk factors, symptom presentation, course of illness, and current treatment approaches. In Chap. 5, Larson and McGraw discuss the importance of providing high-quality health care for women with multiple morbidities (e.g., a combination of several chronic mental and somatic disorders). This chapter provides a succinct overview of the most common somatic conditions in women with mental disorders and focuses on important opportunities for care improvement linked to appropriate and timely detection and treatment of physical health problems for women with serious mental disorders.

In Part II of this text, *Selected Disorders* (Chaps. 6–10), the authors discuss specific mental disorders that are unique or of particular concern to women, including depression and postpartum disorders (Chap. 6—Flynn), eating disorders (Chap. 7—De Bate, Blunt, and Becker), menopause (Chap. 8—Wroolie and Holcomb), substance abuse (Chap. 9—Barry and Blow), and HIV/AIDS (Chap. 10—Frank, Knox, and Wagganer). In addition to discussing the relevant epidemiologic information, the authors provide thorough reviews of the current research and best practices regarding effective treatment and prevention strategies that must be adapted to ensure these strategies work for all women. The authors of the chapters appearing in Part II also discuss the importance of advocacy and involving women in policy development for prevention, care, treatment, and research concerning mental disorders.

Part III of this text, *Services Delivery and Emerging Research* (Chaps. 11–20) covers topics specifically selected to be complementary with each other. The authors of each chapter integrated relevant and current information to illustrate the complex interaction of the different aspects of services delivery and emerging research. The combination and wealth of information provided in Part III of this text provides a clear understanding of the strengths and challenges facing current services delivery systems and the potential impact of emerging research on future systems of care. Part III is composed of chapters covering diverse topics critical to research and the effective provision of mental health services for women.

In Chap. 11, Merrick and Reif address the insurance and financing mechanisms and approaches to quality improvement by analyzing the organization, financing, and delivery of women's mental health services in the current managed care environment. In Chap. 12, Perez, Dixon, and Kelly explore the impact of evidence-based medicine on the quality of mental health services provided to women. Veysey (Chap. 13) presents the specific mental health service needs of women who are incarcerated in US jails. The chapter documents the magnitude of this significant problem and discusses in detail the need for trauma-informed mental health services for incarcerated female populations.

In Chap. 14 (Dugan and Magley), Chap. 15 (Bloom), and Chap. 16 (Mulder, Jackson, and Jarvis) the authors examine the workplace, organization stress, and mental health services for women living and working in rural America. The authors of these chapters also discuss ways in which these settings may support or hinder accessing treatment at the community level for mental disorders.

In Chap. 17, Burke-Miller examines other social and community contexts for women's mental health. Jang, Chiriboga, and Becker (Chap. 18) present information on racial and ethnic disparities and emphasize the importance of cultural, social, economic, and geographic factors commonly associated with unique behavioral presentations that require culturally appropriate, multidimensional, and interdisciplinary responses. Burke-Miller reminds readers of the relevance of race and ethnicity and place to practice, policy, and establishing future research agendas.

In the final two chapters in this text, Nicholson (Chap. 19) and Hanson and Levin (Chap. 20) explore topics frequently missing in prior literature on women's mental health. In Chap. 19, Nicholson provides an ecological perspective on parenting and recovery for mothers with mental disorders and describes these mothers, their experiences, and needs. She extrapolates from the existing literature key components and processes of relevant interventions for mothers and their implications for mental health policy and services delivery. In the last chapter of this text (Chap. 20), Hanson and Levin present critical information on how best to navigate the diversity of knowledge that constitutes women's mental health. The authors also discuss the implications that emerging technologies and information-seeking behaviors have on women's mental health research, services delivery, and policy.

Although space does not permit an examination of all relevant topics and issues in women's mental health, this text emphasizes the importance of establishing a public health perspective for the study of women's mental health. We hope that this multidisciplinary framework will assist individuals from various disciplines to join in future research, services delivery, and policy making efforts in women's mental health.

Acknowledgements

We would like to thank some of the individuals who have provided encouragement, support, and consultation throughout the preparation of this text. In particular, we would like to express our gratitude to Mario Hernandez, Larry Schonfeld, Tom Massey, and Junius Gonzales at the University of South Florida for their ongoing encouragement of our work. We also owe a great deal of appreciation to Ardis Hanson at the University of South Florida who created the subject index for this text. We would also like to extend a special thanks to Diana Lima and Annie DeMuth at the University of South Florida for their tremendous assistance in the preparation of this text as well as Bill Tucker, Khristine Queja, and Ian Marvinney at Springer Publications for their valuable suggestions during the editing of this text.

Finally, we would like to express our deep appreciation and thanks to our families and friends for their love, understanding, and support, particularly throughout the preparation of this text. We dedicate this text to our families and friends, with a special dedication to Sophie Anne Levin.

Bruce Lubotsky Levin
Marion Ann Becker

Contents

Editors and Contributors

Bruce Lubotsky Levin, DrPH, MPH

Bruce Lubotsky Levin is Associate Professor and Head of the Graduate Studies in Behavioral Health Program at the Louis de la Parte Florida Mental Health Institute and at the College of Public Health (COPH), both at the University of South Florida (USF). Dr. Levin is Editor-in-Chief of the *Journal of Behavioral Health Services & Research* and Director of the USF Graduate Certificate in Mental Health Planning, Evaluation, and Accountability Program. He is the Senior Editor of *Mental Health Services: A Public Health Perspective, Third Edition* (Oxford University Press, 2010), *Introduction to Public Health for Pharmacists* (Jones & Bartlett, 2007), *Mental Health Services: A Public Health Perspective, Second Edition* (Oxford University Press, 2004), *Women's Mental Health Services: A Public Health Perspective* (Sage Publications, 1998), and *Mental Health Services: A Public Health Perspective* (Oxford University Press, 1996). He is also Co-Editor of the text *Building a Virtual Library* (Information Science Publishing, 2003). In 2001, Dr. Levin received the Harold C. Piepenbrink Award for outstanding contributions to behavioral health services from the Association of Behavioral Healthcare Management. Dr. Levin earned his undergraduate degree from the University of Wisconsin-Madison and his graduate degrees from the University of Texas. His research interests include managed behavioral health care, mental health policy, graduate behavioral health education, and mental health informatics. He currently teaches graduate behavioral health courses at the USF COPH.

Marion Ann Becker, PhD, MA, RN

Marion Ann Becker is a Professor in the Department of Aging and Mental Health Disparities at the University of South Florida (USF) Louis de la Parte Florida Mental Health Institute. She also holds appointments in the USF School of Social Work, USF College of Public Health, and USF College of Nursing, where she teaches a number of graduate-level courses, including the epidemiology of mental disorders, women's mental health, and case management. Dr. Becker is a psychiatric nurse with a doctorate in Social Welfare from the University of Wisconsin-Madison. Her research focuses on the problems of providing high quality, cost-effective behavioral health services and quality of life outcomes for vulnerable populations.

Dr. Becker is the developer of the Wisconsin Quality of Life Index (W-QLI), a core development in quality of life outcomes research in mental health. In 1997, she received the National Alliance for the Mentally Ill (NAMI) Research Award for her quality of life outcomes research. Dr. Becker has served as Principal Investigator and Co-Principal Investigator on numerous outcome studies. Most recently, she served as Co-Principal Investigator and Lead Evaluator for the Triad Women's Project, a multimillion dollar competitive federal grant designed to create and evaluate specialized interventions for women with alcohol and drug abuse problems and mental disorders who have histories of interpersonal violence. Dr. Becker continues her research focus on women's mental health, quality of life outcomes across the life span, and linking outcomes research to clinical practice.

Mary Jane Alexander, PhD
Mary Jane Alexander is a senior research scientist in the Statistics and Health Services Division of the Nathan Kline Institute in Orangeburg, NY. She is the Director and Principal Investigator of the National Institute of Mental Health funded Center to Study Recovery in Social Contexts. She has worked in collaboration with service users and survivors in research on social recovery, including opportunities for parenting, measures of well-being, and models of healing from trauma, and with public policy makers and foundations to develop strategies and tools to integrate services for co-occurring mental health and substance use problems.

Kristen Lawton Barry, PhD
Kristen Lawton Barry is a Research Associate Professor in the Department of Psychiatry and an investigator at the Department of Veterans Affairs (VA) National Serious Mental Illness Treatment Research and Evaluation Center. She has a number of active and pending National Institutes of Health university-based grants and VA grants. Dr. Barry's primary research foci include substance use screening and brief interventions in emergency and primary care medical care settings, substance use problems in older adults, and treatment efficacy for adults with co-occurring mental health and substance use disorders. She was the Chair of the Substance Abuse and Mental Health Services Administration Treatment Improvement Protocol "Brief Interventions and Brief Therapies for Substance Abuse". She has extensive experience developing curriculum for research and training projects. She has developed curriculum on substance use for the National Institute on Alcohol Abuse and Alcoholism, targeting training of medical personnel and social workers.

Sandra L. Bloom, MD
Sandra L. Bloom is a Board-Certified psychiatrist and is an Associate Professor of Health Management and Policy at Drexel University School of Public Health. She is President of Community Works, an organization committed to the development of nonviolent environments. Dr. Bloom served as Founder and Executive Director of the Sanctuary: inpatient psychiatric programs for the treatment of trauma-related emotional disorders.

Frederic C. Blow, PhD

Frederic C. Blow is Professor and Director of the Mental Health Services Outcomes and Translation Section in the Department of Psychiatry at the University of Michigan Medical School, and Director of the National Serious Mental Illness Treatment Research and Evaluation Center for the Department of Veterans Affairs, Ann Arbor, MI. In addition, he is the first National Huss/Hazelden Research Co-Chair for the Butler Center for Research at the Hazelden Foundation. Dr. Blow is a national expert in mental health and substance abuse services research and policy, with a focus on older adults. His areas of research expertise include substance abuse prevention from a lifespan developmental perspective, alcohol screening and diagnosis for older adults, mental disorders and concurrent substance abuse, alcohol and drug abuse brief interventions in healthcare settings, and mental health services research. He was the Chair of the Substance Abuse and Mental Health Services Administration Treatment Improvement Protocol "Substance Abuse in Older Adults." Dr. Blow has been the principal investigator on numerous federal, state, and foundation grants and has published extensively in the areas of substance abuse and alcoholism among the elderly, substance abuse screening/treatment, and mental health.

Heather Blunt, BA, MPH

Heather Blunt received an honors bachelor of arts in psychology from the University of Waterloo in 2005 and continued on to earn an MPH from the University of South Florida (USF). Ms. Blunt is now a doctoral student in the Graduate Studies in Behavioral Health Program in the Department of Community and Family Health at the USF College of Public Health. Ms. Blunt's dissertation and research interests focus on adolescent sexual and emotional health.

Cynthia Bott, LCSW

Cynthia Bott is a doctoral student in the School of Social Welfare at University at Albany. Her experience includes clinical practice with adolescents and families, field supervision of a major research project with BTW Consultants, Inc., and teaching graduate students in social welfare with San Francisco State University.

Jane Burke-Miller, PhD

Jane Burke-Miller has extensive professional experience in mental health services research and statistical methods. Her mental health services research has focused on disabling social structures, in particular, the role of poverty as a barrier to recovery. She is author of numerous peer-reviewed journal articles and book chapters, and has presented at national and international research conferences, federal project meetings, and consumer/advocacy organizations. She is skilled in multilevel statistical analysis, including mixed effects and generalized estimating equation models. Her doctoral dissertation employed multilevel statistical methods to combine census and survey data in an innovative examination of local-area variations in depressive symptomatology among African-American women.

David Chiriboga, PhD
David Chiriboga received his PhD from the University of Chicago in 1972. He has served on the faculty at the University of California San Francisco and the University of Texas Medical Branch in Galveston, TX. Currently, he is a Professor in the Department of Aging and Mental Health Disparities at the University of South Florida Louis de la Parte Florida Mental Health Institute. His work has three overlapping and continuing themes. The first involves the longitudinal study of the significance of stress exposure for mental health over periods of 20 or more years. The second involves the longitudinal study of differential mental health disparities across minority and majority populations. The third involves the use of technologies associated with distance education/telemedicine for healthcare and the training of health professionals. His current work includes a statewide study of mental and physical health disparities in Florida, disparities in service utilization among Medicaid beneficiaries with Alzheimer's disease, as well as a state-contracted study of prevalence and best practices with regard to mental health disparities.

Rita DiGioacchino DeBate, PhD, MPH, CHES
Rita DiGioacchino DeBate is an Associate Professor in the Department of Community & Family Health, College of Public Health, at the University of South Florida. She has a background in health behavior/health education and public health. Her research interests include obesity and eating disorders. She has authored numerous articles on body image, physical activity, and secondary prevention of eating disorders. She is the program evaluator for Girls on the Run, a developmentally focused youth sport program. She is also the Principal Investigator of a National Institutes of Health funded study to develop a training program for dental professionals on secondary prevention of eating disorders.

Lisa B. Dixon, MD, MPH
Lisa B. Dixon is Professor of Psychiatry and Director of the Division of Mental Health Services Research at the University of Maryland School of Medicine. She is also the Associate Director of Research at the VA Capitol Health Care Network Mental Illness Research, Education, and Clinical Center. Dr. Dixon earned her undergraduate degree in economics at Harvard University and her medical degree at the Cornell University Medical College in New York City. She completed her internship and residency in psychiatry at the New York Hospital Payne Whitney Clinic. From 1989 to 1990, Dr. Dixon was a research fellow at Maryland Psychiatric Research Center in Catonsville, Maryland, and subsequently earned a Master's in Public Health from Johns Hopkins Bloomberg School of Public Health. Dr. Dixon has authored/coauthored over 150 peer-reviewed articles concerning schizophrenia and services for families. She has also been Principal Investigator for numerous National Institute of Mental Health, National Institute on Drug Abuse, and Veteran Affairs funded studies concerning optimizing the quality of care for persons with schizophrenia and other mental illnesses. Her research has focused on diabetes, smoking cessation, reducing obesity, hepatitis, HIV, as well as overall

self-management. She has active partnerships with the educational arm of the National Alliance on Mental Illness with whom she studies how to provide services for families. Dr. Dixon previously was Director of Education and Residency Training in the Department of Psychiatry at the University of Maryland, and is currently a Vice Chair of the University of Maryland Institutional Review Board.

Alicia G. Dugan, MA, LMHC

Alicia G. Dugan is currently completing her doctoral work in Industrial/Organizational Psychology at the University of Connecticut, with a concentration in Women's Studies and Occupational Health Psychology. Prior to studying Psychology, she worked as a licensed mental health clinician in employee assistance programs and work–family services. Her current research centers on psychosocial stress and health outcomes associated with overwork, time pressure, work–life conflict, and self-care.

Heather A. Flynn, PhD

Heather A. Flynn is a clinical psychologist and an Assistant Professor in the Department of Psychiatry at the University of Michigan. She is also an adjunct faculty in the Department of Psychology at the University of Michigan. Dr. Flynn's research is focused on improved identification and treatment of depression in women, especially around the time of childbearing. Her research focus is developing and testing psychotherapeutic treatments for depression around the time of pregnancy, and examining the impact of depression remission on obstetric and infant outcomes. She is currently the Director of Psychotherapy Services in Adult Psychiatry at the University of Michigan. Dr. Flynn leads a multidisciplinary clinical team in Psychiatry specializing in the assessment and treatment of mood and related disorders during pregnancy and postpartum.

Linda Rose Frank, PhD, MSN, ACRN

Linda Rose Frank earned her PhD in Higher Education in 1990 and a Master's Degree in Psychiatric Mental Health Nursing in 1983 from the University of Pittsburgh. She is currently an Associate Professor in the Department of Infectious Diseases and Microbiology and Director of the Community and Behavioral Intervention for Infectious Diseases MPH Program at the University of Pittsburgh Graduate School of Public Health. She is also an Associate Professor in the Division of Health and Community Systems at the University of Pittsburgh School of Nursing. Her academic work has focused on HIV/AIDS, mental health, prison and jail health, healthcare system capacity building, and evaluation studies of educational intervention with health professionals.

Talayeh Ghezel

Talayeh Ghezel is a senior at Stanford University majoring in Human Biology. After graduation, she plans on attending medical school. Her research interests involve the genetics–environment interaction in disease processes.

Megan Holcomb, MS, MBA

Megan Holcomb's academic training includes clinical assessment in neuropsychology, women's health, aging, and sleep disturbance. In addition, she has training in business and human resources. Ms. Holcomb earned her Bachelor's and Master's degrees in Business Management from William Woods University, and will receive her PhD in Clinical Psychology in 2010 from Pacific Graduate School of Psychology.

Robert W. Jackson, MA

Robert W. Jackson is a doctoral student in the Marshall University Psy.D. program in Huntington, West Virginia. Mr. Jackson received his Master's degree in clinical psychology from Morehead State University in 1995. Raised in rural, southeastern Kentucky, Mr. Jackson spent several years serving as a mental health professional addressing the needs of the residents of that region before making the decision to continue his education by pursuing his doctorate.

Yuri Jang, PhD

Yuri Jang is an Associate Professor in the Department of Aging and Mental Health Disparities at the Louis de la Parte Florida Mental Health Institute, University of South Florida. Dr. Jang received her doctoral degree in Aging Studies from the University of South Florida in 2001. Dr. Jang was awarded Minority Fellowships from the Gerontological Society of America and the American Psychological Association. Her current areas of interest include positive adaptation in aging, health disparities, and minority mental health and service utilization.

Sarah Jarvis, MA

Sarah Jarvis, a doctoral student enrolled in the Marshall University Psy.D. program in Huntington, West Virginia, was raised and educated in Virginia. Academically and professionally, her interests are in behavioral medicine and geriatrics. She plans to focus on serving the mental and behavioral health needs of residents of underserved, rural areas. Sarah has recently successfully defended her doctoral dissertation and is completing her internship at Charleston Area Medical Center in Charleston, West Virginia.

Deanna L. Kelly, PharmD, BCPP

Deanna L. Kelly is an Associate Professor of Psychiatry and Director of the Treatment Research Program at the Maryland Psychiatric Research Center, University of Maryland School of Medicine. Dr. Kelly is an Associate Editor for the journal *Clinical Schizophrenia and Related Psychoses.* Her research interests include the treatment of schizophrenia, women's health issues, and comorbid health problems in people with mental illness. She has published over 75 articles, books, and book chapters and has presented over 150 invited lectures and scientific posters. She is currently Principal Investigator of a contract with the National Institute on Drug Abuse to study substance use in mental illness.

Heather A. Kenna, MA

Heather A. Kenna is a Senior Research Associate in the Department of Psychiatry and Behavioral Sciences and a clinical psychology doctoral student at Pacific

Graduate School of Psychology. Her primary research interests are in neuroendocrine dysregulation in mood and cognitive disorders and the development of interdisciplinary treatments for depression and cognitive dysfunction.

Michael D. Knox, PhD

Michael D. Knox earned his PhD in psychology from the University of Michigan in 1974. He is currently a Distinguished Professor of Mental Health Law and Policy, Medicine, Global Health, Psychology, and Aging Studies at the University of South Florida (USF). He is Founder and Director of the Florida/Caribbean AIDS Education and Training Center and the USF Center for HIV Education and Research. Dr. Knox is a Fellow of the American Psychological Association and the Association for Psychological Science. His academic work has focused on issues of HIV/AIDS, death and dying, ethics, and peace studies.

Mary Jo Larson, PhD, MPA

Mary Jo Larson is a Senior Scientist at the Institute for Behavioral Health, Schneider Institutes for Health Policy at Brandeis University. She has authored research and evaluation articles on many aspects of women's behavioral health, including the co-occurrence of mental health and substance use disorders, the presence of physical disabilities among women in treatment for mental health or substance use conditions, and the training of clinicians in using effective-based practices.

Rosalynn Carter

Former First Lady Rosalynn Carter has been a driving force in the field of mental health throughout her public service career. She was a member of the Governor's Commission to Improve Services to the Mentally and Emotionally Handicapped when her husband was governor of Georgia. As active honorary chair of the *President's Commission on Mental Health* during President Carter's administration, she helped bring about passage of the Mental Health Systems Act of 1980.

In 1985, she initiated the Rosalynn Carter Symposium on Mental Health Policy, which brings together representatives of mental health organizations nationwide to focus and coordinate their efforts on key issues. Since then, annual symposia held at The Carter Center have investigated such topics as mental illness and the elderly, child and adolescent illness, family coping, financing mental health services and research, treating mental illness in the primary care setting, and stigma and mental illness. Responding to the need for local collaboration, she instituted in 1996 an annual Georgia Mental Health Forum for professionals and consumers statewide. The Carter Center Mental Health Task Force, chaired by Mrs. Carter and comprised of individuals in a position to affect public policy, meets quarterly to identify policy initiatives and set the agenda for The Carter Center Mental Health Program and annual symposia. With the inception of the Rosalynn Carter Fellowships for Mental Health Journalism in 1996, Mrs. Carter launched one of the most successful national programs in combating the stigma associated with mental illnesses.

Mrs. Carter published *Helping Yourself Help Others: A Book for Caregivers* co-authored with Susan Golant in 1994. Following on the success of her caregiving book, Mrs. Carter teamed up with Susan Golant to write *Helping Someone with Mental Illness: A Compassionate Guide for Family, Friends, and Caregivers*. Building on her 25 years' experience in the field, Mrs. Carter discusses the latest treatments and research generated from her symposia and in consultation with the major mental health organizations in the United States. She also addresses how best to help those with illnesses such as depression, schizophrenia, manic depression, panic attacks, and obsessive-compulsive disorders by being an effective, compassionate caregiver and advocate. *Helping Someone with Mental Illness* was selected as the winner of the 1999 American Society of Journalists and Authors Outstanding Book Award in the service category.

Ardis R. M. Hanson, MLS

Ardis R. M. Hanson is the Head of the Research Library at the Louis de la Parte Florida Mental Health Institute at the University of South Florida (USF). She received her bachelor's degree in Fine Arts from the University of Tampa and her Master's Degree in Library Science from the University of South Florida. Interested in the use of technology to enhance research, she developed the web site for the Library and the Institute in 1993 and, as Institute Webmaster, created a number of specialized research resources for Institute and Internet users. Ms. Hanson has co-presented at Internet2 and been a participant in a number of informatics projects, from portal development to resource directories. She is Senior Editor of the text *Building a Virtual Library* (Information Science Publishing, 2003) and co-author of the text *Integrating Geographic Information Systems into Library Services* (IGI Publishing, 2008). Ms. Hanson has published (with Bruce Lubotsky Levin) extensively on mental health services. She currently teaches graduate behavioral health courses at the USF College of Public Health and is pursing her doctoral degree in health and organizational communication.

Vicki J. Magley, PhD

Vicki J. Magley is an Associate Professor in the Department of Psychology at the University of Connecticut in Storrs, CT. The main focus of her research lies within the domain of occupational health psychology and combines organizational and feminist perspectives in the study of workplace mistreatment. Some specific interests include examining the effects of self-labeling experiences as sexual harassment, outcomes that are associated with experiencing sexual harassment (for both men and women), the effectiveness of sexual harassment training programs, the buffering impact of an intolerant climate for sexual harassment on outcomes, and coping with sexual harassment. Complementing her work on sexual harassment, she has more recently been examining the incidence and effects of nonsexualized, yet uncivil work experiences.

Sarah McGraw, PhD

Sarah McGraw is a Principal Research Scientist in the Center for Applied Ethics within the Education Development Center, Inc., an international nonprofit research and development organization. Trained as a medical anthropologist, her work has spanned a range of topics from disease prevention to health services. Dr. McGraw's recent research concerns health disparities and the evaluation of programs serving populations experiencing chronic homelessness as well as primary care for high-risk individuals with a history of substance use and mental illness. Underlying all of Dr. McGraw's work is an interest in health and access to quality care among minority and disenfranchised populations.

Caitlin McMahon, BA
Caitlin McMahon is a Research Associate in the Division of Alcoholism and Drug Abuse in the Department of Psychiatry at the New York University School of Medicine. She is a graduate of the University of Chicago. Her research interests have been in the role of spirituality in medical treatment, in psychotherapeutic approaches for substance use problems, and in the integration of quantitative and qualitative research methods in order to address the mental and physical health needs of underserved populations, particularly women.

Elizabeth Levy Merrick, PhD, MSW
Elizabeth Levy Merrick is Senior Scientist at the Institute for Behavioral Health at Brandeis University's Heller School for Social Policy and Management. Dr. Merrick is a clinical social worker with a doctorate in social policy who has conducted behavioral health services research for the past 15 years. Her research on mental health and substance abuse services includes a focus on managed care in the public and private sectors, treatment access, and quality of care.

Pamela Mulder, PhD
Pamela Mulder is a Professor of Clinical Psychology teaching in the APA accredited Psy.D. program at Marshall University in Huntington, West Virginia and the senior editor of the *Journal of Rural Community Psychology*. Her research interests, publications, and clinical practice are all focused on addressing the mental and behavioral health care needs of women in Appalachia and other rural regions of the USA. Dr. Mulder received her PhD in clinical psychology at California School of Professional Psychology, Fresno in 1991.

Joanne Nicholson, PhD
Joanne Nicholson is a clinical and research psychologist and Professor of Psychiatry at the University of Massachusetts Medical School (UMMS). She directs the Child and Family Research Core of the UMMS Center for Mental Health Services Research. Dr. Nicholson has established an active program of research on parents with mental illnesses and their families in partnership with people in recovery. Dr. Nicholson has received funding from the National Institute on Disability and Rehabilitation Research, the Substance Abuse and Mental Health Services Administration, the National Alliance for Mental Illness Research Institute, private foundations, and industry sources. In 2006, she received the Armin Loeb Award from the U.S. Psychiatric Rehabilitation Association for her significant career contribution to research in psychiatric rehabilitation. Dr. Nicholson was a W.T. Grant Foundation

Distinguished Fellow from 2005 to 2008, and an NIDRR Switzer Distinguished Research Fellow from 2008 to 2009. She was the recipient of the first UMMS Department of Psychiatry Steven M. Banks Award for Outstanding Research Mentoring in October, 2008.

Gina Perez, MD

Gina Perez earned her medical degree from the University of Pittsburgh School of Medicine and continued at Western Psychiatric Institute and Clinic for her residency training in General Adult Psychiatry. Upon completion of her training, she joined the faculty at the University of Maryland School of Medicine, where she now serves as an Assistant Dean for Student Affairs and as an Assistant Professor of Psychiatry. Her clinical focus is helping individuals with severe psychiatric illnesses in inner city settings. She has a passion for medical education and enjoys teaching on several psychiatric and wellness topics within the medical school and the community.

Natalie L. Rasgon, MD, PhD

Natalie L. Rasgon is a Professor of Psychiatry and Behavioral Sciences and Obstetrics and Gynecology at Stanford University School of Medicine and Director of the Stanford Center for Neuroscience in Women's Health. She is a clinical specialist in women-specific mental health, and has published over 200 articles and book chapters. Her research interests are focused on the neuroendocrine pathophysiological pathways in mood and cognitive disorders in women.

Sharon Reif, PhD

Sharon Reif is a Research Scientist and the Deputy Director of the Institute for Behavioral Health at the Brandeis University Heller School for Social Policy and Management. Dr. Reif has nearly 20 years of experience conducting research primarily related to substance abuse treatment focused on the treatment system, what happens to clients during and after treatment, and how that relates to the providers who treat them, as well as access to and financing of both substance abuse and mental health services.

Bonita Veysey, PhD

Bonita Veysey is an Associate Professor in the School of Criminal Justice at Rutgers University-Newark. Prior to her employment at Rutgers, Dr. Veysey was a Senior Research Associate at Policy Research Associates in Delmar, New York. During that time, she was the Director of the Women's Program Core and the Associate Director of the National GAINS Center and a primary researcher in the area of mental health–criminal justice systems interactions. Dr. Veysey's research to date has focused on behavioral health and justice issues, including police interactions with persons with mental illnesses, mental health and substance abuse treatment in jails and prisons, diversion and treatment services for youth with behavioral health problems, and the effects of trauma.

Annie M. Wagganer, MA

Annie M. Wagganer received her MA in Sociology from the University of South Florida (USF). She is a Research Specialist for the USF Center for HIV Education and Research, as well as an Instructor of Sociology at St. Louis Community College. Her sociological research involves issues of gender, identity, and the relationship between health, beauty standards, and manipulation of the body.

Lynn Warner, MPP, MSW, PhD

Lynn Warner is an Associate Professor at the School of Social Welfare, University at Albany-SUNY. She received an MPP from the Kennedy School of Government at Harvard University, and MSW and PhD degrees from the University of Michigan. She was a National Institute of Mental Health postdoctoral research fellow at the Institute for Health, Health Care Policy and Aging Research at Rutgers University. Dr. Warner's research is focused on understanding patterns of psychiatric vulnerability, including substance abuse and mental illness, as well as the comorbidity between them in order to identify strategies for interventions with vulnerable populations such as low-income women and Latinos. Current projects examine developmental patterns in the use of psychotropic medications and organizational influences on the implementation and adoption of regulatory changes in behavioral health services.

Tonita Wroolie, PhD

Tonita Wroolie is a Clinical Instructor at Stanford Center for Neuroscience in Women's Health, Department of Psychiatry & Behavioral Sciences, Stanford University School of Medicine where she leads the Neurocognitive Assessment Clinic. She is also adjunct faculty at Pacific Graduate School of Psychology in Palo Alto, California. She earned her PhD in Clinical Psychology at Pacific Graduate School of Psychology and her MA in Health Psychology at Stanford University. Her postdoctoral fellowship in neuropsychology was at the Veteran's Affairs Palo Alto Health Care System.

Part I
Overview & Epidemiology of Mental Disorders in Women

Chapter 1
Public Health and Women's Mental Health

Marion Ann Becker, Bruce Lubotsky Levin and Ardis R. M. Hanson

Introduction

Mental disorders are significant contributors to the global burden of disease. Worldwide, it is estimated that approximately 450 million people suffer from a mental disorder (World Health Organization 2001). In developing countries, mental disorders are second only to cardiovascular diseases in contributing to lost years of life (World Health Organization 2003). Although mental disorders have a potential impact upon all individuals, it is important to recognize gender differences in the rates, experience, and course of mental disorders. For example, a recent Substance Abuse and Mental Health Services Administration (SAMHSA) report states that:

> Women are nearly twice as likely as men to suffer from major depression, which is associated with problems such as lost productivity, higher morbidity from medical illness, greater risk of poor self-care or poor adherence to medical regimens, and increased risk of suicide. Perinatal depression affects an estimated 8–11 percent of women during pregnancy and 6–13 percent of mothers in the first post partum year. Rates of anxiety disorders are two to three times higher in women than in men; this includes post-traumatic stress disorder, which affects women more than twice as often as men. Women represent 90 percent of all cases of eating disorders, which carry the highest mortality rate of all mental disorders (*Action steps for improving women's mental health* 2009, p. 5).

Furthermore, Pratt and Brody (2008) examined data from the 2005–2006 National Health and Nutrition Examination Survey (NHANES). "NHANES is a continuous cross-sectional survey of the civilian, noninstitutionalized US population designed to assess the health and nutrition of Americans" (Pratt and Brody 2008, p. 5). The sample for 2005–2006 included approximately 5,000 people of all ages. Pratt and Brody (2008) analyzed the survey results and found a higher percentage of women (6.7%) 12 years of age and older with depression compared to men (4%) with depression. In addition, less than a third of NHANES respondents reporting depressive symptoms sought care from a mental health professional.

M. A. Becker (✉)
Department of Aging & Mental Health Disparities, Louis de la Parte Florida Mental Health Institute, University of South Florida, Tampa, FL 33612, USA

B. L. Levin, M. A. Becker (eds.), *A Public Health Perspective of Women's Mental Health*,
DOI 10.1007/978-1-4419-1526-9_1, © Springer Science+Business Media LLC 2010

Women with mental disorders not only have higher morbidity and mortality rates but are also more at risk for the underdiagnosis of major physical illnesses (McCabe and Leas 2008). In response to current epidemiologic data, the principle that "there is no health without mental health" is gaining ground. Efforts to transform America's public mental health delivery systems to ones that are more person-centered, recovery-focused, evidenced-based, and quality-driven are intensifying (Power 2009).

Due, in part, to the Surgeon General's report on mental health (US Department of Health & Human Services 1999), the efforts of the World Health Organization (2001), and the President's New Freedom Commission on Mental Health (2003), a broader framework for health has been advocated, which emphasizes the idea that disease goes beyond its clinical dimensions. This broader framework makes it essential that public health practitioners, policy makers, consumers, and advocates understand the extent and distribution of mental disorders and disability in order to develop policies and practices that reduce health disparities and contribute to people's daily activities and participation in society (President's New Freedom Commission on Mental Health 2003; World Health Organization 2009).

Chapter Objectives

This chapter, as well as this text, examines a number of critical issues in women's mental health and substance abuse from a multidisciplinary, public health perspective. This chapter focuses on the essential elements of a public health perspective, outlines some major concerns in women's mental health, and sets the stage for the presentation of chapters in three basic areas: (1) an overview of the epidemiology of mental disorders throughout the lifespan of women; (2) a discussion of selected mental and substance use disorders of particular concern to women; and (3) the identification of major issues in services delivery and emerging research in women's mental health.

A Public Health Approach

Historically, teaching, research, and academics have been structured around specific disciplines, each with its own nomenclature, conceptual approaches, literature base, target audiences, and application strategies. However, thus far, outside the field of public health, minimal efforts have been devoted to a multidisciplinary approach to solving problems. One of the core concepts underlining a public health approach or perspective is a focus on the health of an entire population or population at risk. Approximately 90 years ago, Winslow (1920) defined public health as:

> The science and art of preventing disease, prolonging life, and promoting health and efficiency through organized community effort for the sanitation of the environment, the

> control of communicable infections, the organization of medical and nursing services for the early diagnosis and prevention of disease, the education of the individual in personal health and the development of the social machinery to assure everyone a standard of living adequate for the maintenance or improvement of health (pp. 6–7).

Accordingly, a public health approach involves an emphasis on health promotion and disease prevention throughout the lifespan. It takes into consideration a multidisciplinary framework for examining health and mental health problems. The World Health Organization (2009) states that a public health approach includes the following four steps:

1. Define the problem through the systematic collection of information about the magnitude, scope, characteristics, and consequences of a disorder;
2. Establish why the disorder occurs using research to determine the causes and correlates of the disorder, the factors that increase or decrease the risk for the disorder, and the factors that could be modified through interventions;
3. Find out what works to prevent the disorder by designing, implementing, and evaluating interventions; and
4. Implement effective and promising interventions in a wide range of settings. The effects of these interventions on risk factors and the target outcome should be monitored, and their impact and cost-effectiveness should be evaluated (p. 1).

Recently in the USA, mental health consumers advocated the following public health framework for organizing and providing mental health services in Massachusetts (*A public health framework for the state mental health authority* 2006): (1) consumer and family participation; (2) a focus on quality of life issues; (3) assuring staff accountability; and (4) collecting and maintaining useful data.

We suggest that a public health perspective that encompasses multidisciplinary approaches to mental health and emphasizes opportunities for prevention and early intervention will be more likely to reduce the burden of mental illnesses in women. This approach is preferred since it is not individually focused but population based and encompasses important social, cultural, economic, and environmental factors that impact women's health.

Selected Issues: Women and Mental Health

In the material that follows in this chapter and in the chapters in this volume, selected issues of particular importance to women's mental health are discussed. All chapters include a discussion of the current challenges facing the treatment of women with mental disorders and suggestions for overcoming these challenges. Finally, each chapter concludes with an "Implications for Women's Mental Health" section, discussing the importance of each chapter topic to the overall field of women's mental health.

Epidemiology and Health Disparities

Despite increased attention and promising advances in the science and practice of women's mental health, disparities based on gender, race, ethnicity, and socioeconomic status persist, and women continue to have a higher risk than men for mental disorders (Schulz and Mullings 2006). While there is now a greater recognition of the role of mental health in the overall health of individuals and considerable progress in our understanding and treatment of mental illnesses, the prevalence of mental disorders reported by women in the USA may actually be increasing (see Chap. 5 in this volume). In fact, in the most recent revised national comorbidity replication study, the profile for persons with any mental disorder in the prior year was being female, Hispanic, or African American, with less than a college education, low income, not currently cohabitating, and living in a rural area (Kessler et al. 2005c).

In addition to being more common, mental disorders are the leading cause of morbidity in women and the second leading cause in men (U.S. Department of Health & Human Services 1999). Furthermore, the negative impact of mental disorders on overall health and life is similar worldwide (Murray and Lopez 1996; World Health Organization 2004). Data show that about one-half (48.5%) of American women report a mental disorder in their lifetime, and about a third (30.9%) report a disorder in the prior year (Kessler et al. 2005b).

According to the SAMHSA, about 44 million adults and 13.7 million children have a diagnosable mental disorder. However, less than half of the adults and only about 33% of the children receive mental health treatment (President's New Freedom Commission 2003; U.S. Department of Health & Human Services 1999). Although prevalence rates vary depending on the study, age of the population, and methods used across the lifespan, researchers have consistently reported higher rates of mental disorder for females compared with males. Researchers note that starting in early adolescence, rates of mental disorder increase for both genders, but the rates for adolescent females double (Kessler et al. 2005a; Hankin and Abramson 2001; Saluja et al. 2004; Twenge and Nolen-Hoeksema 2002; Wade et al. 2002). Explanations for these differences are not fully known and require continued research. For a more thorough discussion of the epidemiology of mental disorders, see Chap. 2 (girls and adolescents), Chap. 3 (adults), and Chap. 4 (older adults) in this volume. Also see Chap. 5 for an additional discussion of the epidemiology of co-occurring disorders in women.

Services Delivery

The President's New Freedom Commission on Mental Health (2003) identified fragmentation of mental health delivery systems as one of the three major obstacles impeding the treatment of mental disorders in the USA. This has direct implications for issues of access and the utilization of effective mental health care for both primary and mental health care providers. In order to improve the access to and quality of mental health care, the New Freedom Commission suggests that a transformation of mental health service systems is needed to eliminate disparities in mental health, provide mental health education and disease prevention initiatives, and develop (and implement) an integrated information technology and communications infrastructure. This would include the integration of medical records and surveillance systems for identifying mental health needs and disparities (*Action steps for improving women's mental health* 2009).

Health Literacy

Health literacy addresses the ability of an individual to understand information (e.g., diagnostic, treatment, medication, protocols, and lifestyle change) provided by a health or mental health care professional (e.g., physician, nurse practitioner, pharmacist, physician's assistant, and rehabilitation specialist). An expanded model of health literacy also includes the ability of consumers to frame questions about, and acknowledge an understanding of, the health information provided. As treatment becomes more complex with evidence-based practices and new psychopharmacological agents, health literacy becomes even more important in the treatment of physical and mental disorders.

Trauma, Violence, and Abuse

There continues to be increasing evidence regarding the high prevalence of trauma, violence, and abuse against women. Emerging areas of concern are the growing population of incarcerated women, female veterans, and active female military personnel who are exposed to trauma, violence, and abuse with limited access to mental health services. These individuals frequently suffer from posttraumatic stress disorder (PTSD). For example, it has been reported that as many as 30% of women were raped during their military services (Tjaden and Thoennes 2000; Zinzow et al. 2007) compounding the heavy burden already experienced by female veterans and their families. Thus, there is a critical need for new initiatives to address both the short- and long-term effects of trauma, violence, and abuse experienced by women.

Action Steps for Improving Women's Mental Health

Collaborative efforts by a number of federal agencies to affect positive changes and promote progress to improve the mental and overall health of the nation's women and girls are detailed in *Action steps for improving women's mental health* (2009). This report, issued by the National Mental Health Information Center, mirrors international action plans suggested by the World Health Organization (2005, 2003). Among other things, the action steps encourage nations to "Promote a recovery-oriented, strengths-based approach to treatment for women …" (*Action steps for improving women's mental health* 2009, p. iii) and "Build resilience and protective factors to promote the mental health of girls and women and aid recovery" (*Action steps for improving women's mental health* 2009, p. iii).

Implications for Women's Mental Health

Despite an increase in life expectancy and a variety of new medications for more effective treatment of mental disorders, women continue to face increased vulnerability and gender-based risks for major depression, PTSD, and anxiety disorders. In addition, women with mental disorders continue to face significant social stigma and discrimination. Since mental and substance use disorders begin in childhood and adolescence, successful efforts in prevention and early intervention should be initiated during this critical time period.

Concurrently, there is a growing need for the provision of mental health services for women who are incarcerated in jails and prisons as well as the increasing number of women in the military. These at-risk populations create an increased demand on communities, states, and federal health care systems to provide greater access to effective and affordable mental health services for women.

As acknowledged by the World Health Organization (2003), we now have an opportunity to improve access to, and the quality of, mental health services for women. However, given the dramatic reductions in state (financial) support for health, education, and social services, it remains to be seen if this opportunity will be realized. Nevertheless, the recommendations of the President's New Freedom Commission (2003) and the *Action steps for improving women's mental health* (2009) have established a blueprint for continued progress. The hope in America and around the world is that health care reform, currently under consideration in America, will lead to positive changes for women's mental health and result in the implementation of the action steps to improve women's mental health that were widely disseminated by SAMHSA in 2009.

References

A public health framework for the state mental health authority. (2006). Roxbury, MA: Consumer Quality Initiatives.

Action steps for improving women's mental health. (2009). Rockville, MD: Office on Women's Health, Substance Abuse and Mental Health Services Administration. Retrieved July 27, 2009, from http://download.ncadi.samhsa.gov/ken/pdf/OWH09-PROFESSIONAL/ActionSteps.pdf

Hankin, B. L., & Abramson, L. Y. (2001). Development of gender differences in adolescent depression: An elaborated cognitive vulnerability-transactional stress theory. *Psychological Bulletin, 127*(6), 773–796.

Kessler, R. C., Berglund, P., Demler, O., Jin, R., Merikangas, K. R., & Walters, E. E. (2005a). Lifetime prevalence and age-of-onset of DSM-IV disorders in the National Comorbidity Survey Replication. *Archives of General Psychiatry, 62*(6), 593–601.

Kessler, R. C., Berglund, P., Demler, O., Jin, R., Merikangas, K. R., & Walters, E. E. (2005b). Lifetime prevalence and age-of-onset: Distributions of DSM-VI disorders in the National Comorbidity Survey Replication. *Archives of General Psychiatry, 62*, 593–602.

Kessler, R. C., Chiu, W. T., Demler, O., & Walters, E. E. (2005c). Prevalence, severity, and comorbidity of 12-month DSM-IV disorders in the National Comorbidity Survey Replication. *Archives of General Psychiatry, 62*, 617–627.

McCabe, M. P., & Leas, L. (2008). A qualitative study of primary health care access, barriers and satisfaction among people with mental illness. *Psychology, Health & Medicine, 13*(3), 303–312.

Murray, C. J. L., & Lopez, A. D. (1996). *The global burden of disease.* Geneva: World Health Organization, Harvard School of Public Health, World Bank.

Power, K. (2009). A public health model of mental health for the 21st century. *Psychiatric Services, 660*(5), 580–584.

Pratt, L. A., & Brody, D. J. (2008, September 3). *Depression in the United States household population, 2005–2006.* NCHS Data Brief, 7:3, September, 2008. Retrieved July 27, 2009, from http://www.cdc.gov/nchs/data/databriefs/db07.pdf

President's New Freedom Commission on Mental Health. (2003). *Achieving the promise: Transforming mental health care in America. Final Report.* Rockville, MD: Department of Health and Human Services Publication Number SMA-03-3832. Retrieved July 27, 2009, from http://www.mentalhealthcommission.gov/reports/FinalReport/toc.html

Saluja, G., Iachan, R., Scheidt, P. C., Overpeck, M. D., Sun, W., & Giedd, J. N. (2004). Prevalence and risk factors for depression among young adolescents. *Archives of Pediatrics Adolescent Medicine, 158*(8), 760–763.

Schulz, A. J., & Mullings, L. (Eds.). (2006). *Gender, race, class & health: International approaches.* San Francisco, CA: Jossey-Bass.

Tjaden, P., & Thoennes, N. (2000). *Full report of the prevalence, incidence, and consequences of violence against women: Findings from the National Violence Against Women Survey.* Washington, DC: National Institute of Justice and Center for Disease Control and Prevention.

Twenge, J. M., & Nolen-Hoeksema, S. (2002). Age, gender, race, socioeconomic status, and birth cohort differences on the children's depression inventory: A meta-analysis. *Journal of Abnormal Psychology, 11*(4), 578–582.

U.S. Department of Health and Human Services. (1999). *Mental health: A report of the surgeon general.* Rockville, MD: U.S. Department of Health and Human Services, Substance Abuse and Mental Health Services Administration, Center for Mental Health Services, National Institutes of Health, National Institute of Mental Health. Retrieved July 27, 2009, from http://www.surgeongeneral.gov/library/mentalhealth/home.html#forward

Wade, T. J., Cainey, J., & Pevalin, D. J. (2002). Emergence of gender differences in depression during adolescence: National panel results from three countries. *Journal of the American Academy of Chile and Adolescent Psychiatry, 4*(2), 190–195.

Winslow, C.-E. A. (1920). The untilled field of public health. *Modern Medicine, 2*, 1–9.

World Health Organization. (2001). *The world health report, 2001: Mental health: New understanding, new hope.* Geneva, Switzerland: World Health Organization. Retrieved July 27, 2009, from http://www.who.int/mental_health/en/investing_in_mnh_final.pdf

World Health Organization. (2003). *Investing in mental health.* Geneva, Switzerland: World Health Organization. Retrieved July 27, 2009, from http://www.who.int/mental_health/en/investing_in_mnh_final.pdf

World Health Organization. (2004). *World health report 2004: Changing history* (pp. 126–131). Geneva, Switzerland: World Health Organization. [Annex Table 3: Burden of disease in DALYs by cause, sex, and mortality stratum in WHO regions, estimates for 2002]. Retrieved July 27, 2009, from http://www.who.int/whr/2004/en/report04_en.pdf

World Health Organization. (2005). *Mental health action plan for Europe: Facing the challenges, building solutions.* Helsinki, Finland: World Health Organization. Retrieved July 27, 2009, from http://www.euro.who.int/Document/MNH/edoc07.pdf

World Health Organization. (2009). *The public health approach.* Geneva, Switzerland: World Health Organization. Retrieved July 27, 2009, from http://www.who.int/violenceprevention/approach/public_health/en/

Zinzow, H. M., Grugaugh, A. L., Monnier, J., Suffoletta-Malerie, S., & Frush, B. C. (2007). Trauma among female veterans. *Trauma, Violence, & Abuse, 8*(4), 384–400.

Chapter 2
Epidemiology of Mental Disorders in Girls and Female Adolescents

Lynn A. Warner and Cynthia Bott

Introduction

Childhood and adolescence are critical periods for the early identification of psychiatric symptoms and prevention of many mental disorders, including disruptive behavior, mood, and anxiety disorders. Substantial evidence is accumulating from longitudinal birth cohort studies and nationally representative surveys to suggest that there are developmental trajectories of psychiatric problems, many of which onset at young ages. Consequently, effective interventions during early life stages have the potential to support the positive neurobiological, cognitive, and psychosocial development that is needed for successful transitions from youth to adulthood. Epidemiologic studies can help inform priorities for service delivery by identifying the extent to which symptoms remit or develop into disorders during childhood and adolescence, the disorders that may be limited to this age range versus those that persist into adulthood, and the disorders that onset in adulthood for which symptoms may have manifested earlier.

The primary purpose of this chapter is to provide an overview of the prevalence and patterns of mental disorders specifically among girls and female adolescents, with special attention to variations across age (see Chaps. 3 and 4 in this volume on the epidemiology of mental disorders in adult women and older adult women, respectively). The epidemiologic focus on one gender is warranted for three reasons: (1) gender differences in rates of mental disorders among adults likely developed at young ages; (2) the influence of gender roles and expectations on the expression and interpretation of externalizing (behavioral) and internalizing (emotional) symptoms, which are believed to be more common among boys and girls, respectively; and (3) gender as a modifier of the illness risk and protective factors that have been identified at genetic, neurobiological, and psychosocial levels. The focus on

L. A. Warner (✉)
School of Social Welfare, University at Albany,
SUNY, 135 Western Avenue,
Richardson Hall, Albany, NY 12222, USA

B. L. Levin, M. A. Becker (eds.), *A Public Health Perspective of Women's Mental Health*,
DOI 10.1007/978-1-4419-1526-9_2, © Springer Science+Business Media LLC 2010

females is needed because, as will become obvious in the rest of the chapter, the preponderance of our knowledge about mental illness in the early stages of the life course is based on samples of males only, or samples of both males and females with the results reported for both genders together.

The chapter begins with a brief description of key epidemiologic research design issues that facilitate interpreting results on children and youth, and highlights methodological concerns of special relevance for girls and female adolescents. This background information establishes the extent to which results from disparate studies can be compared to one another and, by helping evaluate the strengths and limitations of our knowledge base, reveals areas for future research.

The authors then synthesize findings from studies focused on three diagnostic categories (i.e., attention deficit and disruptive behavior, mood, and anxiety) that capture some of the highest prevalence disorders, and most disabling in terms of morbidity and mortality. A fourth category, eating disorders, is included because of its unique relevance for adolescent females. It is beyond the scope of this chapter to summarize knowledge about substance use and disorder among female youth. However, readers are directed to Chap. 9 in this volume as well as to Armstrong and Costello (2002), who review community studies of comorbidity among adolescents with substance use disorders, including studies of gender differences.

In the final portion of this chapter, the authors identify research priorities and implications for the delivery of mental health services to girls, female adolescents, and women.

Epidemiologic Research and Sensitivity to Girls and Female Adolescents

The primary objective of this chapter was to identify studies of nonclinical samples (i.e., household or school samples) that focused exclusively on females or reported estimates separately by gender. While there are many studies based on pediatric and adolescent mental health treatment samples that address issues for girls and female adolescents, youths in these studies are likely to have the most serious problems, and selection effects would skew the estimates upward. Because of the rarity of community-based studies of preschool-aged children, however, the authors retained studies that recruited children from general medical practices.

Given the rapid changes children and adolescents experience as they age and the multiple contexts in which development occurs, there has been increasing recognition that diagnostic schemes need to be sensitive to the ways developmental stage affects symptom manifestation. For example, in 1994 a consensus group of early childhood development and mental health experts published the first Diagnostic Classification of Mental Health and Developmental Disorders of Infancy and Early Childhood, and revised it in 2005 (DC: 0–3R; Zero to Three 2005). Other research evaluates the reliability and validity of assessment tools for disorders in young children (Sterba et al. 2007), including depression (Stalets and Luby 2006), bipolar (Biederman et al. 2003), obsessive-compulsive (Merlo et al. 2005), anxiety (Seligman et al. 2004), posttraumatic stress (Lonigan et al. 2003), and disruptive behavior (Keenan et al. 2007) disorders.

The emphasis in most measurement and assessment studies has been on identifying age-appropriate measurements, with very little attention placed on investigating the possibility that different measures may be needed for boys and girls. Currently, boys and girls are evaluated using identical criteria that have typically been normed on samples of boys. Using this approach to measure symptoms of conduct and behavior disorder may potentially capture only the most serious cases among girls, thus underestimating their rate of disorder. The opposite approach would use completely different criteria for boys and girls, based on the assumption that normative gender differences do manifest in symptoms of disorder. With this approach, a greater number of girls might be screened as having a disorder, but they would be less impaired than boys. Studies that apply impairment criteria along with diagnostic criteria to calculate prevalence estimates essentially exclude the less serious cases, as was the result when inclusion of impairment criteria significantly reduced the prevalence of any mental disorder for both male and female adolescents in a community sample (Romano et al. 2001) and in a large sample of households enrolled in a health maintenance organization (Roberts et al. 2007).

In addition to assessment complexities presented when diagnosing children and youths across different developmental age periods, it has been acknowledged that multiple informants (e.g., parents, teachers, doctors, and youths themselves) may be needed for at least two reasons. First, at very young ages, children are not able to report reliably on their symptoms, especially if they are asked to report on symptoms experienced at times other than the most recent (Angold and Costello 1995). Second, different informants may be needed to provide a comprehensive understanding of symptom presentation and associated level of impairment when children are at home versus in other social settings. However, studies have shown that different informants will yield different estimates (Romano et al. 2001; Fergusson et al. 1993), presenting an ongoing challenge for researchers who seek to capture multiple dimensions of mental illness in one prevalence estimate, and highlighting concerns about who the most reliable reporter may be.

Similar to the orientation toward male standards in the research on measurement and nosology, a modest amount of research has examined the possibility that informants may have their own gender biases. For example, different informants yielded different prevalence rates of disruptive and antisocial behavior for girls (Hipwell et al. 2002), and teachers' ratings systematically identified more male students than female students with disruptive disorders (Reid et al. 2000). Additionally, Manassas (2006) has argued that fearfulness may be underreported by parents of boys because of greater social acceptability and tolerance of fearfulness expressed by girls and gender role expectations regarding femininity.

The operationalization of "age" itself is a final methodological issue that may bear on interpreting estimates from most epidemiologic studies aiming to specify gender-specific rates of disorder at different life stages. Community- and school-based samples most often use chronological age or grade level as criteria on which to select samples or to demarcate important transition stages in analyses. However, the onset of menarche is an additional measurement of age that may be particularly important for girls. For example, the frequency of panic attacks increased after puberty among girls (Hayward and Essau 2001), and higher rates of anxiety symptoms and disorders occur among girls who reach puberty at younger ages than their peers (Caspi and Moffitt 1991). Additionally, analysis of data from the Minnesota Twin Family Study (MTFS) revealed that girls who had an early age of menarche (before age 11) had higher rates of adolescent conduct disorder (CD) symptoms than those with average (age 12–13) or late onset (after 13) menarche (Burt et al. 2006). If data from the same girls had been analyzed according to grade level alone, there may have been no discernable differences in CD symptoms for girls in seventh versus eighth grade.

Overall, substantial data collection investments have been made that are beginning to allow empirical specification of the development of mental illness during childhood and adolescence. Studies of twins and birth cohorts followed longitudinally, sometimes for decades, allow identification of trajectories and continuity, whereas large cross-sectional studies representative of different age groups inform population-based prevalence estimates. Nevertheless, it is not yet possible to provide a comprehensive picture of female-specific developmental patterns of mental illness because of the dearth of studies that focus on girls and female adolescents. For the purposes of this chapter, it was necessary to incorporate findings from studies based on mixed gender samples, and to briefly address gender differences in the epidemiology of mental disorders. However, because of unanswered questions about the potential extent of gender bias in assessments and other methodological criteria as presented here, caution is warranted in assuming that results from mixed gender samples generalize to all-female populations, or that the magnitudes of gender-based prevalence differences are stable.

Prevalence of Disorders Among Girls and Female Adolescents

In this portion of the chapter, the authors present an epidemiologic overview of four specific diagnostic categories: (1) attention-deficit and disruptive behavior; (2) anxiety disorders; (3) affective disorders; and (4) eating disorders. For each specific diagnostic category, information is presented first about age- and gender-related patterns, followed by selected information on comorbidity between the focal disorder and disorders in other diagnostic categories. The comorbidity estimates are provided with an acknowledgment of the uncertainty in measuring comorbidity among youths, given the possibility that it reflects a unique classification of mixed disorders (Angold et al. 1999a) or a disorder of multiple dysfunction (Zoccolillo 1992).

To interpret data on specific diagnoses in the sections below, it is helpful to have basic information about the prevalence of mental illness and onset patterns among youth in general. In terms of overall estimates, Costello and colleagues (1998) compiled seven data sets to estimate rates of serious emotional disturbance (i.e., psychiatric diagnosis with significant impairment), with resulting prevalence of 5.7% and 5.6% for girls and boys, respectively. Analysis of data from the longitudinal Great Smoky Mountains Study (GSMS) indicates that male and female children who have a mental disorder before age 13 compared to those who do not are significantly more likely to have a mental disorder at age 16, but the likelihood is significantly greater for girls than for boys (Costello et al. 2003). This result is consistent with higher rates of any mental disorder among females compared to males (15.5% vs. 8.5%) in another community sample of adolescents between 14 and 17 years (Romano et al. 2001).

There are three additional points that provide a context for understanding the summaries within a developmental epidemiology framework. First, data consistently show that early stages of the life course, from birth to young adulthood, are key periods for the identification, prevention, and treatment of mental illness. Retrospectively reported survey data from the National Comorbidity Survey Replication (NCS-R) indicate that mental disorders began by age 14 for one-half of the people who ever had a mental illness, and by the age of 24 for three-quarters of them (Kessler et al. 2005). Similarly, according to respondents in a prospective longitudinal birth cohort, three-quarters of adults had a diagnosis before age 18 (Kim-Cohen et al. 2003).

Second, lengthy follow-up periods in longitudinal studies allow analysis of the long-term consequences of psychosocial risk and protective factors, as well as the persistence of internalizing and externalizing symptoms. For example, prenatal and postnatal characteristics, such as very low birth weight (LBW) compared to normal birth weight, have been shown to be associated with significantly greater psychopathology in young adulthood (Dawson et al. 2000; Hack et al. 2004). Data from the 1946 British birth cohort, followed at ages 13, 15, 36, 43, and 53, showed that delays in achieving early developmental milestones, such as standing and walking, increased the likelihood of experiencing anxiety and depression symptoms, even controlling for childhood social circumstances and life events (Colman et al. 2007).

Third, each diagnosis has its own extensive literature describing the risk and protective factors that play a role in the etiology of the disorder, with increasing attention to the multiple levels at which the factors are expressed (genetic, hormonal, biological, psychosocial, and environmental). It is beyond the scope of this chapter to provide a comprehensive review of diagnosis-specific risk profiles, but it is worth pointing out that several studies also demonstrate nonspecific associations between risk and psychopathology in general. See, for example, the review of longitudinal studies on the association between childhood trauma and psychopathology (Pine and Cohen 2002), and the twin study that demonstrates genetic and environmental influences on a majority of diagnoses (Ehringer et al. 2006).

As a companion to the information presented in the specific diagnostic categories below, Table 2.1 highlights the studies that offered female-specific prevalence estimates and summarizes their key design features. The entries are listed alphabetically by author rather than by diagnosis because many studies reported on

Table 2.1 Studies on the prevalence of psychiatric disorders in girls and female adolescents: Study details

Study	Location	Sample size & age	Diagnostic system & instrument(s) & informant(s)	Prevalence
Angold et al., 2002	North Carolina Schools	438 9–17 years	DSM-IV/ICD-10 CBCL/CAPA Parent/Child	0.9% P3M ADHD 2.9% P3M CD 2.8% P3M DD 7.1% P3M AD
Bird et al., 1988	Puerto Rico Households	189 4–16 years	DSM-III CBCL/DISC/CGAS Parent/Teacher/Child	9.9% P6M OD 9.5% P6M ADD 5.9% P6M DD 4.7% P6M SAD
Brown et al., 1996[a]	Western Oregon Schools	889 14–18 years	DSM-III-R K-SADS Child	18.4% LT MD 8.4% LT AD 7.3% LT DBD (At Time 1)
Cohen et al., 1993[a]	Upstate New York Households	260 10–13 years 262 14–16 years 224 17–20 years	DSM-III-R DISC Parent/Child	2.3% (10–13); 7.5% (14–16); 2.7% (17–20)—MD 8.5% (10–13); 6.5% (14–16); 6.2% (17–20)—ADD 3.8% (10–13); 9.2% (14–16); 7.1% (17–20)—CD 10.4% (10–13); 15.6% (14–16); 12.5% (17–20)—OD
Costello et al., 2003[a]	Great Smokey Mountains Study	3,005 9–16 years	DSM-IV CAPA Parent/Child	31.0% Any LT disorder 12.1% LT AD 11.7% LT DD 16.1% LT DBD
Dey et al., 2004	United States Households	12,524 under 18 years	NHIS "If ADHD had been reported to family by doctor or other health professional"	4% ADHD
Deykin et al., 1987	Boston area	271 6–19 years	DSM-III-R DIS Child	6.8% LT MD

Table 2.1 (continued)

Study	Location	Sample size & age	Diagnostic system & instrument(s) & informant(s)	Prevalence
Disney et al., 1999	Minnesota Twin Family Study	674 17 years	DSM-III-R DICA-R/CIDI Mother/Child	4.7% LT ADHD 13.1% LT CD 1.2% LT ADHD/CD
Feehan et al., 1994	Dunedin Multidisciplinary Health and Development Study—New Zealand	454 at age 18 years	DSM-III-R DIS Significant other/Child	2.6% PY GA; 1.1% PY PD 14.8% PY Social Phobia; 8.8% PY Simple Phobia 4.8% PY OCD 4.0% PY MD; 4.6% PY Dysthymia 2.2% PY CD
Fergusson et al., 1993	Christchurch Health and Development Study—New Zealand	961 birth – 15 years	DSM-III-R DISC/DIS/RBPC Mother/Child/Teacher	9.7% Mood Disorders 9.5% CD 2.7% ADHD
Hipwell et al., 2002	Pittsburgh, PA Households	2,451 5–8 years	DSM-IV CGAS/CSI/SRA/AS Parent/Teacher/Child	5.4% (5); 4.1% (6); 5.1% (7); 4.3% (8)—PY ADHD 4.3% (5); 3.5% (6); 4.7% (7); 4.0% (8)—PY ODD 2.8% (7); 2.4% (8)—PY CD
Jensen et al., 1995	US Military Households	135 6–17 years	DSM-III-R DISC/CBCL/CES-D/CDI/RCMAS Parent/Child	25.2% P6M AD 4.3% P6M DD 20.0% P6M ADHD 5.2% P6M ODD 1.9% P6M CD
Kashani et al., 1987	Columbia, MO Schools	75 14–16 years	DSM-III DICA Parent/Child	8% CD
Kessler and Walters, 1998	The National Comorbidity Survey—US Households	900 15–24 years (unweighted N)	DSM-III-R CIDI	8.0% PM MD 16.1% PY MD 20.6% LT MD

Table 2.1 (continued)

Study	Location	Sample size & age	Diagnostic system & instrument(s) & informant(s)	Prevalence
Kilpatrick et al., 2003	National Survey of Adolescents—US Households	1,904 12–17 years (unweighted N)	DSM-IV NWS Child	6.3% P6M PTSD
Lahey et al., 2000	MECA New Haven, CT Puerto Rico Atlanta, GA Westchester, NY Households	604 9–17 years	DSM-III-R DISC Parent/Child	5.2% (9–11); 3.5% (12–14); 1.0% (15–17)—PY ODD 1.4% (9–11); 4.5% (12–14); 3.6% (15–17)—PY CD
Leaf et al., 1996	MECA New Haven, CT Puerto Rico Atlanta, GA Westchester, NY Households	1,285 9–17 years	DSM-III-R DISC/CGAS Parent/Child	5.6% (9–12); 7.4% (13–17)—Any P6M DISC diagnosis
Lewinsohn et al., 2000	Oregon Adolescent Depression Project—Schools	T1 = 891 (high school or below age 24) T2 = 810 (high school or below age 24) T3 = 538 (age 24)	DSM-III-R/DSM-IV K-SADS/CES-D Child	1.3% (T1); 2.3% (T2); 4.0 (T3)—PY AN or BN
Offord et al., 1987	Ontario, Canada Households	1,345 4–16 years 721 4–11 years 624 12–16 years	DSM-III CBCL Parent/Child/Teacher	1.8% (4–11); 4.1% (12–16)—P6M CD 3.3% (4–11); 3.4% (12–16)—P6M Hyperactivity
Pine et al., 2001[a]	Upstate New York Households	388 9–18 years 380 11–20 years 358 17–26 years	DSM-III-R DISC Parent/Child	4.7% (9–18); 10.1% (11–20); 17.8% (17–26)—MD 4.2% (9–18); 12.6% (11–20); 8.2% (17–26)—Social Phobia 11.5% (9–18); 9.5% (11–20); 32.1% (17–26)—Specific Phobia

Table 2.1 (continued)

Study	Location	Sample size & age	Diagnostic system & instrument(s) & informant(s)	Prevalence
Romano et al., 2001	Quebec, Canada Community sample	578 14–17 years	DSM-III-R DISC Mother/Child	15.5% Any DSM-III-R Diagnosis
Stice et al., 2004[a]	Southwest US Schools	496 11–15 years	DSM-IV EDE/K-SADS Child	1.6% (T1); 2.4% (T2); 1.8% (T3)—PY BN; 8.1% (T1); 9.7% (T2); 6.5% (T3)—PY MD
Wu et al., 1999	MECA New Haven, CT Puerto Rico Atlanta, GA Westchester, NY Households	604 9–17 years	DSM-III-R DISC/CGAS Parent/Child	4.3% DD 5.0% DBD 2.6% DD & DBD

Sample size is reported for girls and female adolescents only. When multiple informants are noted, the prevalence rates reflect the estimates derived from parents' reports. Unless otherwise specified, the reporting period for diagnoses was not reported. If a study used impairment criteria, estimates are reported based on diagnostic criteria only.

Abbreviations of instruments: AS = Antisocial Behavior Scale; CAPA = Child and Adolescent Psychiatric Assessment; CBCL = Child Behavior Checklist; CES-D = Center for Epidemiologic Studies Depression Scale; CDI = Children's Depression Inventory; CGAS = Children's Global Assessment Scale; CIDI = Composite International Diagnostic Interview; CSI = Child Symptom Inventory; DICA = Diagnostic Interview for Children and Adolescents; DIS = Diagnostic Interview Schedule; DISC = Diagnostic Interview Schedule for Children; EDE = Eating Disordered Examination; K-SADS = Schedule for Affective Disorders and Schizophrenia for School-Age Children; NWS = National Women's Study; RBPC = Revised Behavior Problems Checklist; RCMAS = Revised Children's Manifest Anxiety Scale; SRA = Self-Reported Antisocial Behavior Scale

Abbreviations of reporting periods: PM = past month; P3M = past 3 months; P6M = past 6 months; PY = past year; LT = lifetime

Abbreviations of diagnoses: AD = anxiety disorders; ADD = attention deficit disorder; ADHD = attention deficit hyperactivity disorder; AN = anorexia nervosa; BN = Bulimia Nervosa; CD = conduct disorder; DBD = disruptive behavior disorder; DD = depressive disorder; GA = generalized anxiety; MD = major depression; OCD = obsessive-compulsive disorder; OD = oppositional disorder; ODD = oppositional defiant disorder; PD = panic disorder; PTSD = posttraumatic stress disorder; SAD = separation anxiety disorder

[a] Longitudinal study

more than one disorder. A brief review of the table underscores the wide variability in age ranges and populations represented, assessment tools used, time frame for diagnostic reporting (e.g., past month, lifetime), informants (e.g., parents, teachers, children) and, if longitudinal, in follow-up periods. In particular, there is notable variation in the recall periods used for reporting prevalence estimates, including lifetime, past year, past 6 months, and past 3 months. Some of the variability is to be expected given the age ranges of the study respondents. For example, "lifetime" and "recent" may be a clinically meaningful distinction for an older adolescent, whereas current status (i.e., past month or past 3 months) may be the only meaningful period for a preschooler. The estimates included in the remaining sections of the chapter are "current" prevalence rates, unless otherwise stated. In addition, the chronological ages that correspond to different life stages are not entirely consistent, but in general, "early childhood" covers ages 0–3 years, "preschool" ages 3–5 years, "childhood" ages 5–11 years, and "adolescence" ages 12–18 years.

Attention-Deficit and Disruptive Behavior Disorders

Disruptive behavior disorders include attention deficit/hyperactivity disorder (ADHD), which is marked by inattention and impulsivity, CD, and oppositional defiant disorder (ODD; Rapoport and Ismond 1996). A CD diagnosis is based on persistent patterns of violations of rules, including aggression toward people and animals and destruction of property, whereas an ODD diagnosis speaks of negative, hostile, or defiant behavior. Notably, an ODD diagnosis is not given if a child or adolescent meets criteria for CD.

According to a systematic review of 102 general population and school-based studies of ADHD prevalence around the world, the pooled prevalence estimate for respondents 18 years or younger was 5.3% (Polanczyk et al. 2007). A higher prevalence rate (8.7%) for the USA has been reported based on data from the 8–15-year-old participants, assessed with DSM-IV criteria, in the cross-sectional 2001–2004 National Health and Nutrition Examination Surveys (Froehlich et al. 2007).

ADHD symptoms most likely onset before school age and rates of diagnosis increase as children age, although prospective studies of nonclinical preschool-aged populations are sufficiently rare that these conclusions should be treated tentatively. According to one of the few studies of disorder among a preschool population, the combined estimate for boys and girls between ages 3 and 5 years was 2% (Lavigne et al. 1996). Estimates between 3 and 5% in studies of elementary school students (Shepard et al. 2000) and between 6 and 9% for adolescents (Anderson et al. 1987; Bird et al. 1988) have been reported.

Rates of CD and ODD among very young children are difficult to find. The Environmental Risk Longitudinal Twin Study estimated a CD prevalence rate of 6.6% among 4.5 to 5-year olds (Kim-Cohen et al. 2005). Symptoms of CD occur before adolescence, between 5 and 8 years for both boys and girls (Lahey et al. 1998), with the onset of disorder in late childhood for boys and in early adolescence for girls

(Cohen et al. 1993). CD prevalence estimates for female adolescents have ranged from 4% (Cohen et al. 1993) to 9% (Zoccolillo 1993).

The CD median onset age reported by respondents aged 18 years and older in the NCS-R was 11.6 years, with lifetime CD prevalence of 7.1% among females and 12.0% among males (Nock et al. 2006). Given the mixture of cross-sectional studies of adults retrospectively reporting symptoms of disorder, and longitudinal studies of children of all ages, it is challenging to determine whether early onset CD persists and additional cases occur as people age, or if the early onset cases remit and are replaced by people at older ages, all of whom are new cases. On the other hand, modest evidence about the persistence of externalizing disorders, measured as an aggregate category, comes from a study of children (aged 4–9 years) recruited from pediatric primary care. The disorder persisted for approximately one-third of the girls with a disorder at baseline (Briggs-Gowan et al. 2003). Additionally, there was no change in ODD prevalence in a pediatric sample recruited at ages 2– 5 years and reinterviewed 4–6 years later (Lavigne et al. 2001). By adulthood, the lifetime prevalence of ODD is 9.2% among females and 11.2% among males (Nock et al. 2007).

Studies that provide insight into gender-based patterns in these diagnoses show that ADHD is between two and three times more common in boys than in girls. According to Polanczyk et al. (2007), the pooled ADHD prevalence estimate for females was close to 5% and 10% for males, with substantial variability in both estimates depending on the age ranges studied and diagnostic systems used. A review of research on CD and ODD reports that, like ADHD, rates of CD tend to be higher among boys compared to girls, whereas rates of ODD are roughly comparable (Loeber et al. 2000).

There are also gender-specific patterns in the symptoms that young males and females are likely to experience, although more research in this area appears to have been devoted to ADHD symptoms compared to CD or ODD symptoms. Results of a meta-analysis suggest that girls with ADHD had lower ratings on hyperactivity, inattention, impulsivity, and externalizing problems compared to boys with ADHD, but greater intellectual impairments and more internalizing problems (Gershon 2002). A few exceptions to this pattern have been noted. For example, Reid et al. (2000) reported a no-difference finding in ADHD symptoms among students aged 5–18 years. Greater impairment among girls compared to boys was also found in a small study (Rucklidge and Tannock 2001); among youths between ages 13 and 16 with ADHD, girls were more impaired than boys on the basis of self-reported anxiety, distress, depression, locus of control, and vocabulary scores.

It is somewhat unclear when gender differences emerge, although distinct ADHD trajectories have been noted as starting around age 6 years or upon entrance to school (Shepard et al. 2000), and higher CD prevalence among boys was consistent across 5–15-year olds in the cross-sectional British Child Mental Health Survey (Maughan et al. 2004). Similarly, there is ambiguity about the degree to which male–female disruptive behavior disorder rates continue to diverge during adolescence, or possibly converge during the transition from childhood to adolescence (Loeber et al. 2000). When boys and girls who had subthreshold conduct-related problems at ages

5 through 10 years were compared at ages 8 through 13, boys (25%) were more likely than girls (7%) to have CD (Messer et al. 2006).

Very high rates of comorbidity among the disruptive behavior disorders have been documented. Newcorn and Halperin (2000) estimated that between 40 and 70% of children with ADHD have ODD or CD. All three diagnoses (ADHD, ODD, and CD) are highly comorbid with anxiety disorders, with some variation in strength depending on the specific externalizing–anxiety pair (Marmorstein 2007). For example, approximately one-quarter of youth with ADHD have an anxiety disorder (Biederman et al. 1991). In a sample restricted to female twins, depression was a prevalent diagnosis among those with CD (Marmorstein and Iacono 2001). As expected, given gender differences in prevalence rates of disruptive disorders, comorbidity patterns vary as well (Boylan et al. 2007; Loeber et al. 2000).

Longitudinal studies help specify the temporal patterns among these comorbidity patterns. Early onset and high levels of disruptive behaviors in elementary school girls predicted CD in adolescence (Coté et al. 2001). Similarly, based on the 25-year longitudinal study of a New Zealand birth cohort, conduct problems at ages 7–9 years were associated with higher rates of substance dependence for males and females (Fergusson et al. 2005). Additionally, the MTFS showed that for boys and girls between ages 11 and 14, any symptom of ADHD or CD was a risk for substance use disorder at age 18 (Elkins et al. 2007).

Studies that emphasize girls' comorbidity patterns show that CD increases later risk of anxiety disorder (Zoccolillo 1993), and among girls between ages 6 and 18 recruited from doctors' offices, those with ADHD compared to those without ADHD are more likely to have depression, ODD, substance use disorder, and anxiety 5 years later (Biederman et al. 2006). The GSMS longitudinal survey of children from 9 to 16 years old showed that ODD is not associated with later CD in girls as it was for boys (Rowe et al. 2002). However, patterns among girls showed that there were strong associations between earlier ADHD and later ODD, and earlier CD and later substance abuse (Costello et al. 2003).

Anxiety Disorders

Aggregate anxiety disorder estimates from mixed gender samples of youth in community settings range from 2.4 to 17.7% (Ollendick et al. 2001). Another review of published studies of anxiety disorders in children below 12 years found a range of 2.6–41.2%, and separation anxiety disorder (SAD) appeared to be most prevalent (Cartwright-Hatton et al. 2006). The broad range is due in part to the types of anxiety disorders that a given study evaluated, and usually include some combination of SAD, generalized anxiety disorder (GAD), specific phobia, social phobia, panic disorder (PD), posttraumatic stress disorder (PTSD), and obsessive-compulsive disorder (OCD). Impairment criteria tend to have been applied in studies of anxiety disorder more than in studies of other types of mental disorder. For example, Kashani and Orvaschel (1988) reported an anxiety disorder prevalence of 17.3% without impairment criteria and 8.7% with it. Romano et al. (2001) showed that impairment criteria have the greatest impact on simple and social phobia estimates.

Across studies that examine specific anxiety disorders among youth, estimates are not consistently reported by age or gender. SAD has been estimated as the most prevalent anxiety disorder among children with rates between 3 and 5%, but only 0.01–2.4% among adolescents (Eisen et al. 2001). Rates of both social phobia (Sweeney and Rapee 2001) and PD have been estimated at about 1–2% of adolescents (Hayward and Essau 2001; Wittchen et al. 1998). These rates tend to be higher among adolescents than children and higher among adults than adolescents (Silverman and Carter 2006). Estimates of panic attacks are higher than those for PD, and they range more widely, leading to questions about the relationship between attacks and the course and severity of PD across childhood and through adolescence. Prevalence of OCD in adolescence has been reported between 3 and 4% (Douglas et al. 1995; Thomsen 2001; Valleni-Basile et al. 1994; Zohar 1999), whereas rates of specific phobias have been reported as high as 12.7% among 13–18-year olds (Essau et al. 2001). According to the review by Schechter and Tosyali (2001), the estimates of PTSD in community studies range from 1.2 to 6.3%, with much higher rates found in samples of children and adolescents who have been exposed to specific traumatic events such as witnessing violence, natural disasters, and physical or sexual abuse.

Few gender differences have been reported in rates of most anxiety disorders among children. Among adolescents, however, rates have been reported to be up to three times higher among females compared to males with regard to aggregated categories of anxiety symptoms and disorders (Anderson et al. 1987; Hayward and Essau 2001; Silverman and Carter 2006; Southam-Gerow 2001), as well as specific phobia (Milne et al. 1995) and social phobia (Wittchen et al. 1999). This pattern was confirmed in one of the few epidemiological studies to compare rates of mental disorder by gender and ethnicity: Hispanic females had significantly higher rates of anxiety than other females and than Hispanic males (McLaughlin et al. 2007). OCD presents an exception, with higher rates reported among boys and male adolescents than girls and female adolescents (Geller et al. 1998). Studies of gender differences in PTSD among adolescents in community samples have been inconsistent (Foy et al. 1996; Schechter and Tosyali 2001). However, with data from the National Survey of Adolescents (aged 12–17 years), Kilpatrick and colleagues (2003) estimated that the rate of PTSD was 6.3% for girls and 3.7% for boys; but for both girls and boys with PTSD, rates of comorbidity were high.

Longitudinal studies have documented that externalizing behaviors among youths (recruited between ages 4 and 16 years) were associated with anxiety disorders in adulthood (reinterviewed at ages 18 through 30; Roza et al. 2003), and anxiety disorders in childhood (before age 13) predicted a range of mental disorders in adolescence (age 13–19; Bittner et al. 2007). Based on retrospective reports from respondents of the National Epidemiological Survey on Alcohol and Related Conditions, anxiety disorder before age 19 increases the risk of bipolar disorder later in life (retrospective reports from Goldstein and Levitt 2007). The relationship between anxiety and depression has been studied quite extensively in longitudinal studies, and it is presented below in the section on Mood Disorders (also see Chap. 6 in this volume on Depression and Post Partum Disorders).

Mood Disorders

Many symptoms of mood disorders, including bipolar disorder and depression, may begin in early childhood, although it is uncertain how many children could be considered to have a disorder. More certain is the high risk that childhood symptoms and diagnosis pose for depression throughout the life course, including adolescence (Costello et al. 2002; Roza et al. 2003), young adulthood (Dekker et al. 2007; Fergusson and Woodward 2002), and middle age (Clark et al. 2007).

Examinations of gender-specific patterns suggest that prior to adolescence there are differences in the types of symptoms experienced by boys and girls. In a study of public school children between ages 10 and 12, girls identified more internalizing symptoms and negative self-esteem, and boys identified more externalizing symptoms and more school problems (Bailey et al. 2007). Despite these different symptom patterns, the rate of depression does not appear to differ substantially between boys and girls prior to puberty. However, several studies have found that unipolar depression rates double or triple around the age of 13 for females but not for males (Angold et al. 1999b; Costello et al. 2002). For example, according to data from the Oregon Adolescent Depression Project (Lewinsohn et al. 1993), adolescent females had higher rates than males of major depressive disorder (25% vs. 12%) and dysthymic disorder (4% vs. 2%). One year later, the rate of depression among the females was 32%. When gender differences in nine symptoms were examined, the investigators found approximately 75% of the girls reported weight or appetite problems, and 82% reported feelings of worthlessness or guilt, both more prevalent than among boys with depression (Lewinsohn et al. 1998). Compared to information about depression, there is much less information on bipolar disorder in childhood, although studies show onset ages around 12 years of age, a prevalence of about 1% during adolescence (ages 14–18), and few gender differences (Costello et al. 2002).

A considerable amount of research has aimed to understand the mechanisms behind the substantial gender difference in depression that manifests around the age of puberty. Based on their analysis of data from females in the Virginia twin registry, Silberg et al. (2001) hypothesized that depression that onsets before age 14 may be an etiologically different disorder from depression that onsets after age 14. When male and female twins from that registry were compared, negative life events had a significant effect on depression for both boys and girls, but a strong genetic component was identified only for female adolescent-onset depression (Silber et al. 1999). Experiences of negative life events during adolescence are potentially important risk factors for males and females, but possibly only in conjunction with other genetic risks or the timing of hormonal changes (Cyranowski et al. 2000). Moreover, the importance of early identification of biologic or physiologic risks has been highlighted by studies of the long-term consequences of LBW. Costello et al. (2007) found that LBW was associated with depression but not other diagnoses, in adolescence but not in childhood, and among girls but not boys. By age 16, girls' rates of depression were 38.1% and 8.4% given LBW and normal birth weight, respectively.

Comorbidity among youths with depression is high. It is estimated that between one-third and three-quarters of children and adolescents with depression have an additional disorder (Lewinsohn et al. 1993). The patterns of co-occurring disorder vary with age; ADHD and CD are prevalent among children with depression, and eating disorders and substance abuse are prevalent among adolescents with depression.

According to one review, between one-quarter and one-half of youth with depression have a comorbid anxiety disorder, and approximately one-tenth of youth with anxiety have depression (Axelson and Birmaher 2001). In an adolescent community sample, adolescent girls had higher rates of co-occurring anxiety and depressive disorders than boys, while boys had higher rates of co-occurring ADHD and CD (Romano et al. 2005). Studies that examine the relative timing of the onset ages of these disorders appear to assume similar patterns for males and females, with predictive models including controls for gender rather than separate analyses being run for males and females, or interactions tested between gender and other risk factors.

There is compelling evidence for a relationship between prior anxiety or anxiety symptoms and later onset of mood disorders. Longitudinal community studies in the USA (Avenevoli et al. 2001) and other countries indicate that among youth who have both anxiety and mood disorders, the anxiety disorders typically onset first (Beesdo et al. 2007; Reinherz et al. 2003; Roza et al. 2003). Moreover, in models predicting risk, adolescents (ages 13–14) who reported a greater number of fears had a higher risk of depression when they were in their early twenties compared to adolescents with fewer fears (Pine et al. 2001), and adolescents with anxiety disorders were at increased risk of developing bipolar symptoms in early adulthood (Johnson et al. 2000) as well as depression (Beesdo et al. 2007).

Some nuances to the relationship between anxiety and depression have been identified in other longitudinal studies. Specifically, depression at age 14 increased OCD risk at age 18 (Douglas et al. 1995). Both the GSMS and the Dunedin study suggest that there may be an equally strong relationship between prior depression and later anxiety (Costello et al. 2003; Moffitt et al. 2007).

Eating Disorders

Estimates based on community samples indicate that rates of eating disorders are low relative to the other disorders presented in this chapter. Prevalence rates of anorexia nervosa, bulimia nervosa, and binge eating disorder were 0.04%, 0.3%, and 1.9%, respectively, in a study of middle and high school aged female students

(Ackard et al. 2007). Reports of eating disturbances were as high as 14.7% in another study of girls between ages 9 and 13, but most were of mild severity (Colton et al. 2007). Despite the low prevalence, mortality rates associated with eating disorders overall and anorexia in particular are higher than those associated with most other mental disorders, according to a review of research in this area (Striegel-Moore and Bulik 2007).

It is suspected that most eating disturbances are resolved after adolescence. However, few longitudinal studies include measures of eating disturbances, and few span the peak period of disorder onset (Keel et al. 2007). Retrospectively reported data from the NCS-R suggest that eating disorders onset between the ages of 19 and 25 (Hudson et al. 2007). Thus, developmental trajectories of problematic eating behaviors and their association with eating disorders in adults have not yet been well-specified.

Arguments have been made for the development of better measurement instruments as additional research develops. Diagnostic classifications may be useful in clinical studies but there is concern about their low specificity and positive predictive value in epidemiologic studies (Ackard et al. 2007; Colton et al. 2007). Moreover, concerns about cultural differences in the presentation of eating disorder symptoms have been identified (Striegel-Moore et al. 2005), along with the need to evaluate eating disorder criteria that may be more appropriate for Latinas (Alegria et al. 2007) and African Americans (Taylor et al. 2007).

There is limited epidemiologic data on comorbidity between eating disorders and other mental disorders. Youth with eating disorders tend to have higher than expected rates of anxiety (Swinbourne and Touyz 2007), especially OCD and social phobia (Kaye et al. 2004), depression and substance use disorders (Baker et al. 2007), and bipolar disorder (McElroy et al. 2005). Studies of the temporal ordering of eating disorder onset ages relative to other diagnoses have not yielded consistent results. For additional information on eating disorders, please see Chap. 7 in this volume.

Implications for Women's Mental Heath

To date, female-specific studies appear to have been conducted on an ad hoc rather than systematic basis. On the basis of this chapter presentation, it is recommended that future research attend to girls and female adolescents in a deliberate way. For example, as developmental trajectories, built upon existing data, are used to specify the genetically complex and heterogeneous pathways that seem to be operant, analyses should be run separately for both genders, or theoretically relevant interactions should be tested (i.e., history of childhood maltreatment and gender). Assessments in longitudinal studies, whether samples comprised both genders or only one, should be as frequent as possible to more accurately capture exposure to and timing of risk factors across different age periods, when vulnerability and resilience may be most salient. Moreover, while highlighting the unique influence of gender, it is important to consider that there are likely to be racial–ethnic differences in prevalence and the mechanisms that explain the development of mental disorders. Cultural influences are particularly important for the definitions of the degree and type of symptoms that are considered "abnormal" and the way gender influences those definitions. As Silverman and Carter (2006) observed with regard to anxiety disorders, very limited research has examined the influence of gender across different age periods and for different ethnic and sociodemographic groups.

From a public health perspective, one should not lose sight of social stratification and community level influences upon mental health, and, in fact, this is a potentially critical area for future research. Without consideration of these influences, the range of potential interventions may be increasingly limited to pharmacological treatments. Several recent studies argue for a balance of attention to individual and environmental influences. First, in a study of families and work that included data on children from birth to third grade, socioeconomic status moderated the effect of child and family risks on symptom severity (Essex et al. 2006). Second, a comparison of adolescents (aged 11–17) representing different ethnic groups (i.e., European Americans, African Americans, and Mexican Americans) showed that economic disadvantage rather than ethnic status was a factor in disorder prevalence (Roberts et al. 2006). Third, neighborhood differences accounted for differences in internalizing behavior problem scores in a longitudinal study of children (aged 5–11 years) recruited from 80 neighborhoods in Chicago (Xue et al. 2005).

The last several years have provided advances in knowledge about the epidemiology and etiology of mental illness, particularly regarding the developmental sequencing of symptoms and disorders across childhood and adolescence. Together with sophisticated methods and analytic approaches, these advances hold substantial promise for the development of interventions that may alter illness trajectories, either by early identification and prevention of the onset of mental disorder or by minimizing its severity and chronicity. As the research develops further, issues of particular importance for girls and female adolescents warrant specific attention. Otherwise, interventions will be developed based on findings that to a great extent are gender-neutral or biased toward the experiences of boys and male adolescents, potentially compromising their effectiveness.

References

Ackard, D. M., Fulkerson, J., & Neumark-Sztainer, D. (2007). Prevalence and utility of DSM-IV eating Disorder diagnostic criteria among youth. *International Journal of Eating Disorders, 40*(5), 409–417.

Alegria, M., Woo, M., Zhun, C., Torres, M., Xiao-li, M., & Striegel-Moore, R. (2007). Prevalence and correlates of eating disorders in Latinos in the United States. *International Journal of Eating Disorders, 40*(Suppl. 3), S15–S21.

Anderson, J. C., Williams, S., McGee, R., & Silva, P. A. (1987). DSM-III disorders in preadolescent children. *Archives of General Psychiatry, 44*, 69–76.

Angold, A., & Costello, E. J. (1995). A test-retest reliability of study of child-reported psychiatric symptoms and diagnoses using the Child and Adolescent Psychiatric Assessment (CAPA-C). *Psychological Medicine, 25,* 755–762.

Angold, A., Costello, E. J., & Erkanli, A. (1999a). Comorbidity. *Journal of Child Psychology and Psychiatry, 40,* 57–87.

Angold, A., Costello, E. J., & Wortham, C. M. (1999b). Pubertal changes in hormone levels and depression in girls. *Psychological Medicine, 29,* 1043–1053.

Angold, A., Erkanli, A., Farmer, E. M., Fairbank, J. A., Burns, B. J., Keeler, G., et al. (2002). Psychiatric disorder, impairment, and service use in rural African American and white youth. *Archives of General Psychiatry, 59,* 893–901.

Armstrong, T., & Costello, E. J. (2002). Community studies on adolescent substance use, abuse, or dependence and psychiatric comorbidity. *Journal of Consulting and Clinical Psychology, 70*(6), 1224–1239.

Avenevoli, S., Stolar, M., Li, J., Dierker, L., & Ries Merikangas, K. R. (2001). Comorbidity of depression in children and adolescents: Models and evidence from a prospective high-risk family study. *Biological Psychiatry, 49*(12), 1071–1081.

Axelson, D. A., & Birmaher, B. (2001). Relation between anxiety and depressive disorders in childhood and adolescence. *Depression and Anxiety, 14*(2), 67–78.

Bailey, M. K., Zauszniewski, J. A., Heinzer, M. H., & Hemstrom-Krainess, M. (2007). Patterns of depressive symptoms in children. *Journal of Child and Adolescent Psychiatric Nursing, 20*(2), 86–95.

Baker, J. H., Mazzeo, S. E., & Kendler, K. S. (2007). Association between broadly defined bulimia nervosa and drug use disorders: Common genetic and environmental influences. *International Journal of Eating Disorders, 40*(8), 673–678.

Beesdo, K., Bittner, A., Pine, D. S., Stein, M. B., Höfler, M., Lieb, R., et al. (2007). Incidence of social anxiety disorder and the consistent risk for secondary depression in the first three decades of life. *Archives of General Psychiatry, 64*(8), 903–912.

Biederman, J., Mick, E., Faraone, S. V., Spencer, T., Wilens, T. E., & Wozniak, J. (2003). Current concepts in the validity, diagnosis and treatment of paediatric bipolar disorder. *The International Journal of Neuropsychopharmacology, 6,* 293–300.

Biederman, J., Monuteaux, M. C., Mick, E., Spencer, T., Wilens, T. E., Klein, K. L., et al. (2006). Psychopathology in females with attention-deficit/hyperactivity disorder: A controlled, five-year prospective study. *Biological Psychiatry, 60*(10), 1098–1105.

Biederman, J., Newcorn, J., & Sprich, S. (1991). Comorbidity of attention deficit hyperactivity disorder with conduct, depressive, anxiety and other disorders. *American Journal of Psychiatry, 148,* 564–577.

Bird, H. R., Canino, G., Rubio-Stipec, M., Gould, M. S., Ribera, J., Sesman, M., et al. (1988). Estimates of the prevalence of childhood maladjustment in a community survey in Puerto Rico. *Archives of General Psychiatry, 45,* 1120–1126.

Bittner, A., Egger, H. L., Erkanli, A., Costello, E. J., Foley, D. L., & Angold, A. (2007). What do childhood anxiety disorders predict? *Journal of Child Psychology and Psychiatry, 48*(12), 1174–1183.

Boylan, K., Vaillancourt, T., Boyle, M., & Szatmari, P. (2007). Comorbidity of internalizing disorders in children with oppositional defiant disorder. *European Child and Adolescent Psychiatry, 16*(8), 484–494.

Briggs-Gowan, M. J., Owens, P., Schwab-Stone, M. E., Leventhal, J. M., Leaf, P. J., & Horwitz, S. M. (2003). Persistence of psychiatric disorders in pediatric settings. *Journal of the American Academy of Child and Adolescent Psychiatry, 42*(11), 1360–1369.

Brown, R. A., Lewinsohn, P. M., Seeley, J. R., & Wagner, E. F. (1996). Cigarette smoking, major depression, and other psychiatric disorders among adolescents. *Journal of the American Academy of Child and Adolescent Psychiatry, 35*(12), 1602–1610.

Burt, S. A., McGue, M., DeMarte, J. A., Krueger, R. F., & Iacono, W. G. (2006). Timing of menarche and the origins of conduct disorder. *Archives of General Psychiatry, 63,* 890–896.

Cartwright-Hatton, S., McNicol, K., & Doubleday, E. (2006). Anxiety in a neglected population: Prevalence of anxiety disorders in pre-adolescent children. *Clinical Psychology Review, 26*(7), 817–833.

Caspi, A., & Moffitt, T. E. (1991). Individual differences are accentuated during periods of social change: The sample case of girls at puberty. *Journal of Personality and Social Psychology, 61,* 157–168.

Clark, C., Rodgers, B., Caldwell, T., Power, C., & Stansfeld, S. (2007). Childhood and adulthood psychological ill health as predictors of midlife affective and anxiety disorders: The 1958 British Birth Cohort. *Archives of General Psychiatry, 64*(6), 668–678.

Cohen, P., Cohen, J., Kasen, S., Velez, C. N., Hartmark, C., Johnson, J., et al. (1993). An epidemiological study of disorders in late childhood and adolescence – I. age – and – gender specific prevalence. *Journal of Child Psychology, 34*(6), 851–867.

Colman, I., Ploubidis, G. B., Wadsworth, M. E. J., Jones, P. B., & Croudace, T. J. (2007). A longitudinal typology of symptoms of depression and anxiety over the life course. *Biological Psychiatry, 62,* 1265–1271.

Colton, P. A., Olmsted, M. P., & Rodin, G. M. (2007). Eating disturbances in a school population of preteen girls: Assessment and screening. *International Journal of Eating Disorders, 40*(5), 435–440.

Costello, E. J., Messer, S. C., Bird, H. R., Cohen, P., & Reinherz, H. Z. (1998). The prevalence of serious emotional disturbance: A re-analysis of community studies. *Journal of Child and Family Studies, 7*(4), 411–432.

Costello, E. J., Mustillo, S., Erkanli, A., Keeler, G., & Angold, A. (2003). Prevalence and development of psychiatric disorders in childhood and adolescence. *Archives of General Psychiatry, 60,* 837–844.

Costello, E. J., Pine, D. J., Hammen, C., March, J. S., Plotsky, P. M., Weissman, M. M., et al. (2002). Development and natural history of mood disorders. *Biological Psychiatry, 52,* 529–542.

Costello, E. J., Worthman, C., Erkanli, A., & Angold, A. (2007). Prediction from low birth weight to female adolescent depression. A test of competing hypotheses. *Archives of General Psychiatry, 64,* 338–344.

Coté, S., Zoccolillo, M., Tremblay, R. E., Nagin, D., & Vitaro, F. (2001). Predicting girls' conduct disorder in adolescence from childhood trajectories of disruptive behaviors. *Journal of the American Academy of Child and Adolescent Psychiatry, 40*(6), 678–684.

Cyranowski, J. M., Frank, E., Young, E., & Shear, M. K. (2000). Adolescent onset of the gender difference in lifetime rates of major depression: A theoretical model. *Archives of General Psychiatry, 57,* 21–27.

Dawson, G., Ashman, S. B., & Carver, L. J. (2000). The role of early experience in shaping behavioral and brain development and its implications for social policy. *Development and Psychopathology, 12,* 695–712.

Dekker, M. C., Ferdinand, R. F., van Lang, N. D. J., Bongers, I. L., van der Ende, J., & Verhulst, F. C. (2007). Developmental trajectories of depressive symptoms from early childhood to late adolescence: Gender differences and adult outcome. *Journal of Child Psychology and Psychiatry, 48*(7), 657–666.

Dey, A. N., Schiller, J. S., & Tai, D. A. (2004). *Summary health statistics for U.S. children: National Health Interview Survey, 2002.* Center for Disease Control and Prevention, National Center for Health Statistics. Vital Health Stat 10(221). Hyattsville, Maryland: U.S. Department of Health and Human Services.

Deykin, E. Y., Levy, J., & Wells, V. (1987). Adolescent depression, alcohol and drug abuse. *American Journal of Public Health, 76,* 178–182.

Disney, E. R., Elkins, I. J., McGue, M., & Iacono, W. G. (1999). Effects of ADHD, conduct disorder, and gender on substance use and abuse in adolescence. *American Journal of Psychiatry, 156,* 1515–1521.

Douglas, H. M., Moffitt, T. E., Dar, R., McGee, R., & Silva, P. (1995). Obsessive-compulsive disorder in a birth cohort of 18-year-olds: Prevalence and predictors. *Journal of the American Academy of Child and Adolescent Psychiatry, 11,* 1424–1431.

Ehringer, M. A., Rhee, S. H., Young, S., Corley, R., & Hewitt, J. K. (2006). Genetic and environmental contributions to common psychopathologies of childhood and adolescence: A study of twins and their siblings. *Journal of Abnormal Psychology, 34,* 1–17.

Eisen, A. R., Brien, L. K., Bowers, J., & Strudler, A. (2001). Separation anxiety disorders. In C. A. Essau & F. Petermann (Eds.), *Anxiety disorders in children and adolescents: Epidemiology, risk factors and treatment* (pp. 111–142). New York, NY: Brunner-Routledge.

Elkins, I. J., McGue, M., & Iacono, W. G. (2007). Prospective effects of attention-deficit/hyperactivity disorder, conduct disorder, and sex on adolescent substance use and abuse. *Archives of General Psychiatry, 64*(10), 1145–1152.

Essau, C. A., Aihara, F., Petermann, F., & Al Wiswasi, S. (2001). Specific phobia. In C. A. Essau & F. Petermann (Eds.), *Anxiety disorders in children and adolescents: Epidemiology, risk factors and treatment* (pp. 193–218). New York, NY: Brunner-Routledge.

Essex, M. J., Kraemer, H. C., Armstrong, J. M., Boyce, T., Goldsmith, H. H., Klein, M. H., et al. (2006). Exploring risk factors for the emergence of children's mental health problems. *Archives of General Psychiatry, 63,* 1246–1256.

Feehan, M., McGee, R., Nada, R. S., & Williams, S. M. (1994). DSM-III-R disorders in New Zealand 18-year-olds. *Australian and New Zealand Journal of Psychiatry, 28,* 87–99.

Fergusson, D. M., Horwood, J. H., & Lynskey, M. T. (1993). Prevalence and comorbidity of DSM-III-R diagnosis in a birth cohort of 15 year olds. *Journal of the American Academy of Child and Adolescent Psychiatry, 32*(6), 1127–1134.

Fergusson, D. M., Horwood, J. H., & Ridder, E. M. (2005). Show me the child at seven: The consequences of conduct problems in childhood for psychosocial functioning in adulthood. *Journal of Child Psychology and Psychiatry, 46*(8), 837–849.

Fergusson, D. M., & Woodward, L. J. (2002). Mental health, educational, and social role outcomes of adolescents with depression. *Archives of General Psychiatry, 59,* 225–231.

Foy, D. W., Madvig, B. T., Pynoos, R. S., & Camilleri, A. J. (1996). Etiologic factors in the development of posttraumatic stress disorder in children and adolescents. *Journal of School Psychology, 34*(2), 133–145.

Froehlich, T. E., Lanphear, B. P., Epstein, J. N., Barbaresi, W. J., Katusic, S. K., & Kahn, R. S. (2007). Prevalence, recognition, and treatment of attention-deficit/hyperactivity disorder in a national sample of U.S. children. *Archives of Pediatrics and Adolescent Medicine, 161*(9), 857–864.

Geller, D., Biederman, J., Jones, J., Park, K., Schwartz, S., Shapiro, S., et al. (1998). Is juvenile obsessive-compulsive disorder a developmental subtype of the disorder? A review of the pediatric literature. *Journal of the American Academy of Child and Adolescent Psychiatry, 37*(4), 420–507.

Gershon, J. (2002). A meta-analytic review of gender differences in ADHD. *Journal of Attention Disorders, 5*(3), 143–154.

Goldstein, B. I., & Levitt, A. J. (2007). Prevalence and correlates of bipolar I disorder among adults with primary youth-onset anxiety disorders. *Journal of Affective Disorders, 103*(1–3), 187–195.

Hack, M., Youngstrom, E. A., Cartar, L., Schluchter, M., Taylor, H. G., Flannery, D., et al. (2004). Behavioral outcomes and evidence of psychopathology among very low birth weight infants at age 20 years. *Pediatrics, 114,* 932–940.

Hayward, C., & Essau, C. A., (2001). Panic attacks and panic disorder. In C. A. Essau & F. Petermann (Eds.), *Anxiety disorders in children and adolescents: Epidemiology, risk factors and treatment* (pp. 143–162). New York, NY: Brunner-Routledge.

Hipwell, A. E., Loeber, R., Stouthamer-Loeber, M., Keenan, K., White, H. R., & Kroneman, L. (2002). Characteristics of girls with early onset disruptive and antisocial behaviour. *Criminal Behavior and Mental Health, 12,* 99–118.

Hudson, J. I., Hiripi, E., Pope, H. G., Jr., & Kessler, R. C. (2007). The prevalence and correlates of eating disorders in the National Comorbidity Survey Replication. *Biological Psychiatry, 61,* 348–358.

Jensen, P. S., Watanabe, H. K., Richters, J. E., Cortes, R., Roper, M., & Liu, S. (1995). Prevalence of mental disorder in military children and adolescents: Findings from a two-stage community survey. *Journal of the American Academy of Child and Adolescent Psychiatry, 34*(11), 1514–1524.

Johnson, J. G., Cohen, P., & Brook, J. S. (2000). Associations between bipolar disorder and other psychiatric disorders during adolescence and early adulthood. *American Journal of Psychiatry, 157,* 1679–1681.

Kashani, J. H., Daniel, A. E., Sulzberger, L. A., Rosenberg, T. K., & Reid, J. C. (1987). Conduct disordered adolescents from a community sample. *Canadian Journal of Psychiatry, 32,* 756–760.

Kashani, J. H., & Orvaschel, H. (1988). Anxiety disorders in mid-adolescence: A community sample. *American Journal of Psychiatry, 145,* 960–964.

Kaye, W. H., Bulik, C. M., Thornton, L., Barbarich, N., & Masters, K. (2004). Comorbidity of anxiety disorders with anorexia and bulimia nervosa. *American Journal of Psychiatry, 161*(12), 2215–2221.

Keel, P. K., Heatherton, T. F., Baxter, M. G., & Joiner, T. E., Jr. (2007). A 20-year longitudinal study of body weight, dieting, and eating disorder symptoms. *Journal of Abnormal Psychology, 116*(2), 422–432.

Keenan, K., Wakschlag, L. S., Danis, B., Hill, C., Humphries, M., Duax, J., et al. (2007). Further evidence of the reliability and validity of DSM-IV ODD and CD in preschool children. *Journal of the American Academy of Child and Adolescent Psychiatry, 46*(4), 457–468.

Kessler, R. C., Berglund, P., Demler, O., Jin, R., Merikangas, K. R., & Walters, E. E. (2005). Lifetime prevalence and age-of-onset distributions of DSM-IV disorders in the National Comorbidity Survey Replication. *Archives of General Psychiatry, 62,* 593–602.

Kessler, R. C., & Walters, E. E. (1998). Epidemiology of DSM-III-R major depression and minor depression among adolescents and young adults in the national comorbidity survey. *Depression and Anxiety, 7,* 3–14.

Kilpatrick, D. G., Ruggiero, K. J., Acierno, R., Saunders, B. E., Resnick, H. S., & Best, C. L. (2003). Violence and risk of PTSD, major depression, substance abuse/dependence, and comorbidity: Results from the National Survey of Adolescents. *Journal of Counseling and Clinical Psychology, 71*(4), 692–700.

Kim-Cohen, J., Arseneault, L., Caspi, A., Tomas, M. P., Taylor, A., & Moffitt, T. E. (2005). Validity of DSM-IV conduct disorder in 4½–5-year old children: A longitudinal epidemiological study. *American Journal of Psychiatry, 162*(6), 1108–1117.

Kim-Cohen, J., Caspi, A., Moffitt, T. E., Harrington, H., Milne, B. J., & Poulton, R. (2003). Prior juvenile diagnoses in adults with mental disorder: Developmental follow-back of a prospective-longitudinal cohort. *Archives of General Psychiatry, 60*(7), 709–717.

Lahey, B. B., Loeber, R., Quay, H. C., Applegate, B., Shaffer, D., Waldman, I., et al. (1998). Validity of DSM-IV subtypes of conduct disorder based on age of onset. *Journal of the American Academy of Child and Adolescent Psychiatry, 37,* 435–442.

Lahey, B. B., Miller, T. L., Schwab-Stone, M., Goodman, S. H., Waldman, I. D., Canino, G., et al. (2000). Age and gender differences in oppositional behavior and conduct problems: A cross-sectional household study of middle childhood and adolescence. *Journal of Abnormal Psychology, 109*(3), 488–503.

Lavigne, J. V., Cicchetti, C., Gibbons, R. D., Binns, H. J., Larsen, L., & DeVito, C. (2001). Oppositional defiant disorder with onset in preschool years: Longitudinal stability and pathways to other disorders. *Journal of the American Academy of Child and Adolescent Psychiatry, 40*(12), 1393–1400.

Lavigne, J. V., Gibbons, R. D., Christoffel, K. K., Arend, R., Rosenbaum, D., Binns, H., et al. (1996). Prevelance rates and correlates of psychiatric disorders among preschool children. *Journal of the American Academy of Child and Adolescent Psychiatry, 35*(2), 204–214.

Leaf, P., Alegria, M., Cohen, P., Goodman, S. H., Horwitz, S. M., Hoven, C. W., et al. (1996). Mental health service use in the community and schools: Results from the four-community MECA study. *Journal of the American Academy of Child and Adolescent Psychiatry, 35,* 889–897.

Lewinsohn, P. M., Hops, H., Roberts, R. E., Seeley, J. R., & Andrews, J. A. (1993). Adolescent psychopathology: I. Prevalence and incidence of depression and other DSM-III-R disorders in high school students. *Journal of Abnormal Psychology, 102,* 133–144.

Lewinsohn, P. M., Rohde, P., & Seeley, J. R. (1988). Major depressive disorder in older adolescents: Prevalence, risk factors, and clinical implications. *Clinical Psychology Review, 18,* 765–794.

Lewinsohn, P. M., Striegel-Moore, R. H., & Seeley, J. R. (2000). Epidemiology and natural course of eating disorders in young women from adolescence to young adulthood. *Journal of the American Academy of Child and Adolescent Psychiatry, 39*(10), 1284–1292.

Loeber, R., Burke, J. D., Lahey, B. B., Winters, A., & Zera, M. (2000). Oppositional defiant and conduct disorder: A review of the past 10 years, Part 1. *Journal of the American Academy of Child and Adolescent Psychiatry, 39,* 1468–1484.

Lonigan, C. J., Phillips, B. M., & Richey, J. A. (2003). Posttraumatic stress disorder in children: Diagnosis, assessment, and associated features. *Child and Adolescent Psychiatric Clinics of North America, 12*(2), 171–194.

Manassas, K. (2006). Depression and anxiety in girls. In S. E. Romans & M. V. Seeman (Eds.), *Women's mental health: A life cycle approach* (pp. 53–69). Philadelphia, PA: Lippincott, Williams & Wilkins.

Marmorstein, N. R. (2007). Relationships between anxiety and externalizing disorders in youth: The influences of age and gender. *Journal of Anxiety Disorders, 21*(3), 420–432.

Marmorstein, N. R., & Iacono, W. G. (2001). An investigation of female adolescent twins with both major depression and conduct disorder. *Journal of the American Academy of Child and Adolescent Psychiatry, 40,* 299–306.

Maughan, B., Rowe, R., Messer, J., Goodman, R., & Meltzer, H. (2004). Conduct disorder and oppositional defiant disorder in a national sample: Developmental epidemiology. *Journal of Child Psychology and Psychiatry, 45*(3), 609–621.

McElroy, S. L., Kotwal, R., Keck, P. E., & Akiskal, H. S. (2005). Comorbidity of bipolar and eating disorders: Distinct or related disorders with shared dysregulations? *Journal of Affective Disorders, 86*(2–3), 107–127.

McLaughlin, K., Hilt, L., & Nolen-Hoeksema, S. (2007). Racial/ethnic differences in internalizing and externalizing symptoms in adolescents. *Journal of Abnormal Psychology, 35,* 801–816.

Merlo, L. J., Storch, E. A., Murphy, T. K., Goodman, W. K., & Geffken, G. R. (2005). Assessment of pediatric obsessive-compulsive disorder: A critical review of current methodology. *Child Psychology and Human Development, 36*(2), 195–214.

Messer, J., Goodman, R., Rowe, R., Meltzer, H., & Maughan, B. (2006). Preadolescent conduct problems in girls and boys. *Journal of the American Academy of Child and Adolescent Psychiatry, 45,* 184–191.

Milne, J. M., Garrison, C. Z., Addy, C. L., McKeown, R. E., Jackson, K. L., Cuffe, S. P., et al. (1995). Frequency of phobic disorder in a community sample of young adolescents. *Journal of the American Academy of Child and Adolescent Psychiatry, 34*(9), 1202–1211.

Moffitt, T. E., Harrington, H., Caspi, A., Kim-Cohen, J., Goldberg, D., Gregory, A. M., et al. (2007). Depression and generalized anxiety disorder: Cumulative and sequential comorbidity in a birth cohort followed prospectively to age 32 years. *Archives of General Psychiatry, 64*(6), 651–660.

Newcorn, J. H., & Halperin, J. M. (2000). Attention-deficit disorders with oppositionality and aggression. In T. E. Brown (Ed.), *Attention-deficit disorders and comorbidities in children, adolescents, and adults* (pp. 171–208). Washington, DC: American Psychiatric Press.

Nock, M. K., Kazdin, A. E., Hiripi, E., & Kessler, R. C. (2006). Prevalence, subtypes, and correlates of DSM-IV conduct disorder in the National Comorbidity Survey Replication. *Psychological Medicine, 36*(5), 699–710.

Nock, M. K., Kazdin, A. E., Hiripi, E., & Kessler, R. C. (2007). Lifetime prevalence, correlates, and persistence of oppositional defiant disorder: Results from the National Comorbidity Survey Replication. *Journal of Child Psychology and Psychiatry, 48*(7), 703–713.

Offord, D. R., Boyle, M. H., Szatmari, P., Rae-Grant, N. I., Links, P. S., Cadman, D. T., et al. (1987). Ontario Child Health Study: II. Six-month prevalence of disorder and rates of service utilization. *Archives of General Psychiatry, 44,* 832–836.

Ollendick, T. H., Grills, A. E., & Alexander, K. L. (2001). Fears, worries and anxiety in children and adolescents. In C. A. Essau & F. Petermann (Eds.), *Anxiety disorders in children and adolescents: Epidemiology, risk factors and treatment* (pp. 1–36). New York, NY: Brunner-Routledge.

Pine, D. S., & Cohen, J. A. (2002). Trauma in children and adolescents: Risk and treatment of psychiatric sequelae. *Biological Psychiatry, 51,* 519–531.

Pine, D. S., Cohen, P., & Brook, J. (2001). Adolescent fears as predictors of depression. *Biological Psychiatry, 50,* 721–724.

Polanczyk, G., de Lima, M. S., Horta, L. B., Biederman, J., & Rohde, L. A. (2007). The worldwide prevalence of ADHD: A systematic review and metaregression analysis. *The American Journal of Psychiatry, 164*(6), 942–948.

Rapoport, J. L., & Ismond, D. R. (1996). *DSM-IV training guide for diagnosis of childhood disorders.* Philadelphia, PA: Brunner/Mazel.

Reid, R., Riccio, C. A., Kessler, R. K., DuPaul, G. J., Power, T. J., Anastopoulos, A. D., et al. (2000). Gender and ethnic differences in ADHD as assessed by behavior ratings. *Journal of Emotional and Behavioral Disorders, 4*(1), 38–48.

Reinherz, H. Z., Paradis, A. D., Giaconia, R. M., Stashwick, C. K., & Fitzmaurice, G. (2003). Childhood and adolescent predictors of major depression in the transition to adulthood. *American Journal of Psychiatry, 160,* 2141–2147.

Roberts, R. E., Roberts, C. R., & Xing, Y. (2006). Prevalence of youth-reported DSM-IV psychiatric disorders among African, European, and Mexican American adolescents. *Journal of the American Academy of Child and Adolescent Psychiatry, 45*(11), 1329–1337.

Roberts, R. E., Roberts, C. R., & Xing, Y. (2007). Rates of DSM-IV psychiatric disorders among adolescents in a large metropolitan area. *Journal of Psychiatric Research, 41*(11), 959–967.

Romano, E., Tremblay, R. E., Vitaro, F., Zoccolillo, M., & Pagani, L. (2001). Prevalence of psychiatric diagnoses and the role of perceived impairment: Findings from an adolescent community sample. *Journal of Child Psychology and Psychiatry, 42,* 451–461.

Romano, E., Tremblay, R. E., Vitaro, F., Zoccolillo, M., & Pagani, L. (2005). Sex and informant effects on diagnostic comorbidity in an adolescent community sample. *Canadian Journal of Psychiatry, 50*(8), 479–489.

Rowe, R. Maughan, B., Pickles, A., Costello, E. J., & Angold, A. (2002). The relationship between DSM-IV oppositional defiant disorder and conduct disorder: Findings from the Great Smoky Mountains Study. *Journal of Child Psychology and Psychiatry, 43*(3), 365–373.

Roza, S. J., Hofstra, M. B., van der Ende, J., & Verhulst, F. C. (2003). Stable prediction of mood and anxiety disorders based on behavioral and emotional problems in childhood: A 14-year follow-up during childhood, adolescence, and young adulthood. *American Journal of Psychiatry, 160,* 2116–2121.

Rucklidge, J. J., & Tannock, R. (2001). Psychiatric, psychosocial, and cognitive functioning of female adolescents with ADHD. *Journal of the American Academy of Child & Adolescent Psychiatry, 40*(5), 530–540.

Schechter, D. S., & Tosyali, M. C., (2001). Posttraumatic stress disorder. In C. A. Essau & F. Petermann (Eds.), *Anxiety disorders in children and adolescents: Epidemiology, risk factors and treatment* (pp. 285–322). New York, NY: Brunner-Routledge.

Seligman, L. D., Ollendick, T. H., Langley, A. K., & Baldacci, H. B. (2004). The utility of measures of child and adolescent anxiety: A meta-analytic review of the Revised Children's Manifest Anxiety Scale, the State-Trait Anxiety Inventory for Children, and the Child Behavior Checklist. *Journal of Clinical Child and Adolescent Psychology, 33*(3), 557–565.

Shepard, B. A., Carter, A. S., & Cohen, J. E. (2000). Attention-deficit/hyperactivity disorder and the preschool child. In T. E. Brown (Ed.), *Attention-deficit disorders and comorbidities in children, adolescents, and adults* (pp. 407–436). Washington, DC: American Psychiatric Press.

Silber, J., Pickles, A., Rutter, M., Hewitt, J., Simonoff, E., Maes, H., et al. (1999). The influence of genetic factors and life stress on depression among girls. *Archives of General Psychiatry, 56,* 225–232.

Silberg, J. L., Rutter, M., & Eaves, L. (2001). Genetic and environmental influences on the temporal association between earlier anxiety and later depression in girls. *Biological Psychiatry, 49,* 1040–1049.

Silverman, W. K., & Carter, R. (2006). Anxiety disturbance in girls and women. In J. Worell & C. D. Goodheart (Eds.), *Handbook of girls' and women's psychological health* (pp. 60–68). New York, NY: Oxford University Press.

Southam-Gerow, M. A. (2001). Generalized anxiety disorder. In C. A. Essau & F. Petermann (Eds.), *Anxiety disorders in children and adolescents: Epidemiology, risk factors and treatment* (pp. 219–260). New York, NY: Brunner-Routledge.

Stalets, M. M., & Luby, J. L. (2006). Preschool depression. *Child and Adolescent Psychiatric Clinics of North America, 15*(4), 899–917.

Sterba, S., Egger, H. L., & Angold, A. (2007). Diagnostic specificity and nonspecificity in the dimensions of preschool psychopathology. *Journal of Child Psychology and Psychiatry, 48*(10), 1005–1013.

Stice, E., Burton, E. M., & Shaw, H. (2004). Prospective relations between bulimic pathology, depression, and substance abuse: Unpacking comorbidity in adolescent girls. *Journal of Consulting and Clinical Psychology, 72,* 62–71.

Striegel-Moore, R. H., & Bulik, C. M. (2007). Risk factors for eating disorders. *American Psychologist, 62*(3), 181–198.

Striegel-Moore, R. H., Franko, D. L., Thompson, D., Barton, B., Schreiber, G. B., & Daniels, S. R. (2005). An empirical study of the typology of bulimia nervosa and its spectrum variants. *Psychological Medicine, 35,* 1563–1572.

Sweeney, L., & Rapee, R. M. (2001). Social phobia. In C. A. Essau & F. Petermann (Eds.), *Anxiety disorders in children and adolescents: Epidemiology, risk factors and treatment* (pp. 163–192). New York, NY: Brunner-Routledge.

Swinbourne, J. M., & Touyz, S. W. (2007). The co-morbidity of eating disorders and anxiety disorders: A review. *European Eating Disorders Review, 15*(4), 253–274.

Taylor, J. Y., Caldwell, C. H., Baser, R. E., Faison, N., & Jackson, J. S. (2007). Prevalence of eating disorders among blacks in the National Survey of American Life. *International Journal of Eating Disorders, 40,* S10–S14.

Thomsen, P. H. (2001). Obsessive-compulsive disorder. In C. A. Essau & F. Petermann (Eds.), *Anxiety disorders in children and adolescents: Epidemiology, risk factors and treatment* (pp. 261–284). New York, NY: Brunner-Routledge.

Valleni-Basile, L. A., Garrison, C. Z., Jackson, K. L., Waller, J. L., McKeown, R. E., Addy, C. L., et al. (1994). Frequency of obsessive-compulsive disorder in a community sample of young adolescents. *Journal of the American Academy of Child and Adolescent Psychiatry, 33*(6), 782–791.

Wittchen, H. U., Reed, V., & Kessler, R. C. (1998). The relationship of agoraphobia and panic in a community sample of adolescents and young adults. *Archives of General Psychiatry, 55,* 1017–1024.

Wittchen, H. U., Stein, M. B., & Kessler, R. C. (1999). Social fears and social phobia in a community sample of adolescents and young adults: Prevalence, risk factors and co-morbidity. *Psychological Medicine, 29*(2), 309–323.

Wu, P., Hoven, C. W., Bird, H. R., Moore, R. E., Cohen, P., Alegria, M., et al. (1999). Depressive and disuptive disorders and mental health service utilization in children and adolescents. *Journal of the American Academy of Child and Adolescent Psychiatry, 38*(9), 1081–1090.

Xue, Y., Leventhal, T., Brooks-Gunn, J., & Earls, F. J. (2005). Neighborhood residence and mental health of 5- to 11-year olds. *Archives of General Psychiatry, 62,* 554–563.

Zero to Three. (2005). *Diagnostic classification of mental health and developmental disorders of infancy and early childhood, revised (DC:0-3R).* Washington, DC: Author.

Zoccolillo, M. (1992). Co-occurrence of conduct disorder and its adult outcomes with depressive and anxiety disorders: A review. *Journal of the American Academy of Child & Adolescent Psychiatry, 31,* 547–556.

Zoccolillo, M. (1993). Gender and the development of conduct disorder. *Development and Psychopathology, 5,* 65–78.

Zohar, A. H. (1999). The epidemiology of obsessive-compulsive disorder in children and adolescents. *Child and Adolescent Psychiatric Clinics of North America, 8*(3), 445–460.

Chapter 3
Mental Conditions in Adult Women: Epidemiology and Impact

Mary Jane Alexander and Caitlin McMahon

Introduction

Thinking about the impact of illness has evolved over the past 50 years to encompass both the physiology of disease and the personal experience of illness. The signs and symptoms evident in bodily structures and functions (impairment) have become disentangled from the personal impact and understanding of them (disability), and their social consequences (handicap; Susser and Watson 1961; World Health Organization (WHO) 1980). More recently, political and social movements have begun to pose the idea that outcomes of care should move beyond well-being and personal satisfaction to include the many aspects of actual participation. In their view, it is essential that public health and social policy and practice support disabled individuals to achieve and sustain practical opportunities or "capabilities" in multiple and valued areas of their lives. In the public mental health arena, the President's New Freedom Commission envisions recovery as the process by which people are able to "live, work, learn and participate fully in their communities" (Hogan 2003, p. 1467). This vision takes the idea of disease beyond its clinical dimensions (WHO 2001), making it essential that public mental health practitioners, policy makers, and advocates understand the extent and distribution of both disability and disorder in order to develop policies and practices that contribute to people's activity and ability to participate in society throughout their lives.

Epidemiology provides information about patterns of disease and the factors that influence them (Lilienfeld and Stolley 1994). In this chapter we provide an overview of the scope of major mental and substance use conditions among adults in the USA, their severity, the disability associated with those conditions for women, and the ways in which social factors contribute to *women's* vulnerabilities and resilience. Particular conditions covered in this chapter include depression, post traumatic stress disorder (PTSD), other anxiety disorders, substance use disorders (SUDs),

M. J. Alexander (✉)
Center to Study Recovery in Social Contexts Statistics and Services Research Division, Nathan Kline Institute, 140 Old Orangeburg Road, Orangeburg, NY 10962, USA

B. L. Levin, M. A. Becker (eds.), *A Public Health Perspective of Women's Mental Health*, DOI 10.1007/978-1-4419-1526-9_3, © Springer Science+Business Media LLC 2010

and physical comorbidities. The implications of these findings for public mental health services are discussed. Information on the scope and impact of mental and substance use conditions is presented in order to better understand the challenges that women face and to suggest policy and practice foci that target their needs and mobilize their strengths.

Epidemiology of Women's Mental Health

Women's health and mental health are basic human rights that in concert develop and thrive, and alternatively, are at risk, over the course of their lives. An effective conceptual framework for mental health must incorporate dynamic interactions between women's personal capacities for resilience and the social factors that work to buffer them from environmental and personal risks for developing mental conditions. From a public mental health perspective, it is essential to take seriously how policy, law, custom, research, and practice can enable women to participate fully in their own lives and in their families and communities, or prevent them from doing so.

While this framework is beyond the scope of this chapter, we try here to place the data of epidemiology in the context of how mental conditions impact women's ability to participate fully in their own lives. We use the disability model of disease to differentiate the presence of a condition from the impairment a woman experiences as a consequence, things like feeling suicidal, or being unable to work, or to parent (Albrecht et al. 2001; Mitra 2006). We add Sen's capabilities framework (Sen 1999) to the disability model's focus on the impact of a condition on a woman's individual capacity, in order to emphasize the social barriers that impede her ability to accomplish what she values (Ware et al. 2007). About three-quarters of the adults surveyed in the most comprehensive, recent national US household survey experienced no mental condition or impairment, but their enduring consequences among the one-quarter who did experience them are substantial. The prevention and effective treatment of these disabling conditions, and the collaborative work with afflicted communities to restore to them opportunities to participate fully in their lives, are among the most important and urgent public health issues of our time.

As a multidimensional approach, the disability model provides a richer understanding of the specific areas in a woman's life that are affected by her condition and to what extent. The capabilities approach, used extensively in international development (Sen 1999), and now being applied to disability (Mitra 2006) and public mental health (Ware et al. 2007, 2008; Hopper 2007), goes farther. Both require a holistic perspective: a woman's practical opportunities to do and be what she values depend on how well she is able to convert resources into a doing or being she values (Sen 1999). Her ability to do so depends on her personal capacity (including, but not limited to, her impairment), her environmental resources, and in critical ways for public mental health, the customs, laws, and policies that affect her access to real opportunities. Current knowledge about the epidemiology of women's mental health—the scope, distribution, and impact of mental conditions—allows us to identify points of traction in practice and policy where significant change can enable women to fully participate in society in ways they value.

Overview

Scope of Mental Disorder and Disability

Mental disorders are among the most prevalent and impairing chronic conditions (Kessler 2000; Kessler et al. 2008). In 2001–2003, almost half (46%) of all adult Americans had experienced a mental condition in their lifetime (Kessler et al. 2005c), and about a quarter (26%) of the total population had experienced a current (in the prior 12 months) mental condition (Kessler et al. 2005a). Women are at higher risk than men. The most common profile of a person with any current mental condition was a single Hispanic or African-American woman with less than a college education and low income, living in a rural area (Kessler et al. 2005c). A decade earlier, half (48%) of American women had a lifetime experience of a mental condition, with almost a third (31%) reporting a current condition (Kessler et al. 1994). These highly prevalent conditions have a substantial impact on people's lives. They are the leading cause of disability for American women, and their impact on women's health and life is similar worldwide (Murray and Lopez 1996; WHO 2004), profoundly limiting women's opportunities to participate fully in the life of their cultures. The most serious among them cost the US economy at least $193 billion annually in lost earnings alone (Kessler et al. 2008).

The most recent comprehensive and representative US national household survey of mental and substance use disorders, the National Comorbidity Survey—Replication (NCS-R), was undertaken between 2001 and 2003. In the first of two phases, lay interviewers administered a structured diagnostic interview to over 9,000 individuals to identify mood, anxiety, impulse control, and SUDs according to the diagnostic criteria in the Diagnostic and Statistical Manual IV-R (DSM-IV-R) of the American Psychiatric Association (American Psychiatric Association (APA) 2000; Kessler et al. 2005a). In the second phase they queried those who met criteria for any condition in Phase 1, and a sample of those who did not, about physical conditions and risk factors. A random subsample of these respondents was also screened for conditions that rarely occur: nonaffective psychosis, schizophrenia, schizoaffective disorder, delusional disorder, and psychosis not otherwise specified (Kessler et al. 2005b). Published findings to date from this survey that pertain to gender are roughly comparable to earlier large-scale community-based epidemiological surveys in the USA, including the original National Comorbidity Study (Kessler et al. 1994) and the Epidemiological Catchment Area Study (Regier et al. 1998), although NCS-R analyses to date focus on profiles of risk and comorbidity, rather than directly on the effects of gender.

Table 3.1 Prevalence of the most frequently occurring mental conditions (NCS-R)

Disorder category	1 year prevalence (%)	Lifetime prevalence (%)
Anxiety	18.1	29
Mood	9.5	21
Impulse control	8.9	25
Substance use	3.8	15
Nonaffective psychoses	0.03	0.05

Overall, the most prevalent current and lifetime conditions identified in the NCS-R were anxiety disorders, followed by mood, impulse control, and SUDs (Table 3.1; Kessler et al. 2005c). Nonaffective psychoses (NAP) were very rare (Kessler et al. 2005b). Women were more likely than men to have mood and anxiety disorders and were less likely to have impulse control and SUDs, but rates of SUDs are increasing among both younger cohorts of women and women over 40 years of age (SAMHSA 2007; Kessler et al. 2005a; Kessler 2000). Key findings of these epidemiological studies, with implications for women's mental health, center on the early ages when women first meet criteria for a mental condition, the ways in which multiple conditions are concentrated within individuals, and the significant impairment associated with these factors, including suicidality, work disability, repeated violent victimization, and days when she is unable to fulfill her normal work, family, or social responsibilities (Sheehan et al. 1996).

Onset, Severity and Multiple Conditions

Mental conditions have been called the chronic conditions of the young because first episodes typically occur during adolescence and young adulthood. In the NCS-R, half of all those who met criteria for any condition in their lifetime did so by age 14, and three-quarters by age 24 (Kessler et al. 2005a). These are the years when young people negotiate critical transitions to adulthood (Modell 1989). They complete their educations, launch careers, establish intimate and social relationships, marry, and make decisions about having children (Kessler et al. 1995a, 1997, 1998). Disruption of these essential life tasks affects their resilience to other stressors, their coping strategies, and their ability to participate fully in the remainder of their lives.

Multiple and severe conditions are key impediments to participation, health, and life expectancy (Dickey et al. 2000, 2002; Parks et al. 2006). Of those NCS-R respondents with any current condition, 55% had one, 22% had two, and 23% had three or more conditions. Over half of those with *any* current condition were also moderately or seriously impaired; however, serious impairment and the most severe conditions were most often paired when a person had multiple lifetime mental conditions (Kessler et al. 1994, 2005c). Only one-tenth of those with a single condition were seriously impaired, whereas one-quarter of those with two, and half of those with three diagnoses were. Virtually all of those with serious impairment reported more than two diagnoses. The NCS-R reveals, through sophisticated and detailed statistical analysis, particular profiles or "clusters" of conditions that shed light on the ways that impairment and disability concentrate among those with multiple conditions, and on how these profiles of co-occurring conditions differ for men and women. As these clusters delineate the complexity of impairment and disability, they highlight the need for holistic, person-centered approaches to practice and changes in policy to facilitate social recovery.

Two seriously disabling clusters together comprise about one-fifth of those with any current condition, and women figure strongly in both (Kessler et al. 2005c). Women who fit these profiles are likely to use public sector services if they seek treatment at all. The more disabling profile was characterized diagnostically by major depression that co-occurs with other conditions, and consisted of unmarried, ethnically non-Hispanic, non-Black women with low education, low to middle income, living in urban and suburban areas. Virtually all the people in this cluster (95%) had three or more conditions, and almost three-quarters were seriously disabled.

A second profile was characterized diagnostically by multiple, internalizing conditions, such as specific and social phobias, major depression, and dysthymia, and was likely to consist of divorced, separated, or widowed women residing in suburban or outlying nonrural areas. Over three-quarters of those in this cluster (85%) had two or more conditions, and about one-third were severely disabled. A third cluster of less diagnostically complex internalizing conditions—mostly major depression or dysthymia (41%)—was characterized by college educated, married women residing in small metropolitan suburbs. Although the individuals with this profile were substantially less disabled, the profile accounts for almost half of those with any condition in the NCS-R study, so practitioners are likely to encounter these women frequently.

Four additional clusters that comprised more externalizing conditions were more strongly associated with male profiles, but women can certainly experience these configurations as well. It is worth noting that the diagnostic categories in the DSM are based on symptom clusters and do not reflect an underlying, currently known pathophysiology of mental condition, so that a person who meets diagnostic criteria for multiple DSM-IV diagnoses does not necessarily have five distinct illnesses. Another approach to mental condition is to take a dimensional, rather than a categorical, view of symptoms and distress (First 2002), as in the clusters described earlier. In conjunction with the capabilities approach and the disabilities model, the clusters provide more contextualized information on the far-reaching effects of mental conditions on everyday life, providing purchase for action that spans the clinical, social, and policy dimensions of public mental health.

Impact of Mental Conditions: Impairment and Disability

Mental conditions are among the most disabling of chronic diseases, with consequences that go well beyond individuals' lives to affect families and society (Murray and Lopez 1996; Olesen and Leonardi 2003; Kessler 2000). In order to make comparisons across conditions and populations, injuries and risks, a measure is used that reflects time or life lost due to a condition: Disability-adjusted life years (DALYs; Murray and Lopez 1996). DALYs are the sum of years of life lost due to premature mortality plus years of life lost due to disability, with each year of life lived weighted by a disability factor arrived at by a panel of nonafflicted individuals. This measure provides a much more accurate and detailed picture of impairment and the broader impact illness has on a person's life than simple mortality rates.

Worldwide, mental conditions account for 15% of the total burden of illness (indirect + direct costs) in advanced economies such as the USA (Murray and Lopez 1996). This is second to the burden from heart disease and is slightly higher than the burden from all types of cancer. Having a serious mental illness not only reduces predicted annual income by an average of about $16,000, but also decreases the likelihood that a person has any income at all (Kessler et al. 2008). In one nationwide study, about half of the respondents with one or more of a wide range of current physical or mental conditions were completely unable to work or carry out their usual activities as a result of these problems for an average of almost 7 days in the prior month (Kessler et al. 2001). Mental conditions alone have a greater disabling impact than chronic physical conditions alone, but comorbid physical–mental conditions are the most disabling combination, accounting for more than four times as many work loss days than either condition alone (Kessler et al. 2003). Other studies have similar findings (Merikangas et al. 2007; Wells et al. 1996; Michaud et al. 2001). Mental conditions cost the US economy $193 billion a year in lost earnings, an underestimate, since it does not include women's uncompensated household work (Kessler et al. 2005c, 2008). Afflicted US citizens were unable to engage in their normal daily activities an average of 88 days in a year (Kessler et al. 2005b). Indirect costs, lost productivity at work, school, and home due to premature death or disability due to affective diagnoses alone were estimated at $78.6 billion in 1990 (Rice and Miller 1996). Because these data exclude the impact of schizophrenia, the most disabling of the mental conditions, they underestimate the individual and social costs of mental conditions.

This view of the broad and substantial impact of mental conditions on our society's well-being is new. Large-scale surveys of disability in the US population only rarely include questions about mental conditions. In 1994, 70% of people in the USA with a mental condition—16.4 million people—were disabled, defined by serious life limitations, work impairment, self-perception, or participation in a disability program such as Supplemental Security Income (SSI) or Social Security Disability Insurance (SSDI; Jans and Stoddard 1999). Their report includes data from an earlier unpublished survey in which roughly two-thirds of women with mental conditions reported that these conditions limited them in nonwork domains and in their ability to cope with daily stress. More specifically, about half experienced limited ability to function socially and to concentrate, and about a fifth were limited in their ability to perform daily instrumental tasks such as shopping or money management. Paradoxically, although women appear in these surveys to be less impaired than men by mental conditions, they are more likely to report actual problem days related to medical, employment, family, psychological, and social problems (Mangrum et al. 2006). Women may have some added resilience because they begin to experience mental conditions (schizophrenia, depression) at later ages, which allows them more time to accomplish the social tasks of adolescence and young adulthood described above (Moldin 2000). They can then rely on the social tools they forged during these earlier periods of high functioning to continue to perform daily and instrumental tasks.

Mood Disorders

Among mental conditions, mood disorders pose the greatest societal burden because of the high prevalence and severe impairment associated with them. About one-fifth (21%) of US adults meet criteria for any lifetime, and one-tenth for any current mood disorder. Their median age of onset is 30 years, and at all ages, women are one and a half times more likely than men to have had a mood disorder in their lifetime (Kessler et al. 2005c). In an earlier national survey, almost one-quarter of women (24%) met criteria for any mood disorder in their lifetime and 14% met criteria currently (Kessler et al. 1994). Mood disorders are seriously disabling, producing serious impairment among almost half (45%) of those who met criteria in the NCS-R. The probability of serious impairment depends on the type of mood disorder: 83% of those with bipolar disorder, 50% of those with dysthymia, and 30% of those with major depressive disorder (MDD) were seriously impaired (Kessler et al. 2005c).

Major Depression

MDD requires a period of 2 weeks of either dysphoria or loss of interest or pleasure, as well as four additional symptoms lasting at least 2 weeks that include weight loss or gain, insomnia or hypersomnia, psychomotor agitation or retardation, fatigue or loss of energy, feelings of worthlessness or inappropriate guilt, impairment in concentration, or recurrent suicidal ideation or a suicide attempt (APA 2000). The lifetime prevalence of MDD is 17%, with women about one and a half times more likely than men to experience this condition in their lifetime and in any given year. In the original NCS (Kessler et al. 1994), 21% of adult women had lifetime, and 13% had current MDD.

Major depression is highly comorbid, with almost three-quarters of individuals with lifetime MDD having another condition queried in the NCS-R. Over half (59%) of those with lifetime MDD had also experienced a lifetime anxiety disorder, about one-third (30%) an impulse control disorder, and about one-quarter (24%) an SUD, controlling for gender, age, and race/ethnicity (Kessler 2003). MDD is episodic and recurrent, with a median age of onset of 32 years (Kessler et al. 2005a), and is highly likely to occur in conjunction with physical disabilities (Turner et al. 2006).

Depression affects women and men differently. In early adolescence, rates of depression begin to increase for girls, but not for boys (Kessler 2003), possibly according to a complex model that includes the different social pressures that girls experience as gender roles emerge, self-esteem issues associated with the physical changes of adolescence, and girls' cognitive and attribution styles (Kessler 2000; Hyde et al. 2008).

The incidence of depression appears to have increased dramatically over the past five decades (Kessler et al. 2005a), possibly due to changing sociodemographic factors, especially weakening social support networks (Eaton et al. 2007). In the USA, successively younger cohorts of women show increased rates of depression at later ages, through midlife, suggesting persistence, and therefore increased prevalence (Kessler 2003; Eaton et al. 2007). If this trend continues, as is likely (WHO 2007), by 2020 depression will be the second leading cause of disability worldwide, for women and men, and across the lifespan.

Women with MDD experience atypical and somatic symptoms of depression and are more likely than men to develop depression after a major life stressor; they are also more likely to report recent stressful life events (Burt and Stein 2002). Some studies indicate that women's reactions to life stress are different from men's, and that they react to stressors that men do not. For instance, women are more likely than men to attempt, though men are more likely to complete, suicide (Moscicki 2001; U.S. Public Health Service 1999), and they are more likely to experience depression in association with financial strain and debt, possibly because they are more acutely affected by economic and educational disparities (Muntaner et al. 2004). Lack of a social network compounds the impact of any of these difficulties, and women with MDD, who are more likely to come from families with histories of psychiatric conditions, may have more fragile family and social networks. Since greater impairment is associated with multiple conditions, women with depression who are seriously impaired are also highly likely to be coping with additional mental conditions and social problems.

Almost all (95%) individuals in the most impaired, highly comorbid cluster of conditions described earlier met criteria for current MDD or for dysthymia. Recall that this cluster is likely to be female, unmarried, White/other non-Hispanic, non-Black race/ethnicity, with low education and low to middle incomes, living in nonrural areas. Besides a mood disorder, this group is also likely to suffer from attention deficit/hyperactivity disorder (56%), a manic or hypomanic episode in the prior year (54%), alcohol abuse or dependence (42%), social phobia (41%), and intermittent explosive disorder (40%; Kessler et al. 2005c).

In the second cluster, described earlier in this chapter, characterized more by anxiety than mood disorders, the likely profile highlights women—divorced, separated, or widowed, living in suburban or outlying nonrural areas—with a comorbid but less impaired clinical profile than the cluster just described. MDD plays a key role in this cluster as well. Over half of those in this anxiety–MDD cluster also currently met criteria for specific phobia (53%) or social phobia (51%), and two-fifths

(41%) met criteria for MDD/dysthymia. Other anxiety disorders figured in this cluster as well, including panic disorder (33%), agoraphobia (24%), and generalized anxiety disorder (23%).

People with MDD experience serious impairment across a broad spectrum of dimensions, including days out of role, self-care, mobility, cognition, productivity, and social relationships, and their impairment increases as the severity of their depression symptoms increases. In the USA in 1996, depression was the second leading cause of disability for women, accounting for almost 7% of total DALYs (Michaud et al. 2001). In developed economies more generally, depression is the fourth leading cause of disability for women, accounting for almost 6% of total DALYs (Ustun et al. 2004). The average time in role activity lost by people with MDD is 35.1 days (Kessler et al. 2003) compared to fewer than 15 days lost by people with most other chronic conditions (Kessler et al. 2001). Among mental conditions, MDD accounts for the largest number of total days—387 million—out of role. Among all mental and physical conditions, it is second only to chronic neck–back pain in accounting for days out of role (Merikangas et al. 2007; also see Chap. 6 in this volume on Depression and Postpartum Disorders).

Anxiety Disorders

Anxiety disorders affect more people than any other category, and women are more likely than men to suffer from these conditions. In the NCS-R study, over a quarter (30%) of US adults met criteria for any anxiety disorder in their lifetime, and about one-fifth (18%) met criteria currently. The median age of onset for anxiety disorders is 11 years, and at all ages, women are 1.6 times more likely than men to have met the criteria for any anxiety disorder in their lifetime (Kessler et al. 2005c). In the earlier NCS, over one-quarter of women (31%) met lifetime criteria for any anxiety disorder, and 23% met criteria currently (Kessler et al. 1994).

Anxiety disorders as a whole are associated with the least impairment. Fewer than one-quarter (23%) of persons with a lifetime anxiety disorder were seriously impaired, but it is worth noting that half (51%) of those with obsessive-compulsive disorder were seriously impaired (Kessler et al. 2005c). Because anxiety disorders occur prior to adolescence, afflicted individuals may have some difficulty navigating adolescence and may develop other conditions with more impairment over time. These conditions frequently co-occur with mood disorders, and among women, when they pair with MDD and dysthymia, result in severe and moderate impairment (Kessler et al. 2005c). Mood disorders, rather than anxiety disorders, bring women into treatment, perhaps because some anxiety disorders are comparatively mild. Over 90% of women with bipolar disorder or dysthymia received treatment, compared to about 80% of those with generalized anxiety disorder, and only about one-quarter (27%) of those with social anxiety disorder (Wang et al. 2005a).

Posttraumatic Stress Disorder

To meet DSM-IV diagnostic criteria for PTSD, an individual must be exposed to an event, either by direct experience or by witnessing, that he or she experiences as life-threatening or potentially life-threatening and is accompanied by intense fear, helplessness, or horror. The traumatic event is followed by intrusive reexperiencing of the event either waking or in nightmares. This may include flashbacks; avoidance of aspects of the event and numbing of general responsiveness, including dissociation; or increased arousal, including sleep difficulties, hypervigilance, irritability, or outbursts of anger (APA 2000). Symptoms generally emerge within 3 months of exposure to the traumatic event, but sometimes do not surface for many years. Once present, symptoms must persist for more than a month to meet diagnostic criteria for PTSD. In simple PTSD, recovery occurs within 6 months. If symptoms persist for longer than 6 months, the diagnosis is considered chronic PTSD.

Exposure to events experienced as life-threatening is not rare. Among the general US population, all but a small minority (90%) have experienced such an event (Breslau 1998). The NCS (Kessler 1995b) probably estimated the lower range of exposure to traumatic events and prevalence of PTSD because it used the earlier, more conservative DSM-III-R criteria for exposure, and limited symptom descriptions to the single most traumatizing event experienced. Using these criteria, over half (60%) of US adults had been exposed to at least one traumatic event in their lifetime. The most frequently reported events were witnessing death or serious injury, experiencing a life-threatening accident, and being threatened with a weapon. Women reported lower rates of exposure to any traumatic event (51%) than men (61%) and experienced fewer events as well. Despite high rates of exposure, only 10% of women and 5% of men who experienced a traumatic event developed PTSD. But conditional risk, that is, the likelihood of developing PTSD given a traumatic experience, was more than twice as likely for women (20%) as for men (8%).

Epidemiological evidence suggests that women's heightened exposure to interpersonal and violent traumatic events such as rape or sexual assault (21%) is key to this increased risk for PTSD. Men are more likely to witness a traumatic event, to be in a life-threatening accident, to have experienced a natural disaster, to be threatened with a weapon, or to be the victim of a physical attack. But men who experience intimate violence are highly likely to develop PTSD as well. Most dramatically, almost half (46%) of women and two-thirds (65%) of men developed PTSD following rape (Kessler et al. 1995b). PTSD, though frequently underdiagnosed, has particular relevance for women's public health agenda, given the clear role of environmental risks and women's vulnerability to them.

PTSD occurs in combination with other conditions and with severe impairment. The vast majority (79%) of people with a lifetime diagnosis of PTSD in the NCS had at least one additional condition, but it was the small, severely impaired group of respondents with three or more conditions (14%) who were most likely to have had a lifetime diagnosis of PTSD (Kessler et al. 1995b). Almost half (44%) of the women with PTSD fell into that severely impaired group. Women with existing PTSD were four times more likely than those without to also have MDD or dysthymia. They were two to three times as likely to have anxiety disorders, including generalized anxiety disorder, panic disorder, social phobia, simple phobia, or agoraphobia, and they were two to four and a half times as likely to have an SUD (Kessler 2000).

Questions remain about whether preexisting other conditions increase the likelihood of exposure to trauma, raising the risk for developing PTSD, whether the prior other conditions directly increase vulnerability for PTSD and whether PTSD increases risk for other conditions when women use alcohol or other substances to cope with the distress of PTSD symptoms. Cross-sectional studies rely on recall to tease out the onset of each co-occurring condition and to develop hypotheses about causal relationships. Prospective studies provide better information on temporal relationships among other conditions, exposure to traumatic events, and development of PTSD symptoms. One such prospective study of a large community sample ($n = 1,007$) of young adults in the Midwest supports the self-medication hypothesis. New cases of SUD were four times higher among those with a history of PTSD at entry into the study, compared to those without a baseline diagnosis, whereas exposure was equivalent over the follow-up period for both groups (Chilcoat and Breslau 1998). In studies of natural disasters among both men and women, those who developed PTSD subsequently had higher prevalence of MDD, panic, generalized anxiety disorder, and SUDs (63%), compared to those with no PTSD (9%; North et al. 1999).

The risk profiles for MDD and PTSD are similar: women with a family history of MDD, a history of childhood trauma, and preexisting anxiety or depressive disorders (Breslau et al. 2000). Exposure to childhood abuse and neglect increase the risk for MDD. In one prospective study (Widom et al. 2007), children with adjudicated cases of childhood physical and sexual abuse were matched with nonabused children on age, race, sex, and social class ($n = 1,196$). In this sample, the neglected children had one and a half times the risk for MDD as the matched controls. They also had earlier onset, more lifetime symptoms, and more episodes of MDD. Although there was no difference in rates of lifetime MDD, the abused and neglected children had more lifetime depression symptoms and more episodes of MDD than the controls. They had earlier onset of MDD, with the groups beginning to diverge at around age 10, just prior to the divergence of male and female rates in early puberty reported above from the NCS-R. Among those with MDD, comorbidity was also higher for abused and neglected individuals: almost all of the abused and neglected group (96%) met criteria for at least one other diagnosis, compared to 83% of the controls. Such studies provide insight into the lifetime histories of those who develop PTSD, and how their early childhood experiences and personal environments may differ from those who do not.

Based on studies with clinical samples, people with severe mental illness have very high rates and unique patterns of exposure to traumatic experiences throughout their lives. Reported rates of exposure to sexual or physical abuse among female psychiatric patients range from 31 to 77% and sexual revictimization in adulthood is very common (Goodman et al. 1997; Mueser et al. 2002; Muenzenmaier et al. 1993). The most frequent traumatic events reported in a sample of outpatients with severe mental illness were sexual assault as adults, sexual assault as children, a car or work accident, and being attacked with a weapon, with an average of 3.5 lifetime traumatic events experienced. In this study, the prevalence of current PTSD was 43%, and predictors of PTSD consisted of a number of different types of trauma in addition to an experience of childhood sexual assault (Mueser et al. 1998). The picture that emerges makes it clear that highly comorbid profiles characterize this population as well. In one clinical study, over half of those who met DSM-III-R criteria for PTSD also met criteria for MDD (58%) and for bipolar disorder (54%), and a substantial proportion also met criteria for other psychotic disorders (40%), schizoaffective disorder (37%), and schizophrenia (28%; Mueser et al. 2002).

Comorbidity can exacerbate the severity of PTSD, and some conditions are characterized by high-risk behaviors that lead to continued exposure to traumatic experiences. PTSD is also characterized by a prolonged stress response that can produce medical conditions, such as chronic fatigue syndrome and fibromyalgia through the deleterious effects of chronic stress on the immune system. Individuals with PTSD can be retraumatized in institutional environments that can, in many ways, be reminiscent of the original event. Recognition of PTSD in these settings is essential for good outcomes and humane management.

Nonaffective Psychoses (NAP), Including Schizophrenia

The Diagnostic and Statistical Manual (APA 2000) groups schizophrenia and other psychotic disorders as NAP. Disorders in this category include schizophrenia, schizoaffective, delusional, and psychotic disorder not otherwise specified. These conditions are frequently treated in public sector settings. It is important to note that although an illicit or prescribed substance or a medical condition may also produce symptoms that characterize an NAP, criteria for an NAP require that the disturbance not be due to these causes. Symptoms of schizophrenia include two or more of the following characteristics: hallucinations, delusions, disorganized speech, disorganized thinking, negative symptoms (e.g., flattened affect or avolition), and social or occupational dysfunction (i.e., below a preonset level). Symptoms must be present for 6 months in order to meet diagnostic criteria for an NAP. This includes prodrome, 1 month of psychotic symptoms and a residual phase. Schizoaffective disorder includes an episode of major depression, a manic episode, or a mixed episode during which there are delusions or hallucinations for at least 2 weeks in the absence of prominent mood symptoms. Mood symptoms must be present for a substantial portion of active and residual periods of the illness. A delusional disorder is characterized by nonbizarre delusions, especially in relation to being persecuted, cheated, poisoned, or harassed. The person does not have impaired or odd and bizarre behavior and has never met criteria for the characteristic symptoms of schizophrenia.

Although rates of NAP, including schizophrenia, are very low, over the long term schizophrenia is one of the most disabling and costliest of diagnoses in terms of public health resources and loss of productivity. Such rare conditions require an extremely large screening sample that would include non-English speakers, street populations, and institutions such as psychiatric hospitals, prisons, and jails. Accomplishing this is complicated by the tendency of individuals with NAP to refuse to participate in surveys about mental conditions (Kessler et al. 2005b). For these reasons, estimates of societal burden and costs do not include this most severe condition. The NCS-R does include NAP and accounts for the sampling difficulties involved. The Structured Clinical Interview for Diagnosis (SCID; First et al. 1997) was administered to those who screened positive for NAP in Phase 2, who endorsed symptoms that were likely to meet criteria for an NAP diagnosis ($n = 73$). Lifetime prevalence of NAP was estimated at 5 per thousand, and 1 year rates at 3 per thousand (Kessler et al. 2005b). The median incidence rate of schizophrenia alone is 0.16 per thousand, based on a review of inpatient and outpatient studies since 1985 where diagnoses were made by a psychiatrist (Eaton 1999).

Rates of schizophrenia do not appear to differ for women and men, although diagnostic criteria, access to health care, geography, and inclusion/exclusion criteria, especially of migrants and homeless people, can greatly alter gender-specific results (Bhugra 2005; McGrath 2005; Kirkbride et al. 2006). But there are consistent gender differences in course and outcomes of these conditions (Grossman et al. 2006). Women with schizophrenia generally have a later age of onset than men, typically in their late 20s to mid-30s, and are more likely to experience depressive symptoms, auditory hallucinations, and paranoia. Many studies have shown that women experience fewer negative symptoms, respond better to antipsychotic medications, and generally follow a less severe course of illness than do men. It is possible that women have more developed social skills and are more intimately involved with family and social networks which provide greater support and can improve outcomes. Another explanation is that specific sex hormones are protective for psychotic symptoms (Grossman et al. 2006).

Individuals with NAP are likely to have additional conditions. Those who met criteria for NAP in their lifetime were 18 times as likely (79%) as those who did not to meet criteria for any other condition. Those who met criteria for a current NAP were six times as likely (64%) as those who did not to meet criteria for another condition. Individuals with lifetime NAP were most likely to also have bipolar disorder and obsessive-compulsive disorder, while those with a current NAP were most likely to also meet criteria for substance use dependence. Almost half of those with lifetime NAP met criteria for three or more conditions, as did almost a third of those with a current NAP (Kessler et al. 2005b).

Substance Use Disorders (SUDs)

SUDs are defined by patterns of use of alcohol or illicit substances that lead to clinically significant impairment or distress. A person meets criteria for substance abuse if in the past year their recurrent use results in one or more of the following at any time during the same 12-month period: (1) recurrent use results in failure to fulfill major work, school, or home obligations; (2) use occurs in situations where it is physically hazardous (driving, operating machinery); (3) recurrent substance-related legal problems; or (4) continued use despite persistent or recurrent social or interpersonal problems caused or exacerbated by the effects of substances (e.g., arguments with spouse about intoxication, physical fights). The criteria for the more serious category of substance dependence are met if in the past year their use results in three or more of the following: (1) tolerance (greater amounts required to achieve the same effect, or same amount produces a diminished effect); (2) physical withdrawal; (3) use of larger amounts or for longer periods than intended; (4) persistent desire or unsuccessful efforts to cut down or control use; (5) a great deal of time spent to obtain, use, or recover from use; (6) interference with involvement in social, occupational, or recreational activities; or (7) continued use despite knowledge that use causes or exacerbates physical or psychological problems (APA 2000).

An annual national probability sample of households and groups, but not institutions such as jails or hospitals, shows that while over half of Americans drank in the prior year, fewer than 10% had done so for 20–30 days in the prior month (SAMHSA 2005b). In the NCS study, about a quarter of American adults met criteria for any substance abuse or dependence in their lifetimes, and about a tenth did currently (Kessler et al. 1994). The median age of onset of SUDs is 20 years (SAMHSA 2006).

For many years SUD treatment, policy, and the research to develop new approaches were driven by the view that SUDs predominantly affect men. Over the past decade, however, more research and practice development have focused on risk factors, use patterns, consequences, treatment, and motivation for sustained recovery that are specific to women (e.g., National Center on Addiction and Substance Abuse (CASA) 2006).

In general, women are less likely than men to drink or use substances, are less likely to drink heavily or to binge drink, and are less likely to have an SUD, but, among recent cohorts, women's rates of substance use are more similar to men's (Kessler et al. 2005c; SAMHSA 2005b). In the past 15 years, there has been a marked drop in the age when young women take their first drink. This is particularly worrisome because women are more likely to develop alcohol-related problems the younger they are when they start drinking, and to develop symptoms of alcohol-related disorders more rapidly than men, a phenomenon known as "telescoping" (Kessler et al. 2005a; Zilberman et al. 2003).

Women's abuse of prescription drugs is similar to men's and is growing among girls, young women, and women over the age of 60. Since women are one and a half times more likely than men to be prescribed a narcotic, antianxiety, or other potentially abusable drug (CASA 2006), the ready accessibility and acceptability of these substances make them a serious threat to the health of women across the lifespan (Volkow 2006). In a national random household survey, nearly one-tenth of girls aged 12–17 said they used a prescription drug—especially psychotherapeutic drugs, including stimulants—to get high at least once in the past year, and about 2% of girls in this age group met criteria for dependence or abuse of prescription drugs (CASA 2006). Adolescents who are pregnant are more likely to abuse stimulants, sedatives, and tranquilizers than other adolescents, although in general, pregnant women are less likely to abuse prescription drugs than their nonpregnant counterparts. Women account for slightly over half of emergency room (ER) visits that involve prescription drug abuse but for only about one-third of street-drug-related ER visits (SAMHSA 2005a). Although absolute numbers are small, women make up almost three-quarters of those receiving treatment for dependence on sedatives (some antidepressants) and on tranquilizers such as Valium or Xanax (SAMHSA 2001).

On an annual basis, substance abuse, including alcohol, illicit drugs, and tobacco, costs the US economy over $414 billion and is the cause of more deaths (one in four), illness, and disabilities than any other preventable health condition (Horgan et al. 2001). In combination with depression and anxiety, which are most prevalent among women, substance abuse is a key risk factor in suicide, and also places women at increased risk for victimization (robbery, physical, or sexual assault); contact with the criminal justice system; sanctions in public systems (e.g., loss of child custody); engagement in high-risk sexual behaviors and contracting sexually transmitted diseases, including HIV/AIDS (Alexander and Muenzenmaier 1998; Teplin et al. 2005; Klinkenberg and Sacks 2004; Stoskopf et al. 2001; Brunette and Dean 2002; Brunette and Drake 1998; SAMHSA 2006). Substance use and abuse also affects women's intimate relationships. Women with an SUD are more likely to be separated or divorced, and those who are married or living under common law are more likely than men to have a partner with a substance-related problem (Zilberman et al. 2003).

Substance abuse is a key feature in complex profiles of mental illness. Overall, almost half of those with a current SUD have another mental condition. Individuals with any mental condition are about twice as likely as those without to have an alcohol use disorder, and about five times as likely to have a drug use disorder (Kessler et al. 1994). Together, SUD and depression constitute the number one cause of lost years of productive life for women (Wenzel et al. 2000), reflected in the role played by alcohol use disorders and MDD in one of the most impairing, complex clusters of conditions associated with women in the NCS-R (Kessler et al. 2005c).

Consistently, people who have a mental condition that results in serious impairment, including NAP and MDD, are at the highest risk for a co-occurring SUD. In 1 month, they are three times more likely to use illicit drugs, and twice as likely to drink heavily (more than five drinks on five or more occasions in a month) than others (SAMHSA 2005b). Based on a national probability sample, these severely impairing mental conditions and SUDs occur together in about 2 million women and about 2 million men (SAMHSA 2003). Studies conducted in mental health settings consistently find slightly lower rates of co-occurring SUD for women (Brunette and Drake 1998; Drake et al. 1989; Mueser et al. 1992, Zilberman et al. 2003), underscoring how important the composition of a study sample is to understanding results: more women are present in mental health treatment settings, and more men in addiction treatment settings.

Few women access treatment for SUD—fewer than 20% of women in a representative national household survey who met criteria for needing treatment received it. Very few (5%) of the women who did not receive treatment thought they needed it, and they cited cost and inadequate insurance, stigma of treatment, and not being ready to stop as access barriers (SAMHSA 2007). They are more likely than men to be referred to chemical dependency treatment by social service or medical providers rather than through the criminal justice system, and are most likely to cite alcohol (40%), cocaine (22%), or heroin/opiates (20%) as their primary substance of abuse (SAMHSA 2001).

In mental health specialty treatment settings, women with co-occurring severe mental illness and substance use problems experience impairment that is as severe as that experienced by men with similar problems, but women have distinct profiles of vulnerability and need (Alexander 1996; Brunette and Drake 1998). Their exposure to trauma and victimization and to messages that diminish self-esteem make them especially vulnerable to SUD: women report that they use alcohol and drugs to increase their confidence, to cope with many of the difficulties of PTSD, and to lose weight (Ullman et al. 2005; Dams-O'Connor et al. 2006). They need access to information and coping strategies around sexuality, including family planning and sexually transmitted diseases (Miller and Finnerty 1996), and education in how to negotiate difficult and complex arrangements for the care and custody of their children (Nicholson et al. 1998). It is to be hoped that recently developed treatment approaches that address women's histories and life circumstances (Ouimette and Brown 2002; Najavits 2003), and federal initiatives to integrate mental health and substance abuse treatment (SAMHSA 2006) will make recovery more accessible to women. For additional information on substance abuse, see Chap. 9 in this volume.

Limitations on Women's Freedom to Participate

A framework currently used in international development, the capabilities approach (Sen 1999) includes local communities in identifying what they value, and focuses on those aspects of social participation, such as income, education/literacy, work, security, and citizenship, to assess what individuals are capable of achieving in a given culture. The capabilities approach, widely used to develop women's participation in developing economies (Alkire 2005), is beginning to be applied to public mental health (Davidson et al. 2008; Hopper 2007; Ware et al. 2007; Alexander and Hopper 2007).

Opportunities for a healthy and normal lifespan that includes participation in family and community life are substantially diminished for women with psychiatric disabilities. Worldwide, disability is associated with poverty and disadvantage (Peat 1998), and regardless of the causal direction, there is little doubt that disadvantage is cumulative and contributes to degraded quality of life, including higher rates of illness and early mortality (Corso et al. 2008; Leeb et al. 2008; Felitti et al. 1998; Draine et al. 2002; Dube et al. 2003; Dickey et al. 2003; Link and Phelan 1995; Kawachi et al. 1997; Hahn 1987; MacIntyre et al. 1993). The high rates of victimization associated with mental conditions compound these quality of life disparities (Felitti et al. 1998; Dube et al. 2003; Teplin et al. 2005). Finally, their limited access to participation in parenting and family life diminishes their ability to fully express aspects of identity that they value. Key life domains are affected. About half of the adults with current MDD experience severe or very severe impairment in their social lives (50%), at home (46%), and in close relationships (43%), and about a third do at school, or work (36%; SAMHSA 2005b).

Disabling mental conditions translate into substantial handicap when those afflicted have limited access to resources and when their ability to convert the resources they can access into real opportunities is further limited by law, custom, and social policies. For instance, while people with psychiatric disorders constitute the largest working-age disability group receiving public income support, 3 years following the work of the President's New Freedom Commission, one-quarter of women with a disabling mental illness were unemployed, as opposed to 7% of women who had a physical disability but no mental illness diagnosis (Cook 2006). Since there is little data available on recovery and participation for people with mental disorders, we focus here on topics of personal disablement and their consequences for women. The challenge for women's public mental health is to promote and sustain policies and social conditions that will foster their recovery and participation. There is much work to be done.

Health

Mental conditions have a serious impact on health and life. Both men and women with severe mental disorders are likely to die 25 years earlier than their age-matched peers (Parks et al. 2006; Colton and Manderscheid 2006). Women in the general population have lower rates of mortality than men from heart disease, cerebrovascular disease, chronic lower respiratory disease, diabetes, hypertension, and elevated blood pressure. Approximately 36% of women in the general population were of healthy weight in 2004 (National Center for Health Statistics 2006). In striking contrast, men and women with serious mental conditions appear to have similar, elevated rates of cardiovascular disease, cancers, smoking and respiratory ailments, diabetes, and metabolic syndrome (Parks et al. 2006). Among Medicaid beneficiaries, they are three times more likely to be treated for diabetes and heart disease, and about twice as likely to be treated for hypertension, asthma, and respiratory disorders as those without a mental condition (Dickey 2005). Indeed, in one study women had higher cause-specific years of potential life lost, except for homicides, pneumonia/influenza, and heart disease (Miller et al. 2006). Women with a mental disorder are almost twice as likely to have HIV/AIDS as women without, although mental illnesses do not increase risk of infection for men (Stoskopf et al. 2001). Although SUDs are relatively low among women, their health consequences are severe. Over half (57%) of AIDS cases among women are associated with intravenous drug-use-related factors, which especially affect African-American (26%) and Hispanic (31%) women (Klinkenberg and Sacks 2004). In the same study, 35% of the women with HIV/AIDS met criteria for PTSD (Klinkenberg and Sacks 2004). We know a good deal about the causes of these health inequities and now need to develop policy and practice to support the social and personal factors that secure and promote healthy lives.

Security

The failure of cultures across the world to provide for children's security and safety, reflected especially in their exposure to violence, undermines their opportunities to live healthy lives. A study of over 9,500 adult HMO enrollees examined the relationships between childhood adversity, risk factors, and adult health and social consequences up to 50 years later (Felitti et al. 1998; Leeb et al. 2008). More than half of the respondents had experienced at least one, and one-quarter had experienced two or more types of adverse childhood events that included psychological, physical, or sexual abuse and witnessing violence against their mothers. Health risks and the likelihood of poor health outcomes were amplified as the number and severity of events increased. Those exposed to four or more types of adverse events had four to twelve times the risk for alcoholism, drug abuse, depression, and suicide attempts. They were two to four times more likely to smoke, to have poor self-rated health, more than 50 sexual partners and sexually transmitted diseases; about one and a half times as likely to have low levels of physical activity and to be severely obese; and had elevated risk of heart disease, cancer, chronic lung disease, fractures, and liver disease. In a slightly different sample, both men and women whose adverse event profiles included childhood sexual abuse had similar elevated rates of substance use and abuse, mental illness, and marital and family problems in later life (Dube et al. 2005). A population-based twin study, where family background factors were similar, suggests a causal relationship between childhood sexual abuse and increased risk for mental and substance use disorders (Kendler et al. 2000). In this study, in which about one-third of the sample reported any childhood sexual abuse, increasingly severe forms of abuse (genital abuse and intercourse) placed the exposed twin at roughly three times the risk for MDD, generalized anxiety disorder, panic, and bulimia, four times the risk for alcohol dependence, and five times the risk for drug dependence and for having two or more mental conditions.

Exposure to violence in childhood increases the risk for homelessness among adults with persistent mental illness, which in turn limits their ability to participate in a stable and cohesive family and community life. High rates of childhood and adult physical and sexual abuse among both men and women who are homeless and mentally ill (Goodman et al. 1995; North and Smith 1993; Caton et al. 1995) suggest that this is a population with few or no social supports or housing options when they leave an abusive home situation. Homeless women have especially high rates of serious mental conditions (50–60%) compared to homeless men (20–40%), to housed, low-income women, and to the general population (6%; Brunette and Drake 1998; Smith et al. 1993; Kessler et al. 2002). In general, homeless women with and without other mental disorders face the same risks for SUDs as men, but sheltered homeless women with SUDs stay homeless longer than other sheltered homeless women (Caton et al. 1995).

Although the media frequently associates mental conditions with committing acts of violence and endangering the safety and security of others, in fact, adults with severe mental illness have quadruple the risk for being a crime victim, especially of a violent crime, compared to other poor people in urban areas. Both men and women are at elevated risk, but women are especially likely to be victims of rape/sexual assault, robbery and assault, simple and aggravated assault. Reports from one study using the National Crime Victims' Survey sampling protocol for this population found that women with serious mental illness were significantly more likely than men (27% vs. 23%) and about 16 times more likely than women in the general population to be victims of violent crime. In addition, 4% of women with serious mental illness reported having been victims of rape or sexual assault, making them about 19 times more likely than women in the general population to be victims of sexual violence (Teplin et al. 2005).

Parenting

Women with mental illness are at least as likely to give birth to children as other US women (Thrasher and Mowbray 1995), but their opportunities to participate in the safe bearing, rearing, and raising of their children are limited. In part, this exclusion is related to the few treatment options available to pregnant and nursing women. The lack of research about the safety of most psychotropic medications for pregnant women increases the risk for women with mental conditions for serious disorders during their pregnancies and following childbirth. Many high-risk women feel they have no choice but to suspend their medication regimen during and sometimes beyond pregnancy, when they are already at increased risk for episodes of depression and bipolar disorder. Depressed women who discontinue medication during pregnancy increase their risk of relapse by 75% (Brunette and Dean 2002; Burt and Stein 2002), and half of the women with untreated bipolar disorder experience postpartum mania, compared to only 10% of those who receive treatment (Brunette and Dean 2002).

Many women with mental disorders who are not visibly with their children are indeed mothers whose identities are deeply embedded in that role and relationship. Mothers with serious mental disorders, particularly in combination with substance abuse, are frequently separated from their children, sometimes having lost custody (Crystal 1984; Cowal et al. 2002; Barrow and Lawinski 2009). The public systems they encounter rarely take into account that these women expect and wish to reunite with their children (Moynihan et al. 2001; Roberts 1999) who are frequently cared for by extended family during these separations (Katz 2002; Barrow 2002; Koegel 1987; Ware et al. 1999; see also Chap. 19 in this volume on "Parenting and Recovery for Mothers with Mental Disorders").

Treatment

Women, as they face elevated lifetime risks for mental conditions, are highly likely to seek and receive treatment. In the NCS-R, receiving any treatment is significantly related to being female, less than 60 years old, of non-Hispanic White ethnicity, previously married, not living in a rural area, and not having low average family income. This profile of women resembles some of the most impaired groups discussed earlier in this chapter who are likely to be unmarried women of non-Hispanic, non-Black ethnicity, with low education and low to middle incomes, living in nonrural areas (Kessler et al. 2005c). Women are more likely than men to receive treatment for their mental conditions in medical settings, with a high likelihood of receiving a prescription for psychotropic medication (Mangrum et al. 2006). However only one-third of treatments in the NCS-R were minimally adequate, according to evidence-based treatment guidelines (Wang et al. 2005b). Effective treatment is scarce, and women's access to it is further limited by difficulties in obtaining transportation and providing care for their children. Furthermore, women, especially those who are most impaired, frequently fear they may lose custody of their children if they engage with mental health or chemical dependency services (Rosen et al. 2004).

Implications for Women's Mental Health

Traditionally, the course of research in public health begins with identifying a problem and ends with ensuring access to treatment and, more recently, access to recovery—a life beyond treatment and treatment systems (Hogan 2003). When women seek professional help for their problems, they should be offered a comprehensive and holistic assessment and access to competent, effective, and recovery-focused services. In a broader sense, the capabilities approach provides a bridge between epidemiological data points, statistical clusters, and the real-life women who struggle to cope daily with the impairment, disability, and handicap of mental conditions. It frames quality of life and well-being within a social context, including a woman's personal characteristics, her environment, and the resources available to her. Capabilities focus on her ability to be and do the things she values—her self-agency (Ware et al. 2007), helped or hindered by law, custom, and policy. Epidemiologic data show us how multiple, interconnected mental conditions and poor health cause significant disability for women. Both can be traced to economic disadvantage and to environments and behaviors that compromise their safety and security. Public health can focus its attention again on malleable social conditions—intimate and family violence, poverty, access to work, criminalization of substance abuse—and on effective and engaging treatment options to provide women and girls with real and practical opportunities to fully realize their potential.

References

Albrecht, G., Seelman, K., & Bury, M. (Eds.). (2001). *The handbook of disability studies.* London: Sage.

Alexander, M. J. (1996). Women with co-occurring addictive and mental disorders: An emerging profile of vulnerability. *American Journal of Orthopsychiatry, 66*(1), 61–70.

Alexander, M. J., & Hopper, K. (2007). *Capabilities and psychiatric disability: Rethinking public mental health.* Paper prepared for the Human Development and Capability Association 2007 Annual Meeting.

Alexander, M. J., & Muenzenmaier, K. (1998). Trauma, addiction and recovery: Addressing public health epidemics among women with severe mental illness. In B. Levin, A. Blanch, & A. Jennings (Eds.), *Women's mental health services: A public health perspective.* Beverly Hills, CA: Sage.

Alkire, S. (2005). Why the capability approach? *Journal of Human Development, 6*(1), 115–135.

American Psychiatric Association (APA). (2000). *Diagnostic and statistical manual of mental disorders, fourth edition, text revision (DSM-IV-TR).* Washington, DC: American Psychiatric Association.

Barrow, S. (2002). *Issues of motherhood for women in homeless shelters for single adults.* Paper presented at the Annual Meeting of the American Public Health Association, Philadelphia.

Barrow, S. M., & Lawinski, T. (2009). Contexts of mother-child separations in homeless families. *Analyses of Social Issues and Public Policy.* doi: 10.1111/j.1530-2415.2009.01171.x.

Bhugra, D. (2005). The global prevalence of schizophrenia. *PLoS Medicine, 2*(5), e151.

Breslau, N. (1998). Epidemiology of trauma and post-traumatic stress disorder. In R. Yehuda (Ed.), *Psychological Trauma.* In J. M. Oldham & M. B. Riba (Eds.), *Review of Psychiatry* (Vol. 17, pp. 1–29). Washington, DC: APA.

Breslau, N., Davis, G. C., Peterson, E. L., & Schultz, L. R. (2000). A second look at comorbidity in victims of trauma: The posttraumatic stress disorder-major depression connection. *Biological Psychiatry, 48*(9), 902–909.

Brunette, M. F., & Dean, W. (2002). Community mental healthcare for women with severe mental illness who are parents. *Community Mental Health Journal, 38*(2), 153–165.

Brunette, M. F., & Drake, R. (1998). Gender differences in homeless persons with schizophrenia and substance abuse. *Community Mental Health Journal, 34*(6), 627–642.

Burt, V. K., & Stein, K. (2002). Epidemiology of depression throughout the female life-cycle. *Journal of Clinical Psychiatry, 63*(Suppl. 7), 9–15.

Caton, C. L. M., Shrout, P. E., Dominguez, B., Eagle, P. F., Opler, L. A., & Cournos, F. (1995). Risk-factors for homelessness among women with schizophrenia. *American Journal of Public Health, 85*(8), 1153–1156.

Chilcoat, H. D., & Breslau, N. (1998). PTSD and drug use disorders: Testing the causal pathways. *Archives of General Psychiatry, 55,* 913–917.

Colton, C. W., & Manderscheid, R. W. (2006). Congruencies in increased mortality rates, years of potential life lost, and causes of death among public mental health clients in eight states. *Preventing Chronic Disease, 3*(2), A42–A56.

Cook, J. A. (2006). Employment barriers for persons with psychiatric disabilities: Update of a report for the President's Commission. *Psychiatric Services, 57*(10), 1391–1405.

Corso, P. S., Edwards, V. J., Fang, X., & Mercy, J. A. (2008). Health-related quality of life among adults who experiences maltreatment during childhood. *American Journal of Public Health, 98*(6), 1094–1100.

Cowal, K., Shinn, M., Weitzman, B. C., Stojanovic, D., & Labay, L. (2002). Mother-child separations among homeless and housed families receiving public assistance in New York City. *American Journal of Community Psychology, 30,* 711–730.

Crystal, S. (1984). Homeless men and homeless women: The gender gap. *Urban and Social Change Review, 17,* 2–6.

Dams-O'Connor, K., Martens, M. P., & Anderson, D. A. (2006). Alcohol-related consequences among women who want to lose weight. *Eating Behaviors, 7*(3), 188–195.

Davidson, L., Schmutte, T., Dinzeo, T., Andres-Hyman, R. (2008). Remission and recovery in schizophrenia: Practitioner and patient perspectives. *Schizophrenia Bulletin, 34,* 5–8.

Dickey, B. (2005). The social gradient of health: A mental health services research agenda based on principles of economic and social justice. *Harvard Health Policy Review, 6*(2), 22–34.

Dickey, B., Azeni, H., Weiss, R., & Sederer, L. (2000). Schizophrenia, substance use disorders and medical co-morbidity. *Journal of Mental Health Policy and Economics, 3,* 27–33.

Dickey, B., Dembling, B., Azeni, H., & Normand, S. L. (2003). Externally caused death rates for adults with mental illness and co-morbid substance use disorders. *Journal of Behavioral Health Services and Research, 1,* 75–85.

Dickey, B., Normand, S.-L. T., Weiss, R. D., Drake, R. E., & Azeni, H. (2002). Medical morbidity, mental illness and substance use disorders. *Psychiatric Services, 53*(7), 861–867.

Draine, J., Salzer, M. S., Culhane, D. P., & Hadley, T. R. (2002). Role of social disadvantage in crime, joblessness, and homelessness among persons with serious mental illness. *Psychiatric Services, 53,* 565–73.

Drake, R. E., Osher, F. C., & Wallach, M. A. (1989). Alcohol use and abuse in schizophrenia: A prospective community study. *Journal of Nervous and Mental Disorders, 177*(7), 408–414.

Dube, S. R., Anda, R. F., Whitfield, C. L., Brown, D. W., Felitti, V. J., Dong, M., & Giles W. H. (2005). Long-term consequences of childhood sexual abuse by gender of victim. *American Journal of Preventive Medicine, 28*(5), 430–438.

Dube, S. R., Felitti, V. J., Dong, M., Giles, W. H., & Anda, R. F. (2003). The impact of adverse childhood experiences on health problems: Evidence from four birth cohorts dating back to 1900. *Preventive Medicine, 37,* 268–277.

Eaton, W. W. (1999). Evidence for universality and uniformity of schizophrenia around the world: Assessment and implications. In W. F. Gattaz & H. Hafner (Eds.), *Search for the Causes of Schizophrenia, Vol. 4: Balance of the Century* (pp. 21–33). New York, NY: Springer.

Eaton, W. W., Kalaydjian, A., Scharfstein, D. O., Mezuk, B., & Ding, Y. (2007). Prevalence and incidence of depressive disorder: The Baltimore ECA follow-up, 1981–2004. *Acta Psychiatrica Scandinavica, 116*(3), 182–188.

Felitti, V. J., Anda, R. F., Nordenberg, D., et al. (1998). Relationship of childhood abuse and household dysfunction to many of the leading causes of death in adults. The adverse childhood experiences (ACE) study. *American Journal of Preventive Medicine, 14,* 354–364.

First, M. B. (2002). DSM-IV and Psychiatric Epidemiology. In M. T. Tsuang & M. Tohen (Eds.), *Textbook in Psychiatric Epidemiology* (2nd ed.). New York, NY: Wiley.

First, M. B., Spitzer, R. L., Gibbon, M., & Williams, J. (1997). *Structured Clinical Interview for DSM-IV Axis I Disorders.* Washington, DC: American Psychiatric Press.

Goodman, L. A., Dutton, M. A., & Harris, M. (1995). Episodically homeless women with serious mental illness: Prevalence of physical and sexual assault. *American Journal of Orthopsychiatry, 65*(4), 468–478.

Goodman, L. A., Rosenberg, S. D., Mueser, K. T., & Drake, R. E. (1997). Physical and sexual assault history in women with serious mental illness: Prevalence, correlates, treatment, and future research directions. *Schizophrenia Bulletin, 23,* 685–696.

Grossman, L. S., Harrow, M., Rosen, C., & Faull, R. (2006). Sex differences in outcome and recovery for schizophrenia and other psychotic and non-psychotic disorders. *Psychiatric Services, 57,* 844–850.

Hahn, H. (1987). Public policy and disabled infants: A sociological perspective. *Issues in Law and Medicine, 3,* 3–27.

Hogan, M. F. (2003). New Freedom Commission Report: The President's New Freedom Commission: Recommendations to transform mental health care in America. *Psychiatric Services, 54,* 1467–1474.

Hopper, K. (2007). Rethinking social recovery in schizophrenia: What a capabilities approach might offer. *Social Science & Medicine, 65*(5), 868–879.

Horgan, C., Skwara, K. C., & Strickler, G. (2001). *Substance abuse: The nation's number one health problem: Indicators for policy.* Princeton, NJ: The Robert Wood Johnson Foundation.

Hyde, J. S., Mezulis, A. H., & Abramson, L. Y. (2008). The ABC's of depression: Integrating affective, biological, and cognitive models to explain the emergence of the gender difference in depression. *Psychological Review, 115*(2), 291–313.

Jans, L., & Stoddard, S. (1999). *Chart book on women and disability in the United States.* An InfoUse Report. Washington, DC: U.S. Department of Education, National Institute on Disability and Rehabilitation Research.

Katz, L. (2002). Evaluation and services for children of incarcerated parents with co-occurring disorders. In S. Davidson & H. Hills (Eds.), *Series on Women with Mental Illness and Co-Occurring Disorders.* Delmar, NY: National Gains Center.

Kawachi, I., Kennedy, B., & Lochner, K. (1997). Long live community: Social capital as public health. *The American Prospect, 35,* 56–59.

Kendler, K. S., Bulik, C. M., Silberg, J., Hettema, J. M., Myers, J., & Prescott, C. A. (2000). Childhood sexual abuse and adult psychiatric and substance abuse disorders in women. *Archives of General Psychiatry, 57,* 953–959.

Kessler, R. C. (2000). PTSD: The burden to the individual and to society. *Journal of Clinical Psychiatry, 61,* 4–12.

Kessler, R. C. (2003). Epidemiology of women and depression. *Journal of Affective Disorders, 74,* 5–13.

Kessler, R. C., Andrews, G., Colpe, L. J., Hiripi, E., Mroczek, D. K., Normand, S. L., et al. (2002). Short screening scales to monitor population prevalences and trends in non-specific psychological distress. *Psychological Medicine, 31,* 959–976.

Kessler, R. C., Berglund, P., Demler, O., Jin, R., & Walters, E. E. (2005a). Lifetime prevalence and age-of-onset distributions of DSM-IV disorders in the National Comorbidity Survey Replication. *Archives of General Psychiatry, 62,* 593–602.

Kessler, R. C., Berglund, P. A., Foster, C. L., Saunders, W. B., Stang, P. E., & Walters, E. E. (1997). Social consequences of psychiatric disorders, II: Teenage parenthood. *American Journal of Psychiatry, 154*(10), 1405–1411.

Kessler, R. C., Birnbaum, H., Demler, O., Falloon, I. R. H., Gagnon, E., Guyer, M., et al. (2005b). The prevalence and correlates of nonaffective psychosis in the National Comorbidity Survey Replication. *Biological Psychiatry, 58*(8), 668–676.

Kessler, R. C., Chiu, W. J., Demler, O., & Walters, E. E. (2005c). Prevalence, severity, and comorbidity of 12-month DSM-IV disorders in the National Comorbidity Survey Replication. *Archives of General Psychiatry, 62,* 617–627.

Kessler, R. C., Foster, C. L., Saunders, W. B., & Stang, P. E. (1995a). Social consequences of psychiatric disorders, I: Educational attainment. *American Journal of Psychiatry, 152*(7), 1026–1032.

Kessler, R. C., Greenberg, P. E., Mickelson, K. D., Meneades, L. M., & Wang, P. S. (2001). The effects of chronic medical conditions on work loss and work cutback. *Journal of Occupational and Environmental Medicine, 43,* 218–225.

Kessler, R. C., Heeringa, S., Lakoma, M. D., Petukhova, M., Rupp, A. E., Schoenbaum, M., et al. (2008). Individual and societal effects of mental disorders on earnings in the United States: Results from the NCS-R. *American Journal of Psychiatry, 165*(6), 703–711.

Kessler, R. C., McGonagle, K. A., Zhao, S., Nelson, C. B., Hughs, M., Eshelman, S., et al. (1994). Lifetime and 12-month prevalence of DSM-III-R psychiatric disorders in the United States: Results from the National Comorbidity Study. *Archives of General Psychiatry, 51,* 8–19.

Kessler, R. C., Ormel, J., Demler, O., & Stang, P. E. (2003). Comorbid mental disorders account for the role impairment of commonly occurring chronic physical disorders: Results from the National Comorbidity Survey. *Journal of Occupational & Environmental Medicine, 45,* 1257–1266.

Kessler, R. C., Sonnega, A., Bromet, E., Hughes, M., & Nelson, C. B. (1995b). Post traumatic stress disorder in the NCS. *Archives of General Psychiatry, 52,* 1048–1060.

Kessler, R. C., Walters, E. E., & Forthofer, M. S. (1998). The social consequences of psychiatric disorders, III: Probability of marital stability. *American Journal of Psychiatry, 155,* 1092–1096.

Kirkbride, J. B., Fearon, P., Morgan, C., Dazzan, P., Morgan, K., Tarrant, J., et al. (2006). Heterogeneity in the incidence rates of schizophrenia and other psychotic syndromes: Findings from the 3-center AESOP study. *Archives of General Psychiatry, 63*, 250–258.

Klinkenberg, W. D., & Sacks, S. (2004). Mental disorders and drug abuse in persons living with HIV/AIDS. *AIDS Care, 16*(Suppl. 1), 522–542.

Koegel, P. (1987, January). *Ethnographic perspectives on homeless and mentally ill homeless women.* Paper presented at the Homeless and homeless mentally ill women: An ethnographic research colloquium. NIMH.

Leeb, R. T., Paulozzi, L., Melanson, C., Simon, T., & Arias, I. (2008). *Child maltreatment surveillance: Uniform definitions for public health and recommended data elements, version 1.0.* Atlanta, GA: Centers for Disease Control & Prevention (CDC), National Center for Injury Prevention and Control.

Lilienfeld, D. E., & Stolley, P. D. (Eds.). (1994). *Foundations of Epidemiology* (3rd ed., p. 3). New York, NY: Oxford University Press.

Link, B. G., & Phelan, J. (1995). Social conditions as fundamental causes of disease. *Journal of Health and Social Behavior,* Spec No., 80–94.

MacIntyre, S., MacIver, S., & Sooman, A. (1993). Area, class and health: Should we be focusing on places or people? *Journal of Social Policy, 22,* 13–34.

Mangrum, L. F., Spence, R. T., & Steinky-Bumgarner, M. D. (2006). Gender differences in substance abuse treatment clients with co-occurring psychiatric and substance-use disorders. *Brief Treatment and Crisis Intervention, 6,* 255–267.

McGrath, J. J. (2005). Myths and plain truths about schizophrenia epidemiology: The NAPE lecture 2004. *Acta Psychiatrica Scandinavica, 111*(1), 4–11.

Merikangas, K. R., Ames, M., Cui, L., Stang, P. E., Ustun, T. B., Von Korff, M., et al. (2007). The impact of comorbidity of mental and physical conditions on role disability in the U.S. adult household population. *Archives of General Psychiatry, 64,* 1180–1188.

Michaud, C. M., Murray, C. J. L., & Bloom, B. R. (2001). Burden of disease – Implications for future research. *The Journal of the American Medical Association, 285*(5), 535–539.

Miller, B. J., Paschall, B., & Svendsen, D. P. (2006). Mortality and medical comorbidity among patients with serious mental illness. *Psychiatric Services, 57,* 1482–1487.

Miller, L. J., & Finnerty, M. (1996). Sexuality, pregnancy, and childrearing among women with schizophrenia – spectrum disorders. *Psychiatric Services, 47*(5), 502–506.

Mitra, S. (2006). The capability approach and disability. *Journal of Disability and Policy Studies, 16*(4), 236–247.

Modell, J. (1989). *Into one's own: From youth to adulthood in the United States, 1920–1975.* Berkeley, CA: University of California Press.

Moldin, S. O. (2000). Gender and schizophrenia: An overview. In E. Frank (Ed.), *Gender and its effect on psychopathology* (pp. 169–186). Washington, DC: American Association Press.

Moscicki, E. K. (2001). Epidemiology of completed and attempted suicide: Toward a framework for prevention. *Clinical Neuroscience Research, 1,* 310–323.

Moynihan, A., Forgey, M. A., & Harris, D. (2001). Symposium: Fordham interdisciplinary conference achieving justice: Parents and the child welfare system: Forward. *Fordham Law Review, 70,* 287–335.

Muenzenmaier, K., Meyer, I., Struening, E., & Ferber, J. (1993). Childhood abuse and neglect among women outpatients with chronic mental illness. *Hospital and Community Psychiatry, 44,* 666–670.

Mueser, K. T., Goodman, L. B., Trumbetta, S. L., Rosenberg, S. D., Osher, C., Vidaver, R., et al. (1998). Trauma and posttraumatic stress disorder in severe mental illness. *Journal of Consulting and Clinical Psychology, 66*(3), 493–499.

Mueser, K. T., Rosenberg, S. D., Goodman, L. A., & Trumbetta, S. L. (2002). Trauma, PTSD, and the course of severe mental illness: An interactive model. *Schizophrenia Research, 53*(1–2), 123–143.

Mueser, K. T., Yarnold, P. R., & Bellack, A. S. (1992). Diagnostic and demographic correlates of substance abuse in schizophrenia and major affective disorder. *Acta Psychiatrica Scandinavica, 85*(1), 48–55.

Muntaner, C., Eaton, W. W., Miech, R., & O'Campo, P. (2004). Socioeconomic position and major mental disorders. *Epidemiologic Review, 26,* 53–62.

Murray, C. J. L., & Lopez, A. D. (1996). *The global burden of disease and injury series, Vol. 1: A comprehensive assessment of mortality and disability from diseases, injuries, and risk factors in 1990 and projected to 2020.* Harvard School of Public Health on behalf of the World Health Organization and World Bank, Cambridge, MA: Harvard University Press.

Najavits, L. M. (2003). Seeking safety: A new psychotherapy for posttraumatic stress disorder and substance use disorder. In P. Ouimette & P. Brown (Eds.), *Trauma and substance abuse: Causes, consequences, and treatment of comorbid disorders* (pp. 147–170). Washington, DC: American Psychological Association Press.

National Center for Health Statistics. (2006). *Women's health tables.* Retrieved 2007, from Centers for Disease Control and Prevention. http://www.cdc.gov/nchs/products/pubs/pubd/hus/women.htm#deaths

National Center on Addiction and Substance Abuse at Columbia University (CASA). (2006). *Women under the influence.* Baltimore, MD: Johns Hopkins University Press.

Nicholson, J., Sweeney, E. M., & Geller, J. L. (1998). Focus on women: Mothers with mental illness: I. The competing demands of parenting and living with mental illness. *Psychiatric Services, 49,* 635–642.

North, C. S., & Smith, E. M. (1993). A comparison of homeless men and women: Different populations, different needs. *Community Mental Health Journal, 29,* 423–431.

North, C. S., Nixon, S. J., Shariat, S., Mallonee, S., McMillen, J. C., Spitznagel, E. L., et al. (1999). Psychiatric disorders among survivors of the Oklahoma city bombing. *Journal of the American Medical Association, 282,* 755–762.

Olesen, J., & Leonardi, M. (2003). The burden of brain diseases in Europe. *European Journal of Neurology, 10,* 471–447.

Ouimette P., & Brown, P. (Eds.). (2002). *Trauma and substance abuse: Causes, consequences, and treatment of comorbid disorders.* Washington, DC: American Psychological Association Press.

Parks, J., Svendsen, D., Singer, P., & Foti, M. E. (2006). *Morbidity and mortality in people with serious mental illness.* NASMHPD Medical Directors' Council, 13th Technical Report, Alexandria, VA, p. 14.

Peat, M. (1998). Disability in the developing world. In M. A. McColl & J. E. Bickenbach (Eds.), *Introduction to disability and handicap* (pp. 43–53). Canada: WB Saunders.

Regier, D. A., Kaelber, C. T., Rae, D. S., Farmer, M. E., Knauper, B., Kessler, R. C., et al. (1998). Limitations of diagnostic criteria and assessment instruments for mental disorders. *Archives of General Psychiatry, 55,* 109–115.

Rice, D. P., & Miller, L. S. (1996). The economic burden of schizophrenia: Conceptual and methodological issues and cost estimates. In M. Moscarelli, A. Rupp, & N. Sartorious (Eds.), *Handbook of mental health economics and health policy: Vol. 1, schizophrenia* (pp. 321–324). New York, NY: Wiley.

Roberts, D. E. (1999). The challenge of substance abuse for family preservation policy. *Journal of Health Care Law and Policy, 3,* 72–86.

Rosen, D., Tolman, R. M., & Warner, L. A. (2004). Low-income women's use of substance abuse and mental health services. *Journal of Health Care for the Poor and Underserved, 15,* 206–219.

SAMHSA (Substance Abuse and Mental Health Services Administration). (2001). The DASIS report: How men and women enter substance abuse treatment (Office of Applied Studies). Retrieved June 8, 2008, from http://www.DrugAbuseStatistics.samhsa.gov

SAMHSA. (2003). Results from the 2002 National Survey on Drug Use and Health (NSDUH) (Office of Applied Studies, NSDUH Series H-22, DHHS Publication No. SMA 03-3836). Rockville, MD: Author.

SAMHSA. (2005a). Drug Abuse Warning Network, 2004: National Estimates of Drug-Related Emergency Department Visits (Office of Applied Studies, DAWN Series D-28, DHHS Publication No. SMA 06-4143). Rockville, MD: Author.

SAMHSA. (2005b). Overview of Findings from the 2004 NSDUH (Office of Applied Studies, NSDUH Series H-27, DHHS Publication No. SMA 05-4061). Rockville, MD: Author.

SAMHSA. (2006). Results from the 2005 NSDUH: National Findings (Office of Applied Studies, NSDUH Series H-30, DHHS Publication No. SMA 06-4194). Rockville, MD: Author.

SAMHSA. (2007). Results from the 2006 NSDUH: National Findings (Office of Applied Studies, NSDUH Series H-32, DHHS Publication No. SMA 07-4293). Rockville, MD: Author.

Sen, A. (1999). *Development as freedom*. New York, NY: Anchor Books.

Sheehan, D. V., Harnett-Sheehan, K., & Raj, B. A. (1996). The measurement of disability. *International Clinical Psychopharmacology, 11*(Suppl. 3), 89–95.

Smith, E. M., North, C. S., & Spitznagel, E. L. (1993). Alcohol, drugs, and psychiatric comorbidity among homeless women: An epidemiologic study. *Journal of Clinical Psychiatry, 54*(3), 82–87.

Stoskopf, C. H., Kim, Y. K., & Glover, S. H. (2001). Dual diagnosis: HIV and mental illness – a population-based study. *Community Mental Health Journal, 37*(6), 469–479.

Susser, M., & Watson, W. (1961). *Sociology in medicine.* New York, NY: Oxford University Press.

Teplin, L. A., McClelland, G. M., Abram, K. M., & Weiner, D. A. (2005). Crime victimization in adults with severe mental illness. *Archives of General Psychiatry, 62,* 911–921.

Thrasher, S. P., & Mowbray, C. T. (1995). A strengths perspective: An ethnographic study of homeless women with children. *Health and Social Work, 20,* 93–101.

Turner, R. J., Lloyd, D. A., & Taylor, J. (2006). Physical disability and mental health: An epidemiology of psychiatric and substance abuse disorders. *Rehabilitation Psychology, 51*(3), 214–223.

Ullman, S. E., Filipas, H. H., Townsend, S. M., & Starzynski, L. L. (2005). Trauma exposure, posttraumatic stress disorder and problem drinking in sexual assault survivors. *Journal of Studies on Alcohol, 66*(5), 610–619.

U.S. Public Health Service. (1999). *The surgeon general's call to action to prevent suicide*. Washington, DC: Author.

Ustun, T. B., Ayuso-Mateos, J. L., Chatterji, S., Mathers, C., & Murray, C. J. (2004). Global burden of depressive disorders in the year 2000. *British Journal of Psychiatry, 184,* 386–392.

Volkow, N. D. (2006, July 26). *Testimony on prescription drug abuse before the house subcommittee on criminal justice, drug policy, and human resources*. Retrieved June 20, 2008, from http://www.hhs.gov/asl/testify/t060726a.html

Wang, P. S., Berglund, P., Olfson, M., Pincus, H. A., Wells, K. B., & Kessler, R. C. (2005a). Failure and delay in initial treatment contact after first onset of mental disorders in the National Comorbidity Survey Replication. *Archives of General Psychiatry, 62,* 603–613.

Wang, P. S., Lane, M., Olfson, M., Pincus, H. A., Wells, K. B., & Kessler, R. C. (2005b). Twelve-month use of mental health services in the United States. *Archives of General Psychiatry, 62,* 629–640.

Ware, N. C., Hopper, K., Tugenberg, T., Dickey, B., & Fisher, D. (2007). Connectedness and citizenship: Redefining social integration. *Psychiatric Services, 58*(4), 469–474.

Ware, N. C., Hopper, K., Tugenberg, T., Dickey, B., & Fisher, D. (2008). A theory of social integration as quality of life. *Psychiatric Services, 59,* 27–33.

Ware, N. C., Tugenberg, T., Dickey, B., & McHorney, C. A. (1999). An ethnographic study of the meaning of continuity of care in mental health services. *Psychiatric Services, 50,* 395–400.

Wenzel, S. L., Koegel, P., & Gelberg, L. (2000). Antecedents of physical and sexual victimization among homeless women: A comparison to homeless men. *American Journal of Community Psychology, 28*(3), 367–390.

Wells, K. B., Strum, R., Sherbourne, C. D., & Meredith, L. S. (1996). *Caring for depression.* Cambridge, MA: Harvard University Press.

Widom, C. S., DuMont, K., & Czaja, S. J. (2007). A prospective investigation of major depressive disorder and comorbidity in abused and neglected children grown up. *Archives of General Psychiatry, 64*(1), 49–56.

World Health Organization (WHO). (1980). *International classification of impairments, disabilities, and handicaps* (Rev. ed.). Geneva, Switzerland: World Health Organization.

WHO. (2001). *International classification of functioning, disability and health.* Geneva, Switzerland: WHO.

WHO. (2004). Changing History, Annex Table 3: Burden of disease in DALYs by cause, sex, and mortality stratum in WHO regions, estimates for 2002. *The world health report 2004.* Geneva, Switzerland: WHO.

WHO. (2007). *Depression.* Retrieved May, 2008 from, http://www.who.int/mental_health/management/depression/definition/en/

Zilberman, M., Tavares, H., & el-Guebaly, N. (2003). Gender similarities and differences: The prevalence and course of alcohol- and other substance-related disorders. *Journal of Addictive Diseases, 22*(4), 61–74.

Chapter 4
Epidemiology of Mental Disorders in Older Women

Heather A. Kenna, Talayeh Ghezel and Natalie L. Rasgon

Introduction

The epidemiology of mental disorders in older women is complex because of overlapping symptomatology with common chronic medical conditions, including cardiovascular and cerebrovascular disorders. There also exist many overlapping symptoms within specific mental disorders common in older women, such as cognitive impairment and depressed mood as symptoms of both major depressive disorder (MDD) and Alzheimer's disease (AD). Greater understanding of mental disorders in older women is of significant clinical importance, especially given the well-documented demographic imperatives such as the increasingly older age distribution of the population and the disproportionate rise in health care expenditures with increasing age (Martini et al. 2007).

Data suggest that the epidemiology of mental disorders in women changes across age groups. As contrasted with the high prevalence of substance use, anxiety, and personality disorders among younger women, mental disorders in older women are more likely to include mood disorders and cognitive disorders (e.g., dementias; Baker et al. 1992; Koenig and Blazer 1992; Tariot et al. 1993). Clinically, it is noteworthy that compared to younger individuals, older individuals with mental disorders are less likely to be seen in mental health settings, yet they are seen in primary care practice more regularly (Atkisson and Zich 1990; Regier et al. 1993; Sheperd and Wilkinson 1988). This is especially important given the fact that older patients who commit suicide have more often seen their primary care provider shortly before their death (Didham et al. 2006), suggesting underrecognized suicidal ideation at these clinical visits.

This chapter presents estimates of the prevalence and incidence of common mental disorders in older women, focusing primarily on epidemiological community studies. We also include broader data to provide a greater picture of mental health

H. A. Kenna (✉)
Department of Psychiatry and Behavioral Sciences, Stanford Center for Neuroscience in Women's Health, Stanford University School of Medicine, 401 Quarry Road, CA 94305, Stanford, USA

B. L. Levin, M. A. Becker (eds.), *A Public Health Perspective of Women's Mental Health*, DOI 10.1007/978-1-4419-1526-9_4, © Springer Science+Business Media LLC 2010

in older women; for example, depressive symptomatology that does not meet standard criteria for major depression yet is associated with significant disability. Similarly, we review impairment secondary to the misuse of prescription psychotropic medication by older women, an issue that has not been well studied. Our goal is to highlight critical themes in the epidemiology of common mental disorders in older women that are especially pertinent to clinical practice as we face the challenges of aging.

A preemptive note should be made on the epidemiological concepts of *prevalence* and *incidence*. *Prevalence* refers to the proportion of the population that meets the criteria for a disorder within a specific period of time. As duration of illness may be affected by treatment and other factors that influence the course of illness, prevalence rates may also be affected by these factors. In contrast, *incidence* is the rate at which an illness arises among persons previously unaffected.

Major Mood Disorders

Depression

Studies of depression among men and women in late life as a whole have been the focus of much research over the past 20 years. Numerous studies have examined the etiology and prevalence of late-life depression in older adults and the medical outcomes associated with MDD, as well as subclinical depressive symptoms. The differential definition of MDD or major depressive episode (MDE), in terms of strict DSM-IV criteria, compared to presence of clinically notable depressive symptoms that may overlap with comorbid medical conditions, are a major point of limitation and contention with respect to epidemiological and clinical findings.

Although MDD is not prevalent in late life, the prevalence of clinically significant depressive symptamotology in older adults is quite high, with estimates of approximately 14% (Blazer and Williams 1980). Twelve-month prevalence estimates of MDD among older women are reported to vary between approximately 3 and 14%, as outlined below. Estimation of the prevalence of MDD in older women specifically varies depending on the diagnostic criteria, procedure, and community sample. Absence of a common diagnostic interview has hampered cross-national syntheses of epidemiological evidence on MDD.

Data from the U.S. Health and Retirement Study of 1996, 1998, and 2000 showed a 12-month prevalence rate of MDD among women between 50 and 64 years of age to be 8.6% (Mojtabai and Olfson 2004). An earlier study that used the same diagnostic criteria and screening method as in the U.S. Health and Retirement Study, estimated the rate of MDD in a nationally representative sample of Canadian women 45–64 years of age to be 6.3%, with a 4.1% annual incidence of MDD (Patten 2000). The declining trend of 12-month prevalence of MDD was visible across the lifespan, decreasing from 9.6% in ages 12–24, 8.6% in ages 25–44, 6.3% in ages

45–64, to 3.1% in ages ≥65 (Patten 2000). Using the same diagnostic criteria and screening methods, Offord and colleagues reported a smaller 12-month prevalence (4.2%) of MDD among women aged 45–64, and again a clear declining trend in prevalence could be seen in the younger to older age cohorts (Offord et al. 1996). The declining MDD trend was again present in data from the 1997 National Survey of Mental Health and Wellbeing of Adults (NSMHWB) of Australia, which reported that prevalence of all affective disorders decreased from 7.3% in ages 45–54, 6.9% in ages 55–64, to 2.4% in ages ≥65 (McLennan 1997). Finally, in a study of nearly 6,000 Finnish adults, which used the Short Form of the University of Michigan version of the Composite International Diagnostic Interview to classify 12-month prevalence of MDEs, there was no declining trend with age (Lindeman et al. 2000). Rather, women between the ages of 45 and 54 had a higher 12-month prevalence rate (13.6%) than the older age cohorts of 55–64 (8.6%) and 65–75 (8.4%) (Lindeman et al. 2000).

The majority of epidemiological studies suggest that the prevalence of MDD declines with age, though subclinical depressive symptomatology increases at the same time (Romanoski et al. 1992). Estimated rates of subclinical depressive symptoms among physically ill older adults are thought to be even higher (Romanoski et al. 1992). Among older adults (ages 60+) treated for MDD, the so-called double depression (MDD with dysthymia) increases the risk for poor outcome (Hybels et al. 2005). Data suggest that across epidemiological age groups, prevalence of any mood disorder tends to be lowest in individuals aged 65 and older (Regier et al. 1988, 1993). Although the reasons for declining prevalence with age are poorly understood, it is speculated that depression-related mortality, increased prevalence of somatic symptoms of depression (i.e., fatigue, poor appetite), or decreased emotional responsiveness may contribute to the observed trend (Romanoski et al. 1992) (see Chap. 6 in this volume for additional information on depression).

Bipolar Disorder

The prevalence of bipolar disorder in older adults has been studied in several community studies, but identification of data specific to women is difficult. However, population studies suggest an equal prevalence of bipolar disorder among older men and women. Weissman et al. (1984) reported a 0.4% prevalence rate of bipolar disorders in adults aged 45–65 years in the Epidemiological Catchment Area (ECA) multisite study of five US communities. Unützer et al. (1988) examined the treated prevalence of bipolar disorder in a health maintenance organization in western Washington State using automated data about treatment between 1995 and 1996. In patients between 40 and 64 years, a 0.46% prevalence rate was found (Unützer et al. 1988). Mitchell et al. (2004) reported the prevalence of bipolar disorder from the data collected by the Australian NSMHWB. Women between the ages of 45 and 54 reported a 0.3% prevalence of DSM-IV 12-month bipolar disorder and women 55 and older reported a 0.1% rate (Mitchell et al. 2004).

Although bipolar disorder has been found to be equally prevalent among both genders, studies show that women with bipolar illness are more likely than men to develop rapid-cycling bipolar disorder. The ratio of female to male patients with rapid-cycling is approximately 3:1. It is also suggested that bipolar women may have more depressive episodes, whereas bipolar men experience more manic episodes. Mixed mania may also be more likely in women bipolar patients, but the data remain contradictory at this point (Kessing 2004).

Anxiety Disorders

Anxiety disorders are some of the most common psychiatric illnesses found around the world. It has been suggested that anxiety disorders afflict 15.7 million people in the USA each year and 30 million people at some point in their lives (Lépine 2002). The DSM-IV classifies anxiety disorders as including general anxiety disorder (GAD), panic disorder (PD), simple phobia, social anxiety disorder (SAD), and obsessive-compulsive disorder (OCD). Anxiety disorders occur more frequently in women throughout their lifespan until age 65, when evidence suggests that the gender difference narrows (Pigott 2003).

McLennan's study of the Australian 1997 NSMHWB reported rates of all anxiety disorders grouped together. Women 45–54 years of age reported a 15.9% 12-month prevalence rate and women 55–64 reported a 9.5% prevalence rate (McLennan 1997). Data on anxiety disorders from the Longitudinal Aging Study Amsterdam (LASA) reported information on over 3,000 older adults from 11 municipalities in the Netherlands using the Hospital Anxiety and Depression Scale (HDS-A) and the CES-D. Beekman et al. (1998) reported that among women aged 55–64 years, the 6-month prevalence rate of GAD was 5.2%. In women 65–74, the 6-month prevalence rate more than doubled to be 12.6%. Suffering functional limitations had the most consistent association with anxiety disorders in this study (Beekman et al. 1998).

Beekman et al. (1998) also reported rates of OCD from the LASA. Six-month prevalence of OCD in women aged 55–64 years was 0.3%, and for women 65–74, it was reported to be 2.7%. A strong association between OCD and marital status, family history, and chronic diseases was also found (Beekman et al. 1998). Mohammadi and colleagues used the Schedule for Affective Disorders and Schizophrenia on over 25,000 subjects in Iran in 2001. The estimated 6-month prevalence of OCD was 3.5% in women 41–55 years and 2.4% in women 56–65 (Mohammadi et al. 2004). An older survey from the 1980s in Edmonton, Canada, reported a 1.5% 6-month prevalence rate for women aged 45–54 and 0.7% rate for those aged 55–64 (Kolada et al. 1994).

Social anxiety disorder is one of the most generally prevalent anxiety disorders. In the Offord et al. (1996) survey of Ontarians, 5.9% of women between the ages of 45 and 64 were found to present with social phobia in the past 12 months. Arnarson and colleagues found a 2.1% 6-month prevalence of social phobia in Icelandic women using an epidemiological postal survey in the 1990s (Arnarson et al. 1998).

In a different study of nationally representative older adults in Canada, fewer than 10% of respondents reported onset after age 54 (Cairney et al. 2007).

Women are twice as likely as men to meet the diagnostic criteria for simple phobias (Pigott 2003). Most studies suggest that mean onset of simple phobia occurs around age 15 (Magee et al. 1996). Offord and colleagues reported a 6.7% 12-month prevalence in Ontarian women aged 45–64 (Offord et al. 1996). Beekman and colleagues reported a 4.2% 6-month prevalence estimate in Dutch women aged 55–64 and a 4.4% estimate for women aged 65–74 (Beekman et al. 1998). Arnarson et al. (1998) found similar rates in Icelandic women. Their study reported 4.3% 6-month prevalence in women between 45 and 64 years old.

Panic disorder and agoraphobia are closely associated. Data from clinical samples suggest that agoraphobia is usually present in subjects with panic disorder. Population surveys, however, suggest that the reverse is not uncommon (Pigott 2003). Joyce et al. reported rates of panic disorder and agoraphobia from the Christchurch Psychiatric Epidemiology Study in a random community survey of urban adults. Using the Diagnostic Interview Schedule, 2% of 45- to 65-year-old women presented with panic disorder. The data also suggest that patients with moderate agoraphobic avoidance seldom existed without panic disorder or other psychopathology (Joyce et al. 1989). In the Netherlands, a 1.4% 6-month prevalence rate of panic disorder in women aged 55–64 and a 3% rate in women aged 65–74 has been reported (Beekman et al. 1998). Arnarson et al. (1998) observed a 1.1% 6-month prevalence rate of agoraphobia in Icelandic women between 45 and 64 years of age.

Late-Onset Schizophrenia

The existence of late-onset schizophrenia is much debated. Neither DSM-IV nor ICD-10 includes a specific category for this disorder at this time. Swiss psychiatrist Manfred Bleuler was the first to describe the disorder in 1943. He noted that 15% of his schizophrenia cases had an onset between 40 and 60 years of age, while first onset after age 60 was rare (Riecher-Rossler 1999). Harris and Jeste (1988) reported that 23.5% of schizophrenic patients had first onset after age 40. A considerable amount of evidence has spurred an international consensus panel of experts to conclude that there is face and clinical validity to support a diagnosis of late-onset schizophrenia for patients with onset between ages 40 and 60. This same panel suggested the term late-onset schizophrenia-like psychosis for patients with illness beginning after age 60 (Howard et al. 2000).

Although there are no reported gender differences in clinical presentation (Lehmann 2003), women do predominate in cases of late-onset schizophrenia (Bleuler 1978). Both men and women demonstrate a peak of new-onset schizophrenia in the early 20s. The incidence is higher in men, however, until the mid-30s. Women have a second peak in incidence during their late 40s to mid-50s, where most would diagnose as "late-onset schizophrenia". Most studies report a ratio of women to men of 2:1 to 4:1 with this diagnosis (Lehmann 2003). One theory to explain this trend is termed "the estrogen hypothesis," which postulates that estradiol has antidopaminergic properties. These properties somehow protect women to a certain degree from puberty to menopause. Estradiol levels decrease at mid-life, leaving some predisposed women vulnerable to a second illness-onset peak.

Substance Use and Abuse

Alcohol and drug use, prescription, illicit, and otherwise, are prevalent among all age groups. The most attention has been paid to alcohol abuse by older adults. Ten to 20% of older adults report daily consumption of alcohol (Beresford and Gomberg 1995). While use and abuse rates of alcohol are higher in men than women, older women still report substantial prevalence rates. Among women 60 years and older, screened among 5,065 adults in primary care practices in Wisconsin, 3.9% detail problem of alcohol use (Adams et al. 1996). The proportion of older women who meet the criteria for alcohol abuse or dependence does seem to be much smaller, but recognizing and addressing alcohol and drug use disorders in older age is as important as in younger persons. Older adults are more likely to be affected by serious complications as a result of substance abuse. Many older adults have compromised or deteriorating physical health and functioning and often take prescription medications. In the USA, 4% of all mortalities are a result of alcohol consumption (Mokdad et al. 2004).

The results of epidemiological studies on substance abuse disorders are wide and varied, but all indicate that a problem exists in older populations that must be addressed. A study by Adams and colleagues, which assessed substance use in 5,065 primary care patients over the age of 60, reported a high rate of alcohol abuse in women between 61 and 65 years of age, with 11.3% consuming 8–14 drinks per week, 1.8% consuming 15–21 drinks per week, and 2.5% consuming more than 21 drinks per week. Patients aged between 66 and 70 years showed a decreasing prevalence in each category: 7.3%, 1.6%, and 1.9%, respectively. There was a 3% prevalence of binge drinking among 61–65 year olds and 1.3% in the older age cohort, i.e., older than 65 (Adams et al. 1996).

Grant et al. (2004) compared the 12-month prevalence of alcohol abuse and dependence between the past two decades in the USA. Between 1991 and 1992, the National Institute on Alcohol Abuse and Alcoholism (NIAAA) conducted the National Longitudinal Alcohol Epidemiologic Survey (NLAES). Ten years later, the NIAAA conducted a similar survey, the National Epidemiologic Survey on Alcohol and Related Conditions (NESARC). Both the NLAES and NESARC used DSM-IV definitions for alcohol abuse and dependence as diagnostic criteria. In all age groups, an increase in the 12-month prevalence of alcohol abuse was seen. In ten years, the prevalence rate increased from 1.32 to 1.70% in women between 45 and 64 years of age. White and black women exhibited the highest rates of alcohol abuse in this age group as well as the greatest change in prevalence rate. Ten years did not appear to affect rates of alcohol dependence. Women aged 45–64 reported a 1.12% 12-month prevalence rate of alcohol dependence in 1991–1992 and only an insignificant 0.03%

increase ten years later. Native American women demonstrated the greatest change in prevalence with a decrease of more than 2% (Grant et al. 2004).

In 2002, a nationally representative sample of Canadian women was surveyed for alcohol and drug use by Statistics Canada in the Canadian Community Health Survey (CCHS) on mental health and wellbeing. The CCHS used the CIDI-SF to derive an alcohol dependence score for each respondent. In women over age 44, the 12-month prevalence of alcohol dependence was reported to be 0.3% while the rate of alcohol interference was 0.2%. There was a 0% reported prevalence rate of dependence on illicit drugs (Piran and Gadalla 2007). McLennan (1997) reported that similar to previously reported studies, a decrease in the rate of alcohol and drug use disorders was seen with increasing age. The prevalence rates of substance abuse disorders were 3.2% (age 45–54), 1.2% (age 55–64), and 0.2% (age 65 or older).

The nonmedical use and abuse of prescription drugs is a growing and concerning problem. Nonmedical use is defined by the World Health Organization (2008) as, "use of a prescription drug, whether obtained by prescription or otherwise, other than in the manner or for the time period prescribed, or by a person for whom the drug was not prescribed." From 1995 to 2005, the number of Americans abusing controlled prescription drugs increased from 6.2 to 15.2 million (Califano 1997). The female sex is a significant risk factor for problems associated with prescription drug use. Older women are prescribed more psychoactive medications, consume more, and are more likely to be long-term users of these substances (Simoni-Wastila and Yang 2006). A recent review of the literature reported that up to 11% of older women misuse prescription drugs and that nonmedical use of prescription drugs among all adults aged ≥50 years will increase to 2.7 million by the year 2020 (Simoni-Wastila and Yang 2006). The U.S. National Household Surveys on Drug Abuse (NHSDA) reported an estimated 1.3% of women 50 years and older having used prescription psychotherapeutics nonmedically in the past year (Colliver et al. 2006). The authors further projected that by 2020, the rate would increase to 2.2% (Colliver et al. 2006). Becker et al. (2007) used data from the 2002–2004 National Survey on Drug Use and Health (NSDUH) to find that 0.8% of American adults between 50 and 80 years of age reported past-year use of nonmedical sedatives or tranquilizers. The authors reported a decrease in prevalence as age increases, but a large difference in use between genders was not observed (Becker et al. 2007). Furthermore, 1.1% of women over age 50 reported nonmedical use of prescription pain relievers in the 2005 NSDUH (Manchikanti 2007). The medical and economic consequences associated with nonmedical use of prescription drugs emphasize the necessity of collecting more epidemiological data to form a better picture of the problem. For additional information on substance abuse and women, see Chap. 9 in this volume.

Eating Disorders

Eating disorders are frequent subjects of epidemiological studies in younger generations, but data are lacking for older adults. The studies that are available demonstrate that eating disorders are a persistent problem throughout the lifespan and require physician vigilance for detection. The scarcity of literature on eating disorders occurring after menopause might be due to hindered recognition because of age-induced weight loss and other medical conditions.

The DSM-IV recognizes three main eating disorders: anorexia nervosa, bulimia nervosa, and eating disorders not otherwise specified (NOS). Binge-eating disorder, which is relatively common among older women, falls under the latter category. There is a significant overlap between all three, but all individuals who do not meet the full criteria for anorexia or bulimia nervosa are grouped under eating disorders NOS (Mitchell and Bulik 2006).

There is a substantial prevalence of binge-eating disorder in the older population, whereas anorexia nervosa and bulimia nervosa are represented much less frequently. In a survey of 1,000 Tyrolean women using screening questions aimed at identifying eating disorders, Kinzl and colleagues reported 0% rate of anorexia nervosa or bulimia nervosa among women between the ages of 45 and 54; however, there was a 5% prevalence rate of binge-eating disorder (Kinzl et al. 1999). In women between 55 and 64 years of age, there was a 0.8% prevalence rate of bulimia nervosa and a 4.7% rate of binge-eating disorder (Kinzl et al. 1999). Mangweth-Matzek et al. (2006) corroborated this finding with a survey of 475 Austrian women between the ages of 60 and 70 using slightly modified questions from the DSM-IV. In that study, 18 (3.8%) of the women surveyed met the criteria for an eating disorder. Of these, there was a single case of anorexia nervosa (with a late onset in her 50s), two cases of bulimia nervosa, and 15 cases of eating disorder NOS (five of which were cases of binge-eating disorder). Single symptoms of an eating disorder were reported in an additional 21 women (4.4%; Mangweth-Matzek et al. 2006). Studies must focus on older women in order to better measure the prevalence in the community across the entire lifespan (see Chap. 7 in this volume for additional information on eating disorders).

Dementia

Alzheimer's Disease

Alzheimer's disease (AD) is the most common form of dementia and is characterized by a gradual, insidious onset and steady decline in cognitive function. AD is diagnosed after other CNS diseases, systemic conditions known to cause symptoms of dementia, and substance-induced conditions are ruled out. The presence of a major psychiatric disease, such as major depression, must also be ruled out, though major depression does frequently occur in patients with AD (for review, please see Wright and Persad (2007)). Age of onset is a major consideration in AD, with "early onset" referring to cases in which symptoms begin prior to age 65.

Data from studies of AD rather consistently suggest a higher prevalence of AD in women compared to men (Bachman et al. 1992; Corso et al. 1992; Folstein et al. 1991; Canadian Study of Health and Aging Working Group 1994; Manubens et al.

1995). Prevalence rates for AD vary across studies, depending in part on the diagnostic criteria being used. In all studies, the prevalence increases with age beyond 65, with a range of <2% in individuals aged 65–69 to approximately 20% in individuals aged over 85 (for review, please see Badgio and Worden (2007)). The majority of studies report a higher risk of AD in women (Badgio and Worden 2007). Studies from the European Community Concerted Action on the Epidemiology and Prevention of Dementia Group (EURODEM) provide data showing that in individuals aged 65 and older, women are at a higher risk of developing AD, with an adjusted relative risk factor of 1.2 (Andersen et al. 1999). However, data from Ruitenberg et al. (2001) suggest that these gender differences emerge only at an advanced age, with an increased prevalence of AD in women observed only after age 90. Greater educational attainment has frequently been shown to be associated with lower risk of AD in both men and women (for example, please see Ott et al. (1995)). Interestingly, EURODEM data showed that the level of education significantly differentiates risk in women, in that women with a high level of education, compared to women with low and middle levels of educations, had 4.6 and 2.6 times increased risk, respectively, for AD (Letenneur et al. 2000). No such educational effect was observed among men in that particular study (Letenneur et al. 2000). Among other potential explanations for the higher prevalence of AD in women compared to men is greater longevity in women and the inherent age-associated risk of AD (Hebert et al. 2001).

Lewy Body Disease

Lewy body disease is the second most common form of dementia, according to autopsy studies. Lewy bodies refer to the abnormal neuronal protein formations seen in the midbrains of patients suffering from Parkison's disease. Patients with Lewy body disease show a diffuse spread of these formations throughout the cortex. Clinically, Lewy body disease shares features with both AD and Parkinson's disease. The cognitive deficits seen in patients with Lewy body disease are similar to those found in AD, yet in Lewy body disease the symptoms generally vary to a great extent day-to-day, whereas day-to-day variability in AD is much less marked. Mild to moderate Parkinsonian symptoms generally start around the same time as symptoms of cognitive impairment in patients with Lewy body disease. A high incidence of psychotic symptoms distinguishes Lewy body disease from other CNS disorders, most often visual hallucinations. Further, in diffuse Lewy body disease, psychotic symptoms present much earlier than in AD (Ballard et al. 1999). It is important to note that patients with Lewy body disease often have severe adverse reactions to antipsychotic medications (Ballard et al. 1999). Thus, early and accurate diagnosis is critical.

Lewy body disease is not as common in women as it is in men, with men having approximately double the risk (Ballard et al. 1999). Prevalence estimates, depending on case criteria, range from 0 to 5% with regard to the general population, and from 0 to 30.5% of all dementia cases (Zaccai et al. 2005).

Vascular Dementia and Dementias Due to General Medical Conditions

Vascular dementia (also known as multiinfarct dementia) is the third most common type of dementia and occurs in men much more frequently than women across all age groups (Ruitenberg et al. 2001). Compared to the slow and insidious onset of AD, vascular dementia is typically abrupt with a stepwise, fluctuating course. Prevalence of vascular dementia is estimated at approximately 1% in the general population (Sicras et al. 2005).

While the majority of dementia cases are due to AD, Lewy body disease, or vascular disease, there are a number of other medical conditions that may produce cognitive impairment severe enough to warrant a diagnosis of dementia. These conditions include coronary artery bypass surgery, head injury, hypothyroidism, breast cancer treatments, fibromyalgia, chronic fatigue, and menopause (Badgio and Worden 2007). Given the multiplicity of causes, careful assessment and accurate diagnosis are crucial in order to design treatments to slow the progression and/or minimize the negative impact of cognitive symptoms (Badgio and Worden 2007).

Suicidal Behavior

In general, suicide rates among older women have decreased over the past 30 years, but suicide and suicidal ideation remain a significant consequence in older age. However, a recent report by the Centers for Disease Control and Prevention (2007) found that while suicide rates continued to decline in persons aged 65 and over, suicide rates among middle-aged individuals (aged 45–65) increased by approximately 16%. The greatest increase (31%) was observed in women aged 45–54. Unfortunately, resources and research into suicide among middle-aged individuals are severely lacking. The lack of concrete research has given rise to a number of theories for the increase in suicide among menopausal-aged women, including a significant decrease in the use of hormone therapy by menopausal women after the initial Women's Health Initiative findings (Shumaker et al. 2003). Another prime suspect is the skyrocketing use and abuse of prescription drugs, as detailed previously.

Since the 1990s, increasing consideration has been applied by the scientific community. Because of the relatively low rates of suicide per year, many retrospective studies have combined data from previous decades to arrive at total prevalence rates. This approach can be both advantageous and problematic, as some studies show the trends in suicide rates per year while others calculate one mean rate for the entire time period disregarding the trends.

Factors that may be associated with suicidal thoughts in older people include psychiatric disorders, the presence of poor physical health and disability, financial and relationship problems, poor social support, and alcohol misuse (Alexopoulos et al. 1999; Conwell et al. 2002; Yip et al. 2003). As an important indicator of potential future harm, the prevalence of suicidal thought and tiredness of life was reported in a national survey of over 8,500 subjects in Great Britain (Dennis et al. 2007). Men and women between the ages of 55 and 74 displayed a rate of tiredness of life of 4.8%, death wishes of 3.3%, and suicidal thoughts of 1.5% (Dennis et al. 2007). In addition, this study revealed that 4.8% of older adults (men and women combined) aged between 55 and 74 experienced tiredness of life in the year before the interview, 3.3% had death wishes, and 1.5% experienced suicidal thoughts (Dennis et al. 2007). The younger age cohorts in the study reported higher rates in all three categories, establishing a trend of decreasing suicidal ideation with increasing age. Kjøller and Helweg-Larsen (2002) reported slightly higher rates of suicidal ideation in a nationwide, representative survey conducted in 1994 by the Danish Institute for Clinical Epidemiology (DICE), wherein women aged 45–66 were observed to have a 5.4% rate of suicidal ideation. The higher rate of suicidal ideation observed in the DICE study may partly be explained by the different age classification and interview questions (Kjøller and Helweg-Larsen 2002). In the USA, Callahan et al. (1996) estimated the prevalence of suicidal ideation in older primary care patients, gender unspecified, to be between 0.7 and 1.2%.

The DICE study results also indicated that only 50–60% of suicide attempts made by their respondents were known to the health care system (Kjøller and Helweg-Larsen 2002). This statistic suggests that retrospective studies of the prevalence of suicide attempts may report underestimated rates if reporting data collected by health care or federal systems. Langlois and Morrison (2002) reported data on suicide deaths for 1979–1998 obtained from the Canadian Vital Statistics Database. The hospitalization rate for an attempted suicide in Canadian women between 45 and 59 years was 81.3 per 100,000 and for women between 60 and 74 years, 25.2 per 100,000. Though suicide act rates have been reported to be lowest among older adults as compared to younger age cohorts, older cohorts have been found to bear the highest rates of completed suicide (Gallo and Lebowitz 1999; Spicer and Miller 2000).

Suicide rates vary widely due to different survey populations, race, gender, locations, and possibly, identification methods. Langlois and Morrison (2002) found that the suicide rate in Canadian women between 45 and 59 was 7.2 per 100,000 and for women between 60 and 74 it was 5.0 per 100,000. A recent Austrian study examining all registered suicides of persons aged 65 and over found the suicide rate to be 21.4 per 100,000 in women aged 65–69 (Kapusta et al. 2007). The authors found that suicide rates increased with age, as did suicides by poisoning, though the possibility of accidental poisonings in persons who use multiple drugs may have influenced the results (Kapusta et al. 2007). However, overall suicide rates among women in all age groups progressively decreased in that study over the study period, from 1970 to 2004 (Kapusta et al. 2007). The overall rates observed in the Austrian study are higher than those usually reported. Information on suicide counts in the state of Rio de Janeiro was reported by Rodriguez and Werneck (2005) by pooling data from the Mortality Information System of the Brazilian Ministry of Health from 1979 to 1998. Women between the ages of 50 and 70 had suicide rates between 5.13 and 6.06 per 100,000 (Rodriguez and Werneck 2005). The authors mentioned that the values may be underestimated because the quality of coding causes of death is often unsatisfactory (Rodriguez and Werneck 2005). Meehan et al. (1991) examined the change in suicide rates between 1980 and 1986 in the USA compiled by the National Center for Health Statistics (NCHS; Meehan et al. 1991). The overall suicide rate for women over 65 years old showed a small increase over time, but no definite trend emerged for women between 65 and 69. The suicide rate fluctuated between 6.6 and 7.6 per 100,000 (Meehan et al. 1991).

Implications for Women's Mental Health

Older individuals with mental disorders are less likely to be seen in mental health settings than younger patients, yet they are seen in primary care practice more regularly (Atkisson and Zich 1990; Regier et al. 1993; Sheperd and Wilkinson 1988). In light of this, greater outreach should be directed toward older women, especially during the menopausal transition when women are at increased risk of mood disorders and cognitive dysfunction. Older women with psychiatric concerns are more likely to present first to their primary care physician, who may be comfortable initiating first-line treatment or may refer the patient to a psychiatrist if symptoms seem severe. However, as described in this review, psychiatric symptoms in older patients (especially symptoms of depression and anxiety) may be easily mistaken for somatic ailments and the underlying psychiatric condition may go unrecognized or inadequately treated. Proper evaluation and treatment may also be delayed due to psychiatric care biases harbored by older women and their primary care physicians (Lehmann 2003). Greater attention should be given to psychiatric symptoms by primary care physicians. Careful psychiatric evaluation may identify medical conditions, including depression, which can be treated and can lead to improvements in the patient's functioning.

References

Adams, W. L., Barry, K. L., & Fleming, M. F. (1996). Screening for problem drinking in older primary care patients. *Journal of the American Medical Association, 276*(24), 1964–1967.

Alexopoulos, G. S., Bruce, M. L., Hull, J., Sirey, J. A., & Kakuma, T. (1999). Clinical determinants of suicidal ideation and behavior in geriatric depression. *Archives of General Psychiatry, 56*(11), 1048–1053.

Andersen, K., Launer, L., Dewey, M., Letenneur, L., Ott, A., Copeland, J., et al. (1999). Gender differences in the incidence of AD and vascular dementia: The EURODEM Studies. EURODEM Incidence Research Group. *Neurology, 53*(9), 1992–1997.

Arnarson, E. O., Gudmundsdóttir, A., & Boyle, G. J. (1998). Six-month prevalence of phobic symptoms in Iceland: An epidemiological postal survey. *Journal of Clinical Psychology, 54*(2), 257–265.

Atkisson, C., & Zich, J. (1990). *Depression in primary care: Screening and detection*. New York, NY: Routledge.

Bachman, D., Wolf, P., Linn, R., Knoefel, J., Cobb, J., Belanger, A., et al. (1992). Prevalence of dementia and probable senile dementia of the Alzheimer's type in the Framingham Study. *Neurology, 42,* 115–119.

Badgio, P. C., & Worden, B. L. (2007). Cognitive functioning and aging in women. *Journal of Women & Aging, 19*(1–2), 13–30.

Baker, F., Lebowitz, B., Katz, I., & Pincus, H. (1992). Geriatric psychopathology: An American perspective on a selected agenda for research. *International Psychogeriatrics, 4,* 141–156.

Ballard, C., Holmes, C., McKeith, I., Neill, D., O'Brien, J., Cairns, N., et al. (1999). Psychiatric morbidity in dementia with Lewy bodies: A prospective clinical and neuropathological comparative study with Alzheimer's disease. *American Journal of Psychiatry, 156*(7), 1039–1045.

Becker, W. C., Fiellin, D. A., & Desai, R. A. (2007). Non-medical use, abuse and dependence on sedatives and tranquilizers among U.S. adults: Psychiatric and socio-demographic correlates. *Drug and Alcohol Dependence, 90*(2–3), 280–287.

Beekman, A. T., Bremmer, M. A., Deeg, D. J., van Balkom, A. J., Smit, J. H., de Beurs, E., et al. (1998). Anxiety disorders in later life: A report from the Longitudinal Aging Study Amsterdam. *International Journal of Geriatric Psychiatry, 13*(10), 717–726.

Beresford, T., & Gomberg, E. (1995). *Alcohol and aging.* New York, NY: Oxford University Press.

Blazer, D., & Williams, C. (1980). Epidemiology of dysphoria and depression in an elderly population. *American Journal of Psychiatry, 137*(4), 439–444.

Bleuler, M. (1978). *The schizophrenic disorders: Long-term patient and family studies.* New Haven, CT: Yale University Press.

Cairney, J., McCabe, L., Veldhuizen, S., Corna, L. M., Streiner, D., & Herrmann, N. (2007). Epidemiology of social phobia in later life. *American Journal of Geriatric Psychiatry, 15*(3), 224–233.

Califano, J. A. (1997). *High society: How substance abuse ravages America and what to do about it.* New York, NY: Perseus Publishing.

Callahan, C. M., Hendrie, H. C., Nienaber, N. A., & Tierney, W. M. (1996). Suicidal ideation among older primary care patients. *Journal of the American Geriatric Society, 44*(10), 1205–1209.

Canadian Study of Health and Aging Working Group. (1994). Canadian Study of Health and Aging: Study methods and prevalence of dementia. *Canadian Medical Association Journal, 150,* 899–913.

Centers for Disease Control and Prevention (CDC). (2007). Increases in age-group-specific injury mortality – United States, 1999–2004. *MMWR (Morbidity and Mortality Weekly Report), 56*(49), 1281–1284.

Colliver, J. D., Compton, W. M., Gfroerer, J. C., & Condon, T. (2006). Projecting drug use among aging baby boomers in 2020. *Annals of Epidemiology, 16*(4), 257–265.

Conwell, Y., Duberstein, P. R., & Caine, E. D. (2002). Risk factors for suicide in later life. *Biological Psychiatry, 52*(3), 193–204.

Corso, E., Campo, G., Triglio, A., Napoli, A., Reggio, A., & Lanaia, F. (1992). Prevalence of moderate and severe Alzheimer dementia and multi-infarct dementia in the population of southeastern Sicily. *Italian Journal of Neurological Science, 13*(3), 215–219.

Dennis, M., Baillon, S., Brugha, T., Lindesay, J., Stewart, R., & Meltzer, H. (2007). The spectrum of suicidal ideation in Great Britain: Comparisons across a 16–74 years age range. *Psychological Medicine, 37*(6), 795–805.

Didham, R., Dovey, S., & Reith, D. (2006). Characteristics of general practitioner consultations prior to suicide: A nested case-control study in New Zealand. *The New Zealand Medical Journal, 119*(1247), U2358.

Folstein, M., Bassett, S., Anthony, J., Romanoski, A., & Nestadt, G. (1991). Dementia: Case ascertainment in a community survey. *Journal of Gerontology, 46*(4), M132–M138.

Gallo, J., & Lebowitz, B. (1999). The epidemiology of common late-life mental disorders in the community: Themes for the new century. *Psychiatric Services, 50*(9), 1158–1166.

Grant, B. F., Dawson, D. A., Stinson, F. S., Chou, S. P., Dufour, M. C., & Pickering, R. P. (2004). The 12-month prevalence and trends in DSM-IV alcohol abuse and dependence: United States, 1991–1992 and 2001–2002. *Drug and Alcohol Dependence, 74*(3), 223–234.

Harris, M. J., & Jeste, D. V. (1988). Late-onset schizophrenia: An overview. *Schizophrenia Bulletin, 14*(1), 39–55.

Hebert, L., Scherr, P., McCann, H., Beckett, L., & Evans, D. (2001). Is the risk of developing Alzheimer's disease greater for women than for men? *American Journal of Epidemiology, 153*(2), 132–136.

Howard, R., Rabins, P. V., Seeman, M. V., & Jeste, D. V. (2000). Late-onset schizophrenia and very-late-onset schizophrenia-like psychosis: An international consensus. The International Late-Onset Schizophrenia Group. *American Journal of Psychiatry, 157*(2), 172–178.

Hybels, C., Blazer, D., & Steffens, D. (2005). Predictors of partial remission in older patients treated for major depression: The role of comorbid dysthymia. *American Journal of Geriatric Psychiatry, 13*(8), 713–721.

Joyce, P. R., Bushnell, J. A., Oakley-Browne, M. A., Wells, J. E., & Hornblow, A. R. (1989). The epidemiology of panic symptomatology and agoraphobic avoidance. *Comprehensive Psychiatry, 30*(4), 303–312.

Kapusta, N. D., Etzersdorfer, E., & Sonneck, G. (2007). Trends in suicide rates of the elderly in Austria, 1970–2004: An analysis of changes in terms of age groups, suicide methods and gender. *International Journal of Geriatric Psychiatry, 22*(5), 438–444.

Kessing, L. (2004). Gender differences in the phenomenology of bipolar disorder. *Bipolar Disorders, 6*(5), 421–425.

Kinzl, J., Traweger, C., Trefalt, E., Mangweth, B., & Biebl, W. (1999). Binge eating disorder in females: A population-based investigation. *The International Journal of Eating Disorders, 25*(3), 287–292.

Kjøller, M., & Helweg-Larsen, M. (2002). Suicidal ideation and suicide attempts among adult Danes. *Scandinavian Journal of Public Health, 28*(1), 54–61.

Koenig, H., & Blazer, D. (1992). Epidemiology of geriatric affective disorders. *Clinical Geriatric Medicine, 8,* 235–251.

Kolada, J. L., Bland, R. C., & Newman, S. C. (1994). Epidemiology of psychiatric disorders in Edmonton. Obsessive-compulsive disorder. *Acta psychiatrica scandinavica. Supplementum, 376,* 24–35.

Langlois, S., & Morrison, P. (2002). Suicide deaths and suicide attempts. *Health Reports, 13*(2), 9–22.

Lehmann, S. W. (2003). Psychiatric disorders in older women. *International Review of Psychiatry, 15*(3), 269–279.

Lépine, J. (2002). The epidemiology of anxiety disorders: Prevalence and societal costs. *Journal of Clinical Psychiatry, 63*(Suppl. 14), 4–8.

Letenneur, L., Launer, L., Andersen, K., Dewey, M., Ott, A., Copeland, J., et al. (2000). Education and the risk for Alzheimer's disease: Sex makes a difference. EURODEM pooled analyses. EURODEM Incidence Research Group. *American Journal of Epidemiology, 151*(11), 1064–1071.

Lindeman, S., Hämäläinen, J., Isometsä, E., Kaprio, J., Poikolainen, K., Heikkinen, M., et al. (2000). The 12-month prevalence and risk factors for major depressive episode in Finland: Representative sample of 5993 adults. *Acta psychiatrica scandinavica, 102*(3), 178–184.

Magee, W. J., Eaton, W. W., Wittchen, H., McGonagle, K. A., & Kessler, R. C. (1996). Agoraphobia, simple phobia, and social phobia in the National Comorbidity Survey. *Archives of General Psychiatry, 53*(2), 159–168.

Manchikanti, L. (2007). National drug control policy and prescription drug abuse: Facts and fallacies. *Pain Physician, 10*(3), 399–424.

Mangweth-Matzek, B., Rupp, C. L., Hausmann, A., Assmayr, K., Mariacher, E., Kemmler, G., et al. (2006). Never too old for eating disorders or body dissatisfaction: A community study of elderly women. *The International Journal of Eating Disorders, 39*(7), 583–586.

Manubens, J., Martínez-Lage, J., Lacruz, F., Muruzabal, J., Larumbe, R., Guarch, C., et al. (1995). Prevalence of Alzheimer's disease and other dementing disorders in Pamplona, Spain. *Neuroepidemiology, 14*(4), 155–164.

Martini, E., Garrett, N., Lindquist, T., & Isham, G. (2007). The boomers are coming: A total cost of care model of the impact of population aging on health care costs in the United States by Major Practice Category. *Health Services Research, 42*(1 Pt 1), 201–218.

McLennan, W. (1997). *Mental health and wellbeing: Profile of adults, Australia* (Australian Bureau of Statistics, Publication No. 4326.0).

Meehan, P. J., Saltzman, L. E., & Sattin, R. W. (1991). Suicides among older United States residents: Epidemiologic characteristics and trends. *American Journal of Public Health, 81*(9), 1198–1200.

Mitchell, A. M., & Bulik, C. M. (2006). Eating disorders and women's health: An update. *Journal of Midwifery and Women's Health, 51*(3), 193–201.

Mitchell, P. B., Slade, T., & Andrews, G. (2004). Twelve-month prevalence and disability of DSM-IV bipolar disorder in an Australian general population survey. *Psychological Medicine, 34*(5), 777–785.

Mohammadi, M. R., Ghanizadeh, A., Rahgozar, M., Noorbala, A. A., Davidian, H., Afzali, H. M., et al. (2004). Prevalence of obsessive-compulsive disorder in Iran. *BMC Psychiatry, 4*(2).

Mojtabai, R., & Olfson, M. (2004). Major depression in community-dwelling middle-aged and older adults: Prevalence and 2- and 4-year follow-up symptoms. *Psychological Medicine, 34,* 623–634.

Mokdad, A. H., Marks, J. S., Stroup, D. F., & Gerberding, J. L. (2004). Actual causes of death in the United States, 2000. *Journal of the American Medical Association, 291*(10), 1238–1245.

Offord, D., Boyle, M., Campbell, D., Goering, P., Lin, E., Wong, M., et al. (1996). One-year prevalence of psychiatric disorder in Ontarians 15 to 64 years of age. *Canadian Journal of Psychiatry, 41*(9), 559–563.

Ott, A., Breteler, M. M., van Harskamp, F., Claus, J. J., Van Der Cammen, T. J., Grobbee, D. E., et al. (1995). Prevalence of Alzheimer's disease and vascular dementia: Association with education. The rotterdam study. *BMJ (Clinical Research Ed.), 310*(6985), 970–973.

Patten, S. (2000). Incidence of major depression in Canada. *CMAJ, 163*(6), 714–715.

Pigott, T. (2003). Anxiety disorders in women. *The Psychiatric Clinics of North America, 27*(3), 621–672.

Piran, N., & Gadalla, T. (2007). Eating disorders and substance abuse in Canadian women: A national study. *Addiction, 102*(1), 105–113.

Regier, D., Boyd, J., Burke, J., Rae, D., Myers, J., Kramer, M., et al. (1988). One-month prevalence of mental disorders in the United States. Based on five Epidemiologic Catchment Area sites. *Archives of General Psychiatry, 45*(11), 977–986.

Regier, D., Farmer, M., Rae, D., Myers, J., Kramer, M., Robins, L., et al. (1993). One-month prevalence of mental disorders in the United States and sociodemographic characteristics: The Epidemiologic Catchment Area Study. *Acta Psychiatrica Scandinavica, 88*(1), 35–47.

Riecher-Rossler, A. (1999). *Late onset schizophrenia: The German concept and literature*. Petersfield, UK and Philadelphia: Wrightson Biomedical Publishing Limited.

Rodriguez, R., & Werneck, G. (2005). Age-period-cohort Analysis of Suicide Rates in Rio de Janeiro, Brazil, 1979–1998. *Social Psychiatry and Psychiatric Epidemiology, 40,* 192–196.

Romanoski, A., Folstein, M., Nestadt, G., Chahal, R., Merchant, A., Brown, C., et al. (1992). The epidemiology of psychiatrist-ascertained depression and DSM-III depressive disorders. Results from the Eastern Baltimore Mental Health Survey Clinical Reappraisal. *Psychological Medicine, 22*(3), 629–655.

Ruitenberg, A., Ott, A., van Swieten, J., Hofman, A., & Breteler, M. (2001). Incidence of dementia: Does gender make a difference? *Neurobiology of Aging, 22*(4), 575–580.

Sheperd, M., & Wilkinson, G. (1988). Primary care as the middle ground for psychiatric epidemiology. *Psychological Medicine, 18,* 263–267.

Shumaker, S., Legault, C., Rapp, S., Thal, L., Wallace, R., Ockene, J., et al. (2003). Estrogen plus progestin and the incidence of dementia and mild cognitive impairment in postmenopausal women: The Women's Health Initiative Memory Study: A randomized controlled trial. *Journal of the American Medical Association, 289*(20), 2651–2662.

Sicras, A., Rejas, J., Arco, S., Flores, E., Ortega, G., Esparcia, A., et al. (2005). Prevalence, resource utilization and costs of vascular dementia compared to Alzheimer's dementia in a population setting. *Dementia and Geriatric Cognitive Disorders, 19*(5–6), 305–315.

Simoni-Wastila, L., & Yang, H. (2006). Psychoactive drug abuse in older adults *American Journal of Geriatric Pharmacotherapy, 4*(4), 380–394.

Spicer, R. S., & Miller, T. R. (2000). Suicide acts in 8 states: Incidence and case fatality rates by demographics and method. *American Journal of Public Health, 90*(12), 1885–1891.

Tariot, P., Podgorski, C., Blazina, L., & Leibovici, A. (1993). Mental disorders in the nursing home: Another perspective. *American Journal of Psychiatry, 150,* 1063–1069.

Unützer, J., Simon, G., Pabiniak, C., Bond, K., & Katon, W. (1988). The treated prevalence of bipolar disorder in a large staff-model HMO. *Psychiatric Services, 49*(8), 1072–1078.

Weissman, M., Leaf, P., Holzer, C., Myers, J., & Tischler, G. (1984). The epidemiology of depression. An update on sex differences in rates. *Journal Affect Disord, 7*(3–4), 179–188.

World Health Organization. (2008). *Lexicon of alcohol and drug terms.* Retrieved March 20, 2008 from http://www.who.int/substance_abuse/terminology/who_lexicon/en/

Wright, S., & Persad, C. (2007). Distinguishing between depression and dementia in older persons: Neuropsychological and neuropathological correlates. *Journal of Geriatric Psychiatry and Neurology, 20*(4), 189–198.

Yip, P. S., Chi, I., Chiu, H., Chi Wai, K., Conwell, Y., & Caine, E. (2003). A prevalence study of suicide ideation among older adults in Hong Kong SAR. *International Journal of Geriatric Psychiatry, 18*(11), 1056–1062.

Zaccai, J., McCracken, C., & Brayne, C. (2005). A systematic review of prevalence and incidence studies of dementia with Lewy bodies. *Age and Ageing, 34*(6), 561–566.

Chapter 5
Physical Illness and Medical Needs of Women with Mental Disorders

Mary Jo Larson and Sarah McGraw

Introduction

This chapter discusses the importance of providing effective treatment for physical or somatic conditions that co-occur among women with serious mental disorders. Providing high-quality healthcare for women with multimorbidities (e.g., a combination of several chronic mental and somatic conditions) may be particularly challenging for a number of reasons related to numerous risk factors, lifestyle issues, active symptoms of the patients, difficult interactions between unsupported or inadequately trained medical providers and patients, and inadequacies built into a fragmented healthcare system. Even though there is a higher disease burden and treatment need among women with mental disorders compared to other women, too little is known about why these factors lead to premature death, high rates of disability, and undertreatment of somatic conditions. This chapter identifies the most common somatic conditions among women with mental disorders and focuses on several opportunities for care improvement linked to appropriate and timely detection and care of physical health problems for women with serious mental health disorders. As co-occurrence of multiple problems may be the rule, not the exception, there is a need for effective comprehensive treatment models.

Scope of the Problem

The typical woman patient with a mental disorder will also have accompanying physical conditions. This co-occurrence of psychological and physical challenges is more common among women than men, and requires that both the mental health care and primary care providers for women be competent in recognizing, referring, and

M. J. Larson (✉)
Institute for Behavioral Health, Schneider Institutes for Health Policy, Brandeis University, 415 South Street, Mailstop 035, Waltham, MA 02454, USA

B. L. Levin, M. A. Becker (eds.), *A Public Health Perspective of Women's Mental Health*, DOI 10.1007/978-1-4419-1526-9_5, © Springer Science+Business Media LLC 2010

treating conditions that commonly co-occur. The impact of untreated and undertreated co-occurrence may be preventable premature death, increased functional limitations and increased utilization of health services to treat acute symptoms or problems and does not increase the overall quality of life of women with mental disorders.

Premature Death

As a result of higher rates of serious somatic illness and a consequence of under-treatment of psychiatric and physical illnesses, premature death is substantially elevated among women with mental disorders. Extensive mortality studies have been conducted on persons with schizophrenia, and less is known about the impact of other mental disorders. Not all studies separately report on mortality for women and men; however, elevated risk of death appears to affect both genders. Compared to other women, women with schizophrenia (and other mental disorders) have an elevated risk of death from suicide (Palmer et al. 2005) and premature death from comorbid somatic conditions (Brown 1997). Specifically, the elevated mortality risk for adults with schizophrenia compared to the general population, measured as the all-cause standardized mortality ratio, was estimated as 1.5 in two reviews (Brown 1997). A meta-analysis reviewing studies from 25 different nations found that elevated mortality-risk-associated schizophrenia is nearly universal (Lucas et al. 2005). Comparing adults with schizophrenia to the general population, the median of mortality ratios for unnatural causes of death (suicide and accidents) was 7.5 across 37 international studies, and the median of mortality ratios for natural causes was 2.4. The all-cause mortality ratio for women was not statistically different from that of men in these studies (Saha et al. 2007).

Limited data on causes of death among persons with other psychiatric conditions exist. In a study based in the UK, elevated accidental death rates were associated with most psychiatric diagnosis groups. Respiratory and circulatory system disorders accounted for excessive mortality among psychiatric inpatients and others with psychotic illnesses, but no excess deaths were due to neoplasm (Prior et al. 1996). State psychiatric hospitals are the location of deaths and responsible for managing chronic physical disease among many patients with chronic psychiatric illness. Competent medical care is needed for these patients who may have very complex physical health needs. The patients who died in a study of patient deaths in one state hospital had a mean of eight physical illnesses, with over one-half of patients having circulatory and respiratory conditions (Kamara et al. 1998).

Increased Disability and Functional Limitations

Women with mental disorder histories are particularly vulnerable to a host of risk factors associated with increased incidence, inadequate detection, and inappropriate care of physical disability and poor health. These factors may disproportionately affect women's health relative to men, as certain psychiatric conditions have a larger impact on women (Brett and Burt 2001). In the USA, for example, major depression is the second leading cause of disability-adjusted life-years (DALYs) lost in women, whereas it is the tenth leading cause of DALYs in men (Egede 2004). There is a complex interplay of mental disorders with physical illness which leads to disability and functional limitations. For example, this relationship is confounded by the presence of substance use disorders (Katon 2003b; Larson et al. 2007; Saitz et al. 2007) and certain somatic conditions. Chronic pain, for example, has an impact on functional and role disability, particularly when it co-occurs with other chronic diseases and mental disorders (Von Korff et al. 2005). The impact of chronic illness on women with mental disorders may not be uniform across patient subgroups. In general, foreign-born women report better health status, fewer activity limitations, and fewer risk behaviors than their US-born counterparts (Lucas et al. 2005) and are also less likely to report serious psychological distress (Dey and Lucas 2006).

A mental disorder may complicate symptoms and add to functional limitations of common comorbidities. Evidence from a national survey compared adults with neither diabetes nor mental disorder to those with these disorders and found that the odds of functional disability are 3.00 for major depression alone, 2.42 for diabetes alone, and much higher (7.15) when diabetes is comorbid with major depression (Egede 2004). Given that anywhere from 9 to 23% of survey participants with one or more chronic physical disease had comorbid depression, in an international study of world health, the impact of comorbidity on disability is highly relevant (Moussavi et al. 2007). The authors of this world health study concluded that depression produces the greatest decrement in health compared with the chronic diseases angina, arthritis, asthma, and diabetes, and that comorbid depression incrementally worsens health compared with any combination of chronic diseases without depression (Moussavi et al. 2007). Posttraumatic stress disorder (PTSD) is a second common diagnosis in the general population of women and particularly among veterans associated with high levels of short- and long-term disability, even after controlling for accompanying physical and other mental disorders (Sareen et al. 2007).

Viewed another way, health care professionals who treat patients with chronic physical illness, specifically those with multimorbid conditions, will see elevated rates of common psychiatric conditions because of the strong association of mental disorders and chronic illness. Comparing data from two large German epidemiologic surveys, rates of psychiatric disorders were compared across inpatient populations and the general population. In both groups between 42 and 44% of patients with one of the chronic somatic diseases (musculoskeletal, cardiovascular, cancer, or respiratory tract disease) also had a mental disorder, most frequently mood and anxiety disorders, and the adjusted odds ratio was 2.2 compared to healthy controls (Harter et al. 2007). Lifetime severe asthma in a community study of adults in Germany was linked with elevated odds of panic disorder, anxiety disorder, social phobia and bipolar disorder (Clouse et al. 2003; Goodwin et al. 2003b).

High and Unexplained Rates of Medical Service Utilization

Barriers to use of primary care services have been linked to higher rates of emergency department care for preventable exacerbations of chronic conditions (Falik et al. 2001; Oster and Bindman 2003), and women of color, particularly, may receive care in settings and under conditions that contribute to poor quality care overall (Smedley et al. 2003). The high-utilizers of healthcare frequently suffer from psychiatric illnesses comorbid with one or several medical conditions (Farley and Patsalides 2001; Garis and Farmer 2002), but too little is known about the risk factors and the types of care they are receiving. For women with mental disorders and multiple chronic illnesses leading to high-cost patterns of care, the issue may not only be a failure to deliver evidence-based treatments for their conditions, but may also be related to the healthcare system's inability to organize the myriad of care required into a coherent treatment plan when medical, social, mental health, and substance abuse problems co-occur. Women with these complex combinations may also face particular challenges that require assistance in order to maintain their health, including problems of literacy, poverty, housing instability, illness in the family, drug dependency, and abusive relationships (Kertesz et al. 2006). The presence of a mental disorder may affect the women's perceptions and willingness to seek medical care when indicated, to engage in the medical care recommended by a professional, or to be judged suitable for a course of treatment by the professional (Hansen et al. 2002).

Even when ignoring pregnancy-related services, the rate of ambulatory medical care visits for women is 33% higher than that for men, and women are more likely to make primary care visits than men where an antidepressant is prescribed (Brett and Burt 2001). The average annual visit rate for women to an ambulatory medical provider is between four and five visits. Injury-related visits occurred among 46 of 100 women aged 15–44 years, and seeking treatment for a chronic condition accounted for 39% of all visits (Brett and Burt 2001). Only small studies of special populations provide estimates of health care use among women with psychiatric and physical conditions. In a Medicaid managed care sample, men and women with severe mental illness had lower medical costs (exclusive of pregnancy and mental health care) in outpatient offices and hospitals and inpatient settings, but higher costs for emergency care including ambulances; 28% of costs were for emergency care (Berren et al. 1999). The literature presents convincing evidence that women with mental disorders are more likely to have a range of chronic conditions that do require greater utilization of medical care than their counterparts without mental disorders, but those medical needs may go unaddressed.

Pervasive Acute and Chronic Somatic Conditions

In general, there is underdetection and underdiagnosis of acute and chronic illness among women with mental disorders. There is also concern that women with mental disorders will not make use of appropriate care settings for their medical problems, either because of a fragmented healthcare system, provider misunderstanding of this patient population, or because of their personal characteristics. Nevertheless, systematic studies have identified that women (and men) with mental disorders are at high risk of other acute and chronic somatic conditions. Numerous articles have investigated the relationship between mood, anxiety, and physical illness (e.g., asthma, autoimmune disorders, cancer, cardiovascular disease, obesity, and sexual dysfunction). There is growing evidence of an overall negative impact of depression, other mood states, and anxiety on numerous physical illnesses and conditions and disease outcomes (Balon 2006). In a population-based Canadian national health study, the presence of lifetime mood disorder (meeting bipolar or major depressive disorder diagnostic criteria) was associated with elevated odds (1.22) of obesity in women but not in men (McIntyre et al. 2006). In a large US study, obesity was associated with significantly higher rates of mood and anxiety disorders but significantly lower rates of substance use disorder; there were no differences in these associations between men and women in the US study (Katon 2003a; Simon et al. 2006). Reviewed briefly here is literature linking common or serious mental disorders to highly prevalent somatic conditions that generally shorten a lifespan or elevate risk of disability: diabetes, cardiovascular disease, cancer, multimorbidity, and chronic pain.

Risk of Diabetes and Metabolic Syndrome

Much of the depression that co-occurs with diabetes goes unrecognized or untreated by primary care clinicians (Bair et al. 2003). In a review of seven controlled studies of diabetes, the odds of depression were significantly elevated in both women and men with diabetes compared to those without diabetes (odds ratios 1.7 in both groups), and there is some evidence from prospective studies that depression doubles the risk of incident type 2 diabetes (Anderson et al. 2001). Metabolic syndrome is increasingly recognized as an important risk factor for diabetes, cardiovascular disease, and premature mortality, but the clinical investigation of metabolic syndrome in patients with mental disorders is surprisingly scarce (Jakovljevic et al. 2007). A systematic literature review revealed that metabolic syndrome was reported in 12–36% of patients with recurrent depression (and was even higher among patients with other mental disorders), 32–35% of patients with PTSD, 25–50% of patients with bipolar, and 19–63% of patients with schizophrenia (Jakovljevic et al. 2007). Currently the pathophysiologic link among these disorders is unclear. However, a second review also noted that bipolar disorder and metabolic syndrome share features of hormonal, immunologic, and autonomic nervous system dysregulation (Taylor and MacQueen 2006). This suggests a common predisposing physiologic risk not limited to common lifestyle factors. Even before treatment with medications with known adverse metabolic effects, persons with psychosis have a two- to threefold higher prevalence of diabetes (Nasrallah 2003) and risk factors for cardiovascular disease (Birkenaes et al. 2007).

Cardiovascular Disease

Heart disease is often, but not always, linked with diabetes and is also a common reason for visits among adults seeking medical care. In addition, heart disease is associated with increased mental disorders. In a study of cardiovascular disease among adults in primary care with and without psychoses, earlier onset of risk factors and heart disease was noted among individuals with schizophrenia compared to those with affective psychoses and no disabilities. Patients with schizophrenia had increased relative risk for obesity, congestive heart failure, dementia, depression, and death, while patients with affective psychoses had increased risk for dementia and diabetes (McDermott et al. 2005). Furthermore, in 76 diabetic women patients, major depression was an independent risk factor that accelerated the development of chronic heart disease (Clouse et al. 2003). Smoking, obesity, and other cardiovascular risk factors were twice as high among patients in a longitudinal study with bipolar disorder and schizophrenia as the general population in the Oslo (Norway) Health Study (Birkenaes et al. 2007). Thus, primary care clinicians seeing patients with heart disease should carefully screen for the presence of a mental disorder.

Risk of Cancer

A number of small studies provide evidence that individuals with mental disorders may have a higher risk of some cancers. In a nested case–control study of malignancies, individuals diagnosed with schizophrenia and bipolar disorder had markedly higher rates than other patients of colon cancer (OR 2.90), and this ratio increased to 4.08 among patients taking antipsychotics. Breast cancer rates among the patients with schizophrenia were also slightly higher (1.52) while there were no detectable differences in rates of malignancies among patients with bipolar disorders (Hippisley-Cox et al. 2007). Another study suggests the incidence of breast cancer was higher among older women in a psychiatric hospital compared to their counterparts in a general hospital as well as outpatients. Rate differentials among women with mental disorders and other women, while not conclusive, could occur because of patient risk behaviors (smoking and alcohol use), elevated prolactin or hormone levels, medication effects, or other environmental and genetic differences. Thus, it is inconclusive if women with mental disorders are at particular risk for malignancies.

Chronic Pain

Depression and pain share biological pathways and thus simultaneous treatment of both may improve health outcomes (Bair et al. 2003). Among US women in general, the presence of chronic pain is a common symptom that goes underdetected and undertreated. Women appear to have higher rates of disability from chronic pain than men (Smith et al. 2001). In a national survey, 20% of women reported migraines or severe headaches, 29% had pain in the lower back, and 16% reported neck pain (Pleis and Lethbridge-Cejku 2007b). Also, pain may lead to more distress among women than men when combined with psychiatric disorders and other psychosocial factors (McBeth et al. 2002). Unfortunately, depression and chronic pain frequently co-occur in women. Using a high cut-off score for depression based on the Center for Epidemiologic Studies (CES-D), 18% of adults with chronic pain were found to have depression, compared to 8% of adults who did not have chronic pain (Magni et al. 1990). There is also evidence that drinking problems and chronic pain are associated among older women, and this drinking may disproportionately affect the health of older women with mental disorders (Brennan et al. 2005).

When chronic pain co-occurs with depression, its impact may differ among racial/ethnic groups of women. Overall, comorbid pain with depression in a national study was associated with significantly lower physical and mental component health status scores (Bao et al. 2003). Black women with chronic pain experience more physical impairments than White women. Disability mediates the race–depression relationship, such that Black women are more vulnerable to depression as a result of higher disability (Ndao-Brumblay and Green 2005). There are other race/ethnicity differences as well. Within Hispanic Americans, for example, the prevalence rates of chronic abdominal pain were 4.6% in Mexican Americans, 5.8% in Cuban Americans, and 8.3% among Puerto Ricans. Major depression criteria (DSM-III) were met among those with chronic pain in 6.8% of Mexican and Cuban Americans and 12.6% of Puerto Ricans. In this study, chronic abdominal pain occurred more frequently in women than in men (Magni et al. 1992).

The type of chronic pain appears to vary by specific mental diagnosis, and the adverse impact of pain may be higher when combined with a mental disorder. Pain in multiple body locations, rather than a single location, is associated with particularly high odds ratios for mood disorders (3.7) and anxiety disorders (3.6) in an international study conducted in 17 countries. In the same study, mood disorders and anxiety disorders occurred at nearly twice the odds among persons with heart disease than those without (Ormel et al. 2007). In the USA, persons with panic disorder (OR = 4.27) and posttraumatic stress disorder (OR = 3.69) had elevated odds of chronic pain. Regarding pain-related disability, having one psychiatric disorder was not significantly associated with disability, but having multiple psychiatric disorders was significantly associated with increased disability (Kessler et al. 1994; McWilliams et al. 2003).

Multimorbidity

Psychiatric disorder increases the odds of reporting physical symptoms three- to sevenfold, and the relationship is strongest when the outcome studied is multiple symptoms. Population-attributable risk of psychiatric or subsyndromal disorder was linked as a cause to 40% of multiple somatic symptoms (Hotopf et al. 1998). Furthermore, multimorbidity is common; 74% of persons with serious mental disorders had a diagnosis of at least one chronic health problem, and 50% had two or more chronic health problems, with chronic pulmonary illness the most prevalent and the most comorbid. Substance use disorder was a significant predictor of health problem severity (Jones et al. 2004) and may account in part for the higher rates of certain physical disorders with serious mental disorders (Blank et al. 2002).

Comorbidity with Substance Use

Substance use disorders are a common comorbidity with many mental disorders (Breslau et al. 2003; Compton et al. 2005) and contribute to the increased disability and impairment found in women with mental disorders (Johnson et al. 1995; Kessler et al. 2005; Regier et al. 1990). Chronic or heavy substance use is known to independently contribute to serious illnesses, medical complications, and chronic conditions (Leonard et al. 2001; Neiman et al. 2000), and alcohol and drug dependence also substantially increase mortality (Barr et al. 1984; Hulse et al. 1999). For example, women with chronic drug use are at increased risk of injuries and other associated medical complications (Larson et al. 2006; Zavala and French 2003). Cocaine use in one study accounted for up to 25% of heart attacks in patients between the ages of 18 and 45 (Lange and Hillis 2001; Saitz et al. 2007). Alcohol and drug use is associated with high-risk behavior that increases likelihood of HIV transmission, such as unprotected sex and injection of illicit drugs (Anderson et al. 1999). Women with substance use disorders comorbid with mental disorders will frequently end up in jail or prison for drug-related or drug-motivated offenses. Among those with a mental disorder, sexual victimization was three times as high among female inmates (23.4%) as among male inmates (8.3%; Wolff et al. 2007, also see Chap. 9 in this volume for additional information on substance abuse and women).

Plausible Contributory Factors

Women's psychiatric impairments can contribute in various ways to the prevalence and experience of disabling conditions and premature death. There are both individual and environmental risk factors, including violence and iatrogenic effects of treatment, which may result in the presence of one condition increasing the probability of a second.

Individual Risk Factors

The onset of a mental disorder may increase the tendency toward unhealthy lifestyle behaviors (e.g., alcohol, drug use, poor diet) that in turn increase the likelihood of somatic illness. Thus, some of the excessive rates of mortality, morbidity, and disability are associated with these unhealthy behaviors that in turn are more common among women with mental disorders than their peers. For example, studies have linked the increased smoking rates of adults with mental disorders to high incidence of emphysema. These studies have also documented that higher rates of chronic pulmonary disease remained even after controlling for differential smoking rates among adults with and without mental disorders (Sokal et al. 2004). One study found pulmonary illness to be the most frequently occurring comorbid condition (31%) among 147 persons with serious mental illness (Jones et al. 2004). Excessive alcohol consumption is another health behavior associated with mental disorders that is linked to preventable deaths, illness, and injury (Bloss 2005; Rehm et al. 2006). Furthermore, in the presence of serious mental illness, women often have symptoms of inactivity and emotional withdrawal, which may contribute to their limited motivation for positive health behaviors and attention to health problems (Dickerson et al. 2006). Thus, interventions may need to address these behavioral components of mental disorders.

Environmental Risk Factors

The importance of biological vulnerability factors and environment is the subject of emerging research; some argue that a substantial proportion of morbidity may be attributed not to a specific risk for one disorder, but to a few underlying liability factors that influence both somatic and psychiatric disorders (Bondy 2003). Certain mental and somatic disorders may share a common genetic or environmental pathway, and increased comorbid conditions may be downstream expressions of these shared factors (Saha et al. 2007). Even in the absence of shared genetic predisposition, common mental disorders are associated with increased exposure to environmental threats, such as lack of housing, selling sex for drugs, common STDs, and, perhaps most importantly, exposure to violence or abuse.

Violence and Abuse

Interpersonal violence is widespread among women in general (Browne and Bassuk 1997), and childhood physical abuse is estimated at 10–12% among women and childhood sexual abuse at 13–17% among women (*Violence against women* 1992). Among women in treatment for either mental or substance use disorders, the majority will report histories of physical and/or sexual violence (Browne and Finkelhor 1986; El-Bassel et al. 2003; Kessler et al. 1995; Najavits et al. 1997). Furthermore, persons with serious mental disorders are more likely to be victims of a violent crime; one study reported an annual incidence of violent crime in persons with SMI as 168.2 incidents per 1,000 persons, more than four times higher than the general population rates (39.9 incidents per 1,000 persons). Depending on the type of violent crime (rape/sexual assault, robbery, assault, and their subcategories), prevalence was 6–23 times greater among persons with serious mental disorders than among the general population (Teplin et al. 2005).

This exposure to violence, in childhood and repeatedly in adulthood, is a public health concern in the community treatment of women with serious mental disorders as it is associated with a range of physical sequelae that may require medical care. One study documented that childhood sexual and physical abuse was independently associated with serious health problems, and its effects were only partially mediated through participant's psychiatric disorders. Childhood abuse is an important predictor of elevated risk for mental disorders and also increases the likelihood of exposure to adult trauma, to problems with alcohol and drug use, and to emergence of a substance use disorder (Fullilove et al. 1993; Gil-Rivas et al. 1996; Kaplan and Klinetob 2000; MacMillan et al. 2001; McCauley et al. 1997; Miller et al. 1993; Najavits et al. 1997; Yandow 1989; Zierler et al. 1991). Studies have linked exposure to physical and sexual abuse in childhood and adulthood to poor health status in women (Arnow 2004; Campbell et al. 2002; De Alba et al. 2004; Felitti 1991; Kovac et al. 2003), a greater number of medical symptoms (Goodwin et al. 2003a; Walker et al. 1992), and increased report of chronic pain (Bassuk et al. 2001; Romans et al. 2002) and disability. Childhood abuse is also associated with poorer health habits in adulthood such as smoking (Anda et al. 1999), risky sexual behaviors (Zierler et al. 1991), and other high-risk behaviors (Felitti et al. 1998).

Other common consequences are associated with interpersonal violence when accompanied by depression, including self-mutilation and suicide attempts which present to medical sector providers (Beitchman et al. 1991, 1992; Breslau et al. 1997, 2003; Briere et al. 1997). Furthermore, physical sequelae of repeated abuse include chronic stress leading to diseases of body systems, gynecological difficulties, gastrointestinal problems, and headaches (Liebschutz et al. 1997; van der Kolk et al. 1996). A serious consequence of past abuse, particularly repeated experiences, is posttraumatic stress disorder or PTSD (American Psychological Association (APA) 1994), which often presents with other physical and psychiatric comorbidities (Albucher and Liberzon 2002). As PTSD can also contribute to the risk of substance use and substance abuse relapses (Breslau et al. 2003; Chilcoat and Breslau 1998; Clark et al. 2001; Harris and Fallot 2001), it directly and indirectly contributes to increased risk of somatic illness in women. Using cross-sectional data from a midwestern state's Medicaid eligibility and paid-claims data, among young girls and teens, PTSD was associated with adverse health outcomes, and victimization alone was sometimes independently associated with adverse health outcomes. In the adolescent age group, those with PTSD had increased odds for blood disorders, irritable bowel syndrome, sexually transmitted infection, and cervical dysplasia.

The importance of PTSD diagnosis as a predictor of disease or chronic conditions seemed to increase with age (Seng et al. 2005).

Somatic Effects of Psychotropic Medications

Medications which are commonly used to treat certain serious mental disorders, particularly schizophrenia and bipolar disorder, include mood stabilizers, anticonvulsants, and antipsychotic medications. Some of the most commonly used medications in these classes have been linked to risk for adverse metabolic changes in patients with effects on weight gain, type 2 diabetes, and cardiovascular disease (Nasrallah 2003; Newcomer 2005, 2006), obesity (especially with clozapine and olanzapine), and dyslipidemia. The prevalence of type 2 diabetes may be doubled in patients with atypical antipsychotic use relative to people with psychosis not treated with these medications, and increased rates of subclinical hyperglycemia and serious weight gain are important risk factors for disease (Nasrallah 2003). Thus, physicians should take a careful family history and consider the risk of using atypicals as first-line psychiatric treatment. The use of antidepressant medication in one study was an independent risk factor for diabetes onset, while elevated depression scores alone were not. Compared with no use, continuous antidepressant use during the 3-year study was associated with hazard ratios of 2.60 compared to the placebo arm and 3.39 compared to the intensive lifestyle modification arm (Rubin et al. 2008).

Medical Care and Service Delivery Problems

A large group of studies has documented low rates of preventive care among women and patients with mental disorders and provides other evidence that medical care could be improved for persons with psychiatric conditions (Coyle and Santiago 2002). Clearly, detection depends on the intersection of women seeking some care for symptoms and the clinician's ability to diagnose the problems being seen (Kessler et al. 2001). Women may present to primary care providers more frequently than men, given that they have increased risk of highly prevalent mental disorders commonly seen in primary care settings; their risk of depression and anxiety disorders is two to three times greater than it is for men (Kessler et al. 2003, 2005).

Many of the somatic conditions common in women with mental disorders could be managed in part by improved health behaviors if given additional support from their medical providers or other social support. For example, regular walking and exercise are two health behaviors that would improve outcomes; however, persons with severe mental illness are less active than the general population. They report very little confidence in their ability to exercise when feeling sad or stressed, and may have low levels of social support toward exercising. Approximately half or more of the respondents with severe mental illness in one study expressed a belief in the health benefits of exercise, enjoyment of exercise, and a desire to be more active. The majority agreed that they would exercise more if they talked with an exercise instructor or were advised by their doctor (Ussher et al. 2007).

In order to receive adequate care that addresses medical conditions and gives attention to the co-occurring mental disorder, primary care providers and healthcare systems must be able to recognize and treat or refer for the mental disorder as well. However, when women with mental disorders are seen in medical care settings, their mental health problems often go undetected and untreated. This inadequate treatment also implies that the care for the somatic conditions is jeopardized (Fig. 5.1). Two factors may partially explain this problem: (1) lack of training or skill of medical care providers to detect and treat mental health disorders and (2) stereotyping or stigma associated with mental disorders leading providers to minimize their attention to possible disorders. Both inexperience and stereotyping of women with mental disorders may lead providers to interpret certain behaviors and symptoms commonly associated with mental disorders as "difficult" and these behaviors may impede a satisfactory relationship with an untrained or less skillful clinician.

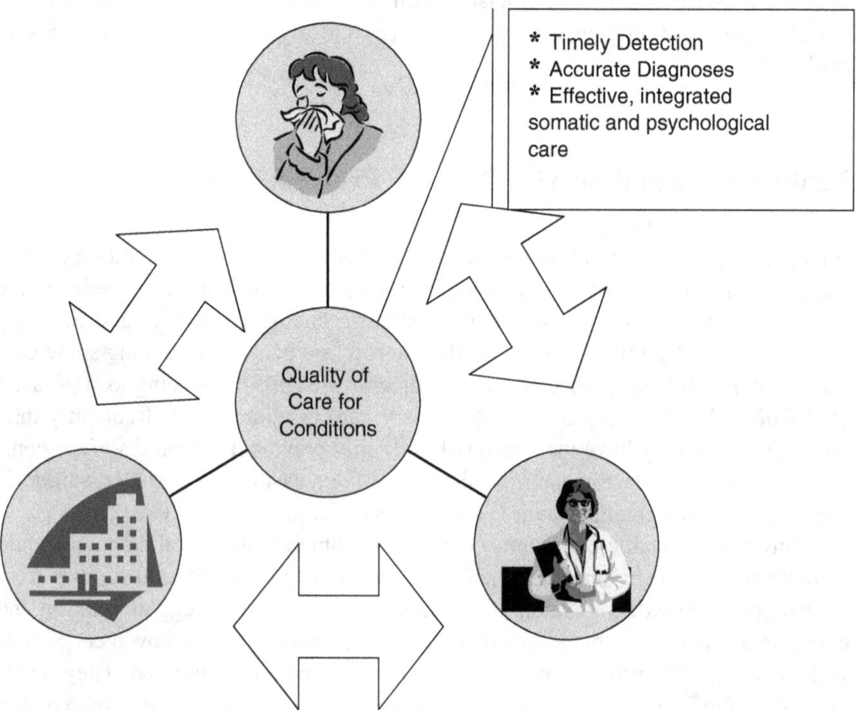

Fig. 5.1 Individual, provider, and system of care factors influence outcomes for women with mental disorders and concurrent acute or chronic somatic conditions

Medical Providers' Lack of Expertise in Mental Health

While mental health conditions are prevalent in the primary care or general practice setting, many providers fail to detect or treat these conditions adequately. Thus, women patients with such disorders may be labeled difficult or challenging rather than seen as in need of additional or a different type of care. For example, most individuals experiencing depression go to primary care providers first, presenting with a somatic complaint (Goldman et al. 1999). Data from the Medical Outcomes study suggest that clinicians fail to recognize half of the depressed patients as such, and only about half of the patients who are recognized to be depressed receive adequate care (Goldman et al. 1999; Institute of Medicine 2001). Data further suggest that even when depression is detected and treated in primary care settings, the key to improved outcomes is the presence of systems to improve follow-up and patient adherence (Katon 2003b).

Somatizing or somatically preoccupied patients make up a substantial portion of patient visits to primary care practitioners. For up to a half of all primary care patients, there are no adequate physical explanations for their symptoms (Institute of Medicine 2006; Kroenke et al. 2000; Righter and Sansone 1999; Ring et al. 2005). Patients with medical symptoms that are difficult to explain are more likely to have anxiety or depressive disorders and more likely to be considered difficult, resulting in inadequate care (Gross et al. 2002). The prevalence of personality disorders is also high among primary care patients labeled as difficult, and estimated to be 20–25% (Gross et al. 2002). In a study of an urban primary care practice, 6.5% of patients were identified as individuals with borderline personality disorders based on structured clinical interviews, but their physicians recognized only half of these individuals as having an emotional or mental health problem (Hackman et al. 2006).

Underutilization of Preventive Gynecologic Care and Contraception

Obstetrician-gynecologists are a dominant source of primary care for women; the majority of women seek their care first and most consistently from the obstetrician-gynecologists. However, obstetrician-gynecologists report limited preparation or confidence in their ability to recognize and treat depression in their patients, and evidence from some studies suggests that the mental health needs of women seeking care in obstetric-gynecologic clinics is substantial (Cassidy et al. 2003). A survey of patients of a gynecologic clinic in a public-sector hospital revealed high rates of major depression (21.5%), anxiety, and a history of sexual trauma (Miranda et al. 1998).

Medical Care Complications of Pregnancy Care

Given the high co-occurrence of mental problems, gynecologic care, contraception, and pregnancy are medical issues that deserve special attention in women with mental disorders. While preventive care is especially critical, the evidence on receipt of pelvic exams and Pap tests among women with severe mental disorders is very limited. While a small study of women with mental disorders drawn from two clinics in one city reported that women with disorders in a mental health clinic were more likely to receive gynecologic exams than were their counterparts in the primary care clinic, women who reported a history of rape or other forms of physical abuse were less likely to receive gynecologic care (Steiner et al. 1998). Women with a diagnosis of schizophrenia were less likely to report receiving a pelvic exam, Pap test, or mammogram in a study of a convenience sample of older women with and without a diagnosis of schizophrenia (Lindamer et al. 2003). Another study suggests that older psychiatric patients are less likely to obtain mammograms than are women without psychiatric illness (Carney and Jones 2006).

There also is evidence that family planning and contraception needs of women with mental disorders remain inadequately addressed. While women with schizophrenia have low rates of fertility, they also experience higher rates of coerced sex and unwanted pregnancies (Miller 1997) and higher STD risk (Coverdale et al. 1997). Rates of contraceptive usage are lower among women with schizophrenia compared to those who do not have a diagnosis of schizophrenia. Women with schizophrenia experience higher risk of preterm delivery, stillbirths, and low birth weight (Miller 1997; Nilsson et al. 2002). These differences are explained, in part, by less prenatal care, poor nutrition, and higher rates of substance use and smoking among women with schizophrenia (Yaeger et al. 2006). In addition, some evidence suggests that psychosis, agitation, and anxiety may have a detrimental impact on the fetus (Nilsson et al. 2002).

Treatment of mental illness during pregnancy also requires careful thought, weighing the risks and benefits of medication use and lack of treatment (Chambers et al. 2007; Ramsay et al. 2001). Decisions about medication use are complicated by the relatively few studies, with small sample sizes, and the lack of randomized controlled trials. A literature review on antipsychotic medication during pregnancy suggests that typical antipsychotic medications can increase perinatal risks, including congenital malformations, signs of neurologic injury, and adverse behavioral outcomes in the child (Howard et al. 2004; Yaeger et al. 2006). There is less evidence of adverse outcomes in studies of atypical antipsychotics during pregnancy; however, the known side effects of atypical antipsychotics (obesity, hypertension, diabetes) are associated with increased risk of poor pregnancy outcomes. Concerns also exist around treatment of mood disorders during pregnancy (Chambers et al. 2007). Recent evidence suggests that serotonin reuptake inhibitors (SSRIs) can increase the risk of congenital heart defects, and there is some limited evidence that SSRIs may be related to neurobehavioral impairment in children. Evidence on the effect on prematurity and birth weight of both SSRIs and untreated depression during pregnancy is equivocal.

Finally, ethical issues surrounding pregnancy and schizophrenia have also been raised in the literature. Since, in some cases, schizophrenia can lead to impaired autonomy or decision-making, Coverdale et al. (2004) propose strategies for handling ethical issues that may arise with pregnancy. They explore concerns about beneficence and patient autonomy in decisions around terminating the pregnancy and the use of antipsychotics. They suggest approaches such as assisted decision making or surrogate decision making.

Other Settings

This underutilization of procedures for women with mental disorders is not limited to conditions specific to women. Women patients in a sample of 200 patients with schizophrenia or mood disorders had higher rates of emergency department use than male patients (44% compared with 28%) and more than the general population (20%). Psychiatric patients had higher use of somatic outpatient services than the comparison national sample (80% compared with 65%), but had comparable rates of somatic hospitalization (13% compared with 9%) (Haas et al. 2005; Hahn et al. 1994, 1996; Jackson et al. 1999).

Another study of Medicaid patients with severe and persistent mental illness found that the patients had access to providers; however, they received unacceptably low levels of preventive care. There were high rates of service use for outpatient services, but very low levels for primary and preventive services. Use of health services for general medical problems differed somewhat by primary diagnosis. Persons with a diagnosis of schizophrenia had lower rates of using office-based services than persons with an anxiety disorder. Also, 69% of persons with schizophrenia had at least one emergency department visit compared to 83% of those with an anxiety disorder. Dental and vision visits and the use of mammograms and pap tests followed the same pattern (Salsberry et al. 2005).

Medical Provider Relationship with Patients with Mental Disorders

A number of studies suggest that in part the medical care of persons with mental disorders is neglected because of stigma related to psychiatric disorders. Existing data suggest that medical providers find 15–30% of their patients to be "difficult," challenging, or troublesome (Groves 1978; Haas et al. 2005; Hahn et al. 1994, 1996; Koekkoek et al. 2006). As noted by Koekkoek et al. (2006), "The so-called difficult patient is always at risk of not being considered a real patient, in need of and deserving care. Illness may be denied or exaggerated, both with detrimental results" (p. 800). Of individuals who had borderline personality disorders based on structured clinical interviews, their physicians recognized only half as having an emotional or mental health problem. When psychiatric symptoms are not recognized, providers tend to label patients with disorders as "difficult," and patients are less likely to receive the care they need (Hall et al. 1996). Patients who are perceived as more emotionally distressed elicit more negative responses from physicians, which can inhibit effective provider–patient communication (Katon 2003b). Thus, untreated or poorly treated mental health conditions among women can compromise the treatment outcomes for medical conditions (Koekkoek et al. 2006). The Institute of Medicine (2006) report highlights that mental health conditions, substance use conditions, and general illnesses are highly interrelated; this interrelatedness is especially close for chronic illness and injury.

Three characteristics of difficult patient “relationships,” all more prevalent among women with mental disorders than their peers, are presented in the literature (Goldman et al. 1999). First, chronicity of the complaint or condition is associated with perceived difficulty. Women patients may appear demanding, clinging, or “unreasonable” when they have chronic complaints, or behavior or symptoms such as paranoia or borderline personality traits. Second, an inexperienced provider may have beliefs or a tendency to blame the patient for her symptoms, may desire to seek cure as opposed to manage chronic problems, or have a belief that certain symptoms are not “real” but rather reflect personal shortcomings (Latour et al. 2007). Finally, there are social norms leading to prejudice, stigma, and labeling that affect most social relationships toward those with mental illness including the patient–provider relationship. Furthermore, rather than build trust with only one provider, women with serious mental disorders and other multiple conditions and illnesses typically must interact effectively with multiple providers and organizations. Patients with multiple comorbidities generally have more providers, which increases care coordination problems, and care is likely to be extremely fragmented (Institute of Medicine 2006).

Thus, given this backdrop, there are persistent problems of underdetection of mental illnesses by the health care providers who treat medical conditions, and misdiagnosis and poor treatment of physical conditions that commonly co-occur with mental conditions. Effective collaboration of mental, substance use, general healthcare, and service providers is one strategy recommended by the Institute of Medicine to improve the quality of care for persons with mental health conditions (Bao et al. 2003; Savoca 1999).

Implications for Women’s Mental Health

The increased rates of medical conditions, disability, and even premature death among women with serious mental disorders underscore the importance of improving our knowledge of health service gaps and understanding each of the factors contributing to these gaps. Women with mental health disorders, when seeking care for physical comorbidities, face a number of difficulties gaining access to needed medical care, have more medically unexplained symptoms than other women, may delay seeking care that they need, and often receive inadequate care (Farley and Patsalides 2001). They rely more heavily on costly emergency departments and less frequently on preventive visits. Thus, women with serious mental disorders are less likely than the general population to receive effective medical procedures and preventive care services. Despite less adequate care, they are more likely than their peers without mental illness to make use of medical services. Ideally, a patient-centered approach would better match medical services to patient medical needs and thus reduce unnecessary medical care.

The complex needs of women with concurrent mental disorders and chronic physical conditions require attention in both behavioral health systems and medical care systems. Providing care to women with a multitude of co-occurring conditions will require additional training and collaboration between specialists and consultation to primary care teams. Reimbursement of primary care providers for care management of these complex cases could increase the incentives for providing good management of physical health burdens confronting this vulnerable group. By addressing chronic care for comorbidity as an urgent public health priority, we might reduce disease burden and disability and improve the overall health of women with serious mental disorders.

There are a range of personal, clinical, institutional, and social factors that are on the pathway between complex symptoms and receipt of appropriate health care. Behavioral service providers should consider the importance of discussing with their patients which aspects of their health hinder participation in ongoing medical and psychological treatment. Group settings for these conditions may facilitate learning from peers and reduce social isolation and stigma. Providers of care for chronic severe pain may redouble their efforts to find sufficient pain solutions as a means to reduce unhealthy reliance on alcohol or other drugs as an analgesic or coping mechanism (Larson et al. 2007). Care teams composed of multiple disciplines are better prepared to address chronic conditions, such as HIV disease or hepatitis that require coordinated medical and behavioral care and careful monitoring of incompatible treatments. The knowledge that the behavioral and medical care needs of women with these multiple morbidities may be complex, overwhelming, and require constant vigilance should be considered in the design of service delivery and in fair reimbursement for comprehensive, integrated services.

There are promising innovations that provide integrated mental health and primary care through on-site or close affiliation with mental health providers; some clinical models use a mental health team in the primary care clinic to rapidly evaluate and stabilize patients and educate the primary care clinical staff (Asarnow et al. 2005; Katon et al. 1997), others offer a chronic disease management intervention that aims at improved functional outcomes as well as decreased disability from mental disorder (Gelber and Dougherty 2005; Neumeyer-Gromen et al. 2004). In these integrated approaches, receipt of mental health services increased, referrals decreased, patients benefit by continuing to be treated by their primary care physicians, and physicians benefit from additional support and training from mental health professionals. In yet another model, primary care may be successfully integrated with psychiatric care in a mental health clinic (Pleis and Lethbridge-Cejku 2007a) which emphasizes preventive measures, patient education, and close collaboration with mental health providers.

There is growing support for the comprehensive, multi-ingredient approach to chronic illness in Wagner's Chronic Care Model (Wagner 1997). An active ingredient of this model that may be particularly salient for women with mental disorders is reliance on self-management support (Institute of Medicine 2006). Self-management support is also essential in a specialized integrated program for behavioral disorders known as Illness Management and Recovery (Mueser et al. 2002, 2003). This program targets individuals with chronic mental disorders, builds on self-management, and aims at recovery—that is, a return to meaningful life activities. When self-management is combined with integrated care teams who aim for recovery, not simply symptom reduction, there is hope that outcomes for both mental and somatic conditions will improve.

References

Albucher, R. C., & Liberzon, I. (2002). Psychopharmacological treatment in PTSD: A critical review. *Journal of Psychiatric Research, 36*(6), 355–367.

American Psychological Association. (1994). Posttraumatic stress disorder. *DSM-IV-TM Diagnostic and statistical manual of mental disorders* (4th ed., Text Revision ed., pp. 424–429). Arlington, VA: American Psychiatric Publishing, Inc.

Anda, R. F., Croft, J. B., Felitti, V. J., Nordenberg, D., Giles, W. H., Williamson, D. F., et al. (1999). Adverse childhood experiences and smoking during adolescence and adulthood. *The Journal of the American Medical Association, 282*(17), 1652–1658.

Anderson, R. J., Freedland, K. E., Clouse, R. E., & Lustman, P. J. (2001). The prevalence of comorbid depression in adults with diabetes: A meta-analysis. *Diabetes Care, 24*(6), 1069–1078.

Anderson, J. E., Wilson, R. W., Barker, P., Doll, L., Jones, T. S., & Holtgrave, D. (1999). Prevalence of sexual and drug-related HIV risk behaviors in the U.S. adult population: Results of the 1996 National Household Survey on Drug Abuse. *Journal of Acquired Immune Deficiency Syndromes, 21*(2), 148–156.

Arnow, B. A. (2004). Relationships between childhood maltreatment, adult health and psychiatric outcomes, and medical utilization. *The Journal of Clinical Psychiatry, 65*(Suppl. 12), 10–15.

Asarnow, J. R., Jaycox, L. H., Duan, N., LaBorde, A. P., Rea, M. M., Murray, P., et al. (2005). Effectiveness of a quality improvement intervention for adolescent depression in primary care clinics: A randomized controlled trial. *The Journal of the American Medical Association, 293*(3), 311–319.

Bair, M. J., Robinson, R. L., Katon, W., & Kroenke, K. (2003). Depression and pain comorbidity: A literature review. *Archives of Internal Medicine, 163*(20), 2433–2445.

Balon, R. (2006). Mood, anxiety, and physical illness: Body and mind, or mind and body? *Depression and Anxiety, 23*(6), 377–387.

Bao, Y., Sturm, R., & Croghan, T. W. (2003). A national study of the effect of chronic pain on the use of health care by depressed persons. *Psychiatric Services, 54*(5), 693–697.

Barr, H. L., Antes, D., Ottenberg, D. J., & Rosen, A. (1984). Mortality of treated alcoholics and drug addicts: The benefits of abstinence. *Journal of Studies on Alcohol, 45*(5), 440–452.

Bassuk, E. L., Dawson, R., Perloff, J., & Weinreb, L. (2001). Post-traumatic stress disorder in extremely poor women: Implications for health care clinicians. *Journal of the American Medical Women's Association, 56*(2), 79–85.

Beitchman, J. H., Zucker, K. J., Hood, J. E., daCosta, G. A., & Akman, D. (1991). A review of the short-term effects of child sexual abuse. *Child Abuse & Neglect, 15*(4), 537–556.

Beitchman, J. H., Zucker, K. J., Hood, J. E., daCosta, G. A., Akman, D., & Cassavia, E. (1992). A review of the long-term effects of child sexual abuse. *Child Abuse & Neglect, 16*(1), 101–118.

Berren, M. R., Santiago, J. M., Zent, M. R., & Carbone, C. P. (1999). Health care utilization by persons with severe and persistent mental illness. *Psychiatric Services, 50*(4), 559–561.

Birkenaes, A. B., Opjordsmoen, S., Brunborg, C., Engh, J. A., Jonsdottir, H., Ringen, P. A., et al. (2007). The level of cardiovascular risk factors in bipolar disorder equals that of schizophrenia: A comparative study. *The Journal of Clinical Psychiatry, 68*(6), 917–923.

Blank, M. B., Mandell, D. S., Aiken, L., & Hadley, T. R. (2002). Co-occurrence of HIV and serious mental illness among medicaid recipients. *Psychiatric Services, 53*(7), 868–873.

Bloss, G. (2005). Measuring the health consequences of alcohol consumption: Current needs and methodological challenges. *Digestive Diseases, 23*(3–4), 162–169.

Bondy, B. (2003). Common genetic risk factors for psychiatric and somatic disorders. In M. Jean-Paul Macher (Ed.), *Dialogues in clinical neuroscience* (Vol. 5, pp. 129–138). Neuilly-sur-Seine, France: Les Laboratoires Servier.

Brennan, P. L., Schutte, K. K., & Moos, R. H. (2005). Pain and use of alcohol to manage pain: Prevalence and 3-year outcomes among older problem and non-problem drinkers. *Addiction, 100*(6), 777–786.

Breslau, N., Davis, G. C., Peterson, E. L., & Schultz, L. (1997). Psychiatric sequelae of posttraumatic stress disorder in women. *Archives of General Psychiatry, 54*(1), 81–87.

Breslau, N., Davis, G. C., & Schultz, L. R. (2003). Posttraumatic stress disorder and the incidence of nicotine, alcohol, and other drug disorders in persons who have experienced trauma. *Archives of General Psychiatry, 60*(3), 289–294.

Brett, K. M., & Burt, C. W. (2001). *Utilization of ambulatory medical care by women: United States, 1997–98*. Atlanta, GA: CDC/Dept. of Health, and Human Services.

Briere, J., Woo, R., McRae, B., Foltz, J., & Sitzman, R. (1997). Lifetime victimization history, demographics and clinical status in female psychiatric emergency room patients. *The Journal of Nervous and Mental Disease, 185*, 95–101.

Brown, S. (1997). Excess mortality of schizophrenia. A meta-analysis. *The British Journal of Psychiatry: The Journal of Mental Science, 171*, 502–508.

Browne, A., & Bassuk, S. S. (1997). Intimate violence in the lives of homeless and poor housed women: Prevalence and patterns in an ethnically diverse sample. *The American Journal of Orthopsychiatry, 67*(2), 261–278.

Browne, A., & Finkelhor, D. (1986). Impact of child sexual abuse: A review of the research. *Psychological Bulletin, 99*(1), 66–77.

Campbell, J., Jones, A. S., Dienemann, J., Kub, J., Schollenberger, J., O'Campo, P., et al. (2002). Intimate partner violence and physical health consequences. *Archives of Internal Medicine, 162*, 1157–1163.

Carney, C. P., & Jones, L. E. (2006). The influence of type and severity of mental illness on receipt of screening mammography. *Journal of General Internal Medicine, 21*(10), 1097–1104.

Cassidy, J. M., Boyle, V. A., & Lawrence, H. L. (2003). Behavioral health care integration in obstetrics and gynecology. *Medscape General Medicine, 5*(2). Accessed December 4, 2009, from http://www.medscape.com/viewarticle/453592

Chambers, C., Moses-Kolko, E., & Wisner, K. L. (2007). Antidepressant use in pregnancy: New concerns, old dilemmas. *Expert Review of Neurotherapeutics, 7*(7), 761–764.

Chilcoat, H. D., & Breslau, N. (1998). Posttraumatic stress disorder and drug disorders: Testing causal pathways. *Archives of General Psychiatry, 55*(10), 913–917.

Clark, H. W., Masson, C. L., Delucchi, K. L., Hall, S. M., & Sees, K. L. (2001). Violent traumatic events and drug abuse severity. *Journal of Substance Abuse Treatment, 20*(2), 121–127.

Clouse, R. E., Lustman, P. J., Freedland, K. E., Griffith, L. S., McGill, J. B., & Carney, R. M. (2003). Depression and coronary heart disease in women with diabetes. *Psychosomatic Medicine, 65*(3), 376–383.

Compton, W. M., Conway, K. P., Stinson, F. S., Colliver, J. D., & Grant, B. F. (2005). Prevalence, correlates, and comorbidity of DSM-IV antisocial personality syndromes and alcohol and specific drug use disorders in the United States: Results from the national epidemiologic survey on alcohol and related conditions. *The Journal of Clinical Psychiatry, 66*(6), 677–685.

Coverdale, J. H., McCullough, L. B., & Chervenak, F. A. (2004). Assisted and surrogate decision making for pregnant patients who have schizophrenia. *Schizophrenia Bulletin, 30*(3), 659–664.

Coverdale, J. H., Turbott, S. H., & Roberts, H. (1997). Family planning needs and STD risk behaviours of female psychiatric out-patients. *The British Journal of Psychiatry: The Journal of Mental Science, 171*, 69–72.

Coyle, C. P., & Santiago, M. C. (2002). Healthcare utilization among women with physical disabilities. *Medscape Womens Health, 7*(4), 2.

De Alba, I., Samet, J. H., & Saitz, R. (2004). Burden of medical illness in drug- and alcohol-dependent persons without primary care. *The American Journal on Addictions, 13*(1), 33–45.

Dey, A. N., & Lucas, J. W. (2006). Physical and mental health characteristics of U.S.- and foreign-born adults: United States, 1998–2003. *Advance Data, 369,* 1–19.

Dickerson, F. B., Brown, C. H., Daumit, G. L., Fang, L., Goldberg, R. W., Wohlheiter, K., et al. (2006). Health status of individuals with serious mental illness. *Schizophrenia Bulletin, 32,* 584–589.

Egede, L. E. (2004). Diabetes, major depression, and functional disability among U.S. adults. *Diabetes Care, 27*(2), 421–428.

El-Bassel, N., Gilbert, L., Witte, S., Wu, E., Gaeta, T., Schilling, R., et al. (2003). Intimate partner violence and substance abuse among minority women receiving care from an inner-city emergency department. *Womens Health Issues, 13*(1), 16–22.

Falik, M., Needleman, J., Wells, B. L., & Korb, J. (2001). Ambulatory care sensitive hospitalizations and emergency visits: Experiences of Medicaid patients using federally qualified health centers. *Medical Care, 39*(6), 551–561.

Farley, M., & Patsalides, B. M. (2001). Physical symptoms, posttraumatic stress disorder, and healthcare utilization of women with and without childhood physical and sexual abuse. *Psychological Reports, 89*(3), 595–606.

Felitti, V. J. (1991). Long-term medical consequences of incest, rape, and molestation. *The Southern Medical Journal, 84*(3), 328–331.

Felitti, V. J., Anda, R. F., Nordenberg, D., Williamson, D. F., Spitz, A. M., Edwards, V., et al. (1998). Relationship of childhood abuse and household dysfunction to many of the leading causes of death in adults. The Adverse Childhood Experiences (ACE) Study. *American Journal of Preventive Medicine, 14*(4), 245–258.

Fullilove, M., Fullilove, R., Smith, M., Winkler, K., Michael, C., Panzer, P., et al. (1993). Violence, trauma and post-traumatic stress disorder among women drug users. *Journal of Traumatic Stress, 6*(4), 533–543.

Garis, R. I., & Farmer, K. C. (2002). Examining costs of chronic conditions in a Medicaid population. *Managed Care, 11*(8), 43–50.

Gelber, S., & Dougherty, R. H. (2005). *Disease management for chronic behavioral health and substance use disorders* (Resource Paper). Princeton, NJ: Center for Health Care Strategies, Inc. (CHCS).

Gil-Rivas, V., Fiorentine, R., & Anglin, M. D. (1996). Sexual abuse, physical abuse, and posttraumatic stress disorder among women participating in outpatient drug abuse treatment. *Journal of Psychoactive Drugs, 28*(1), 95–102.

Goldman, L. S., Nielsen, N. H., & Champion, H. C. (1999). Awareness, diagnosis, and treatment of depression. *Journal of General Internal Medicine, 14*(9), 569–580.

Goodwin, R. D., Hoven, C. W., Murison, R., & Hotopf, M. (2003a). Association between childhood physical abuse and gastrointestinal disorders and migraine in adulthood. *American Journal of Public Health, 93*(7), 1065–1067.

Goodwin, R. D., Jacobi, F., & Thefeld, W. (2003b). Mental disorders and asthma in the community. *Archives of General Psychiatry, 60*(11), 1125–1130.

Gross, R., Olfson, M., Gameroff, M., Shea, S., Feder, A., Fuentes, M., et al. (2002). Borderline personality disorder in primary care. *Archives of Internal Medicine, 162*(1), 53–60.

Groves, J. E. (1978). Taking care of the hateful patient. *New England Journal of Medicine, 298*(16), 883–887.

Haas, L. J., Leiser, J. P., Magill, M. K., & Sanyer, O. N. (2005). Management of the difficult patient. *American Family Physician, 72*(10), 2063–2068.

Hackman, A. L., Goldberg, R. W., Brown, C. H., Fang, L. J., Dickerson, F. B., Wohlheiter, K., et al. (2006). Use of emergency department services for somatic reasons by people with serious mental illness. *Psychiatric Services, 57*(4), 563–566.

Hahn, S. R., Kroenke, K., Spitzer, R. L., Brody, D., Williams, J. B., Linzer, M., et al. (1996). The difficult patient: Prevalence, psychopathology, and functional impairment. *Journal of General Internal Medicine, 11*(1), 1–8.

Hahn, S. R., Thompson, K. S., Wills, T. A., Stern, V., & Budner, N. S. (1994). The difficult doctor-patient relationship: Somatization, personality and psychopathology. *Journal of Clinical Epidemiology, 47*(6), 647–657.

Hall, J. A., Roter, D. L., Milburn, M. A., & Daltroy, L. H. (1996). Patients' health as a predictor of physician and patient behavior in medical visits. A synthesis of four studies. *Medical Care, 34*(12), 1205–1218.

Hansen, M. S., Fink, P., Frydenberg, M., & Oxhoj, M. L. (2002). Use of health services, mental illness, and self-rated disability and health in medical inpatients. *Psychosomatic Medicine, 64*(4), 668–675.

Harris, M., & Fallot, R. D. (2001). Envisioning a trauma-informed service system: A vital paradigm shift. *New Directions for Mental Health Services, 89,* 3–22.

Harter, M., Baumeister, H., Reuter, K., Jacobi, F., Hofler, M., Bengel, J., et al. (2007). Increased 12-month prevalence rates of mental disorders in patients with chronic somatic diseases. *Psychotherapy and Psychosomatics, 76*(6), 354–360.

Hippisley-Cox, J., Vinogradova, Y., Coupland, C., & Parker, C. (2007). Risk of malignancy in patients with schizophrenia or bipolar disorder: Nested case-control study. *Archives of General Psychiatry, 64*(12), 1368–1376.

Hotopf, M., Mayou, R., Wadsworth, M., & Wessely, S. (1998). Temporal relationships between physical symptoms and psychiatric disorder. Results from a national birth cohort. *The British Journal of Psychiatry: The Journal of Mental Science, 173,* 255–261.

Howard, L., Webb, R., & Abel, K. (2004). Safety of antipsychotic drugs for pregnant and breast-feeding women with non-affective psychosis. *British Medical Journal, 329*(7472), 933–934.

Hulse, G. K., English, D. R., Milne, E., & Holman, C. D. (1999). The quantification of mortality resulting from the regular use of illicit opiates. *Addiction, 94*(2), 221–229.

Institute of Medicine. (2001). *Crossing the quality chasm: A new health system for the 21st century*. Washington, DC: The National Academies Press.

Institute of Medicine. (2006). *Improving the quality of health care for mental and substance-use conditions*. Washington, DC: The National Academies Press.

Jackson, J. S., Williams, D. R., & Torres, M. (1999). Perceptions of discrimination, health and mental health: The social stress process: Chapter 8. *Socioeconomic conditions, stress and mental disorders: Toward a new synthesis of research and public policy* (http://www.mhsip.org/nimhdoc/socioeconmh_home2.htm ed.). Institute for Social Research, University of Michigan: Office of the Deputy Administrator of the Substance Abuse and Mental Health Services Administration, NIH Office of Behavioral and Social Science Research, NIH Prevention Office, NIH Fogarty International Center, Mental Health Statistical Improvement Office of the SAMHSA Center on Mental Health Services.

Jakovljevic, M., Crncevic, Z., Ljubicic, D., Babic, D., Topic, R., & Saric, M. (2007). Mental disorders and metabolic syndrome: A fatamorgana or warning reality? *Psychiatria Danubina, 19*(1–2), 76–86.

Johnson, J. G., Spitzer, R. L., Williams, J. B., Kroenke, K., Linzer, M., Brody, D., et al. (1995). Psychiatric comorbidity, health status, and functional impairment associated with alcohol abuse and dependence in primary care patients: Findings of the PRIME MD-1000 study. *Journal of Consulting and Clinical Psychology, 63*(1), 133–140.

Jones, D. R., Macias, C., Barreira, P. J., Fisher, W. H., Hargreaves, W. A., & Harding, C. M. (2004). Prevalence, severity, and co-occurrence of chronic physical health problems of persons with serious mental illness. *Psychiatric Services, 55*(11), 1250–1257.

Kamara, S. G., Peterson, P. D., & Dennis, J. L. (1998). Prevalence of physical illness among psychiatric inpatients who die of natural causes. *Psychiatric Services, 49*(6), 788–793.

Kaplan, M. J., & Klinetob, N. A. (2000). (AB) Childhood emotional trauma and chronic posttraumatic stress disorder in adult outpatients with treatment-resistant depression. *Journal of Nervous Mental Disorders, 188*(9), 596–601.

Katon, W. J. (2003a). Clinical and health services relationships between major depression, depressive symptoms, and general medical illness. *Biological Psychiatry, 54*(3), 216–226.

Katon, W. J. (2003b). Clinical and health services relationships between major depression, depressive symptoms, and general medical illness. *Biological Psychiatry, 54*(3), 216–226.

Katon, W., Von Korff, M., Lin, E., Simon, G., Walker, E., Bush, T., et al. (1997). Collaborative management to achieve depression treatment guidelines. *The Journal of Clinical Psychiatry, 58*(Suppl. 1), 20–23.

Kertesz, S. G., Larson, M. J., Cheng, D. M., Tucker, J. A., Winter, M., Mullins, A., et al. (2006). Need and non-need factors associated with addiction treatment utilization within cohort of homeless and housed. *Medical Care, 44*(3), 225–233.

Kessler, R. C., Berglund, P. A., Bruce, M. L., Koch, J. R., Laska, E. M., Leaf, P. J., et al. (2001). The prevalence and correlates of untreated serious mental illness. *Health Services Research, 36*(6 Pt 1), 987–1007.

Kessler, R. C., Berglund, P., Demler, O., Jin, R., Koretz, D., Merikangas, K. R., et al. (2003). The epidemiology of major depressive disorder: Results from the National Comorbidity Survey Replication (NCS-R). *The Journal of the American Medical Association, 289*(23), 3095–3105.

Kessler, R. C., Chiu, W. T., Demler, O., Merikangas, K. R., & Walters, E. E. (2005). Prevalence, severity, and comorbidity of 12-month DSM-IV disorders in the National Comorbidity Survey Replication. *Archives of General Psychiatry, 62*(6), 617–627.

Kessler, R. C., McGonagle, K. A., Zhao, S., Nelson, C. B., Hughes, M., Eshleman, S., et al. (1994). Lifetime and 12-month prevalence of DSM-III-R psychiatric disorders in the United States. Results from the National Comorbidity Survey. *Archives of General Psychiatry, 51*(1), 8–19.

Kessler, R. C., Sonnega, A., Bromet, E., Hughes, M., & Nelson, C. B. (1995). Posttraumatic stress disorder in the National Comorbidity Survey. *Archives of General Psychiatry, 52*(12), 1048–1060.

Koekkoek, B., van Meijel, B., & Hutschemaekers, G. (2006). "Difficult Patients" in mental health care: A review. *Psychiatric Services, 57*(6), 795–802.

Kovac, S. H., Klapow, J. C., Kroenke, K., Spitzer, R. L., & Williams, J. B. (2003). Differing symptoms of abused versus nonabused women in obstetric-gynecology settings. *American Journal of Obstetrics and Gynecology, 188*(3), 707–713.

Kroenke, K., Taylor-Vaisey, A., Dietrich, A. J., & Oxman, T. E. (2000). Interventions to improve provider diagnosis and treatment of mental disorders in primary care: A critical review of the literature. *Psychosomatics, 41*(1), 39–52.

Lange, R. A., & Hillis, L. D. (2001). Cardiovascular complications of cocaine use. *New England Journal of Medicine, 345*(5), 351–358.

Larson, M. J., Paasche-Orlow, M., Cheng, D. M., Lloyd-Travaglini, C., Saitz, R., & Samet, J. H. (2007). Persistent pain is associated with substance use after detoxification: A prospective cohort analysis. *Addiction, 102*(5), 752–760.

Larson, M. J., Saitz, R., Horton, N. J., Lloyd-Travaglini, C., & Samet, J. H. (2006). Emergency department and hospital utilization among alcohol and drug-dependent detoxification patients without primary medical care. *The American Journal of Drug and Alcohol Abuse, 32*(3), 435–452.

Latour, C. H., Huyse, F. J., de Vos, R., & Stalman, W. A. (2007). A method to provide integrated care for complex medically ill patients: The INTERMED. *Nursing & Health Sciences, 9*(2), 150–157.

Leonard, S., Adler, L. E., Benhammou, K., Berger, R., Breese, C. R., Drebing, C., et al. (2001). Smoking and mental illness. *Pharmacology, Biochemistry, and Behavior, 70*(4), 561–570.

Liebschutz, J. M., Mulvey, K. P., & Samet, J. H. (1997). Victimization among substance-abusing women. Worse health outcomes. *Archives of Internal Medicine, 157*(10), 1093–1097.

Lindamer, L. A., Buse, D. C., Auslander, L., Unutzer, J., Bartels, S. J., & Jeste, D. V. (2003). A comparison of gynecological variables and service use among older women with and without schizophrenia. *Psychiatric Services, 54*(6), 902–904.

Lucas, J. W., Barr-Anderson, D. J., & Kington, R. S. (2005). Health status of non-Hispanic U.S.-born and foreign-born black and white persons: United States, 1992–95. *Vital and Health Statistics, 10*(226), 1–20.

MacMillan, H. L., Fleming, J. E., Streiner, D. L., Lin, E., Boyle, M. H., Jamieson, E., et al. (2001). (AB) Childhood abuse and lifetime psychopathology in a community sample. *American Journal of Psychiatry, 158*(11), 1878–1883.

Magni, G., Caldieron, C., Rigatti-Luchini, S., & Merskey, H. (1990). Chronic musculoskeletal pain and depressive symptoms in the general population. An analysis of the 1st National Health and Nutrition Examination Survey data. *Pain, 43*(3), 299–307.

Magni, G., Rossi, M. R., Rigatti-Luchini, S., & Merskey, H. (1992). Chronic abdominal pain and depression. Epidemiologic findings in the United States. Hispanic Health and Nutrition Examination Survey. *Pain, 49*(1), 77–85.

McBeth, J., Macfarlane, G. J., & Silman, A. J. (2002). Does chronic pain predict future psychological distress? *Pain, 96*(3), 239–245.

McCauley, J., Kern, D. E., Kolodner, K., Dill, L., Schroeder, A. F., DeChant, H. K., et al. (1997). Clinical characteristics of women with a history of childhood abuse: Unhealed wounds. *The Journal of the American Medical Association, 277*(17), 1362–1368.

McDermott, S., Moran, R., Platt, T., Isaac, T., Wood, H., & Dasari, S. (2005). Heart disease, schizophrenia, and affective psychoses: Epidemiology of risk in primary care. *Community Mental Health Journal, 41*(6), 747–755.

McIntyre, R. S., Konarski, J. Z., Wilkins, K., Soczynska, J. K., & Kennedy, S. H. (2006). Obesity in bipolar disorder and major depressive disorder: Results from a national community health survey on mental health and well-being. *Canadian Journal of Psychiatry, 51*(5), 274–280.

McWilliams, L. A., Cox, B. J., & Enns, M. W. (2003). Mood and anxiety disorders associated with chronic pain: An examination in a nationally representative sample. *Pain, 106*(1–2), 127–133.

Miller, L. J. (1997). Sexuality, reproduction, and family planning in women with schizophrenia. *Schizophrenia Bulletin, 23*(4), 623–635.

Miller, B. A., Downs, W. R., & Testa, M. (1993). Interrelationships between victimization experiences and women's alcohol use. *Journal of Studies on Alcohol, 11*(Suppl.), 109–117.

Miranda, J., Azocar, F., Komaromy, M., & Golding, J. M. (1998). Unmet mental health needs of women in public-sector gynecologic clinics. *American Journal of Obstetrics and Gynecology, 178*(2), 212–217.

Moussavi, S., Chatterji, S., Verdes, E., Tandon, A., Patel, V., & Ustun, B. (2007). Depression, chronic diseases, and decrements in health: Results from the World Health Surveys. *Lancet, 370*(9590), 851–858.

Mueser, K. T., Corrigan, P. W., Hilton, D. W., Tanzman, B., Schaub, A., Gingerich, S., et al. (2002). Illness management and recovery: A review of the research. *Psychiatric Services, 53*(10), 1272–1284.

Mueser, K. T., Torrey, W. C., Lynde, D., Singer, P., & Drake, R. E. (2003). Implementing evidence-based practices for people with severe mental illness. *Behavior Modification, 27*(3), 387–411.

Najavits, L. M., Weiss, R. D., & Shaw, S. R. (1997). The link between substance abuse and post-traumatic stress disorder in women. A research review. *The American Journal on Addictions, 6*(4), 273–283.

Nasrallah, H. A. (2003). Factors in antipsychotic drug selection: Tolerability considerations. *CNS Spectrums, 8*(11 Suppl. 2), 23–25.

Ndao-Brumblay, S. K., & Green, C. R. (2005). Racial differences in the physical and psychosocial health among black and white women with chronic pain. *Journal of the National Medical Association, 97*(10), 1369–1377.

Neiman, J., Haapaniemi, H. M., & Hillbom, M. (2000). Neurological complications of drug abuse: Pathophysiological mechanisms. *European Journal of Neurology, 7*(6), 595–606.

Neumeyer-Gromen, A., Lampert, T., Stark, K., & Kallischnigg, G. (2004). Disease management programs for depression: A systematic review and meta-analysis of randomized controlled trials. *Medical Care, 42*(12), 1211–1221.

Newcomer, J. W. (2005). Second-generation (atypical) antipsychotics and metabolic effects: A comprehensive literature review. *CNS Drugs, 19*(Suppl. 1), 1–93.

Newcomer, J. W. (2006). Medical risk in patients with bipolar disorder and schizophrenia. *The Journal of Clinical Psychiatry, 67*(11), e16.

Nilsson, E., Lichtenstein, P., Cnattingius, S., Murray, R. M., & Hultman, C. M. (2002). Women with schizophrenia: Pregnancy outcome and infant death among their offspring. *Schizophrenia Research, 58*(2–3), 221–229.

Ormel, J., Von Korff, M., Burger, H., Scott, K., Demyttenaere, K., Huang, Y. Q., et al. (2007). Mental disorders among persons with heart disease – results from World Mental Health surveys. *General Hospital Psychiatry, 29*(4), 325–334.

Oster, A., & Bindman, A. B. (2003). Emergency department visits for ambulatory care sensitive conditions: Insights into preventable hospitalizations. *Medical Care, 41*(2), 198–207.

Palmer, B. A., Pankratz, V. S., & Bostwick, J. M. (2005). The lifetime risk of suicide in schizophrenia: A reexamination. *Archives of General Psychiatry, 62*(3), 247–253.

Pleis, J. R., & Lethbridge-Cejku, M. (2007a). Summary health statistics for U.S. adults: National Health Interview Survey, 2006. *Vital & Health Statistics, 10*(235), 1–153.

Pleis, J. R., & Lethbridge-Cejku, M. (2007b). *Summary health statistics for U.S. adults: National Health Interview Survey, 2006.* Hyattsville, MD: National Center for Health Statistics. *Vital Health Statistics, 10*(235).

Prior, P., Hassall, C., & Cross, K. W. (1996). Causes of death associated with psychiatric illness. *Journal of Public Health Medicine, 18*(4), 381–389.

Ramsay, R., Welch, S., & Youard, E. (2001). Needs of women patients with mental illness. *Advances in Psychiatric Treatment, 7,* 85–92.

Regier, D. A., Farmer, M. E., Rae, D. S., Locke, B. Z., Keith, S. J., Judd, L. L., et al. (1990). Comorbidity of mental disorders with alcohol and other drug abuse. Results from the Epidemiologic Catchment Area (ECA) Study. *The Journal of the American Medical Association, 264*(19), 2511–2518.

Rehm, J., Patra, J., & Popova, S. (2006). Alcohol-attributable mortality and potential years of life lost in Canada 2001: Implications for prevention and policy. *Addiction, 101*(3), 373–384.

Righter, E. L., & Sansone, R. A. (1999). Managing somatic preoccupation. *American Family Physician, 59*(11), 3113–3120.

Ring, A., Dowrick, C. F., Humphris, G. M., Davies, J., & Salmon, P. (2005). The somatising effect of clinical consultation: What patients and doctors say and do not say when patients present medically unexplained physical symptoms. *Social Science & Medicine, 61*(7), 1505–1515.

Romans, S., Belaise, C., Martin, J., Morris, E., & Raffi, A. (2002). Childhood abuse and later medical disorders in women. An epidemiological study. *Psychotherapy & Psychosomatics, 71*(3), 141–150.

Rubin, R. R., Ma, Y., Marrero, D. G., Peyrot, M., Barrett-Connor, E. L., Kahn, S. E., et al. (2008). Elevated depression symptoms, antidepressant medicine use, and risk of developing diabetes during the diabetes prevention program. *Diabetes Care, 31*(3), 420–426.

Saha, S., Chant, D., & McGrath, J. (2007). A systematic review of mortality in schizophrenia: Is the differential mortality gap worsening over time? *Archives of General Psychiatry, 64*(10), 1123–1131.

Saitz, R., Gaeta, J., Cheng, D. M., Richardson, J. M., Larson, M. J., & Samet, J. H. (2007). Risk of mortality during four years after substance detoxification in urban adults. *Journal of Urban Health, 84*(2), 272–282.

Salsberry, P. J., Chipps, E., & Kennedy, C. (2005). Use of general medical services among medicaid patients with severe and persistent mental illness. *Psychiatric Services, 56*(4), 458–462.

Sareen, J., Cox, B. J., Stein, M. B., Afifi, T. O., Fleet, C., & Asmundson, G. J. (2007). Physical and mental comorbidity, disability, and suicidal behavior associated with posttraumatic stress disorder in a large community sample. *Psychosomatic Medicine, 69*(3), 242–248. Epub 2007 March 2030.

Savoca, E. (1999). Psychiatric co-morbidity and hospital utilization in the general medical sector. *Psychological Medicine, 29,* 457–464.

Seng, J. S., Graham-Bermann, S. A., Clark, M. K., McCarthy, A. M., & Ronis, D. L. (2005). Posttraumatic stress disorder and physical comorbidity among female children and adolescents: Results from service-use data. *Pediatrics, 116*(6), e767–e776.

Simon, G. E., Von Korff, M., Saunders, K., Miglioretti, D. L., Crane, P. K., van Belle, G., et al. (2006). Association between obesity and psychiatric disorders in the U.S. adult population. *Archives of General Psychiatry, 63*(7), 824–830.

Smedley, B. D., Stith, A. Y., & Nelson, A. R. (2003). In A. Y. S. Brian, D. Smedley, & Alan R. Nelson (Eds.), *Unequal treatment: Confronting racial and ethnic disparities in health care.* Washington, DC: National Academy of Sciences.

Smith, B. H., Elliott, A. M., Chambers, W. A., Smith, W. C., Hannaford, P. C., & Penny, K. (2001). The impact of chronic pain in the community. *Family Practice, 18*(3), 292–299.

Sokal, J., Messias, E., Dickerson, F. B., Kreyenbuhl, J., Brown, C. H., Goldberg, R. W., et al. (2004). Comorbidity of medical illnesses among adults with serious mental illness who are receiving community psychiatric services. *The Journal of Nervous and Mental Disease, 192*(6), 421–427.

Steiner, J. L., Hoff, R. A., Moffett, C., Reynolds, H., Mitchell, M., & Rosenheck, R. (1998). Preventive health care for mentally ill women. *Psychiatric Services, 49*(5), 696–698.

Taylor, V., & MacQueen, G. (2006). Associations between bipolar disorder and metabolic syndrome: A review. *The Journal of Clinical Psychiatry, 67*(7), 1034–1041.

Teplin, L. A., McClelland, G. M., Abram, K. M., & Weiner, D. A. (2005). Crime victimization in adults with severe mental illness: Comparison with the National Crime Victimization Survey. *Archives of General Psychiatry, 62*(8), 911–921.

Ussher, M., Stanbury, L., Cheeseman, V., & Faulkner, G. (2007). Physical activity preferences and perceived barriers to activity among persons with severe mental illness in the United Kingdom. *Psychiatric Services, 58*(3), 405–408.

van der Kolk, B. A., Pelcovitz, D., Roth, S., Mandel, F. S., McFarlane, A., & Herman, J. L. (1996). Dissociation, somatization, and affect dysregulation: The complexity of adaptation of trauma. *The American Journal of Psychiatry, 153*(Suppl. 7), 83–93.

Violence against women: Relevance for medical practitioners. (1992). *The Journal of the American Medical Association, 267*(23), 3184–3189.

Von Korff, M., Crane, P., Lane, M., Miglioretti, D. L., Simon, G., Saunders, K., et al. (2005). Chronic spinal pain and physical-mental comorbidity in the United States: Results from the national comorbidity survey replication. *Pain, 113*(3), 331–339.

Wagner, E. (1997). Managed care and chronic illness: Health services research needs. *Health Services Research, 32*(5), 702–714.

Walker, E. A., Katon, W. J., Hansom, J., Harrop-Griffiths, J., Holm, L., Jones, M. L., et al. (1992). Medical and psychiatric symptoms in women with childhood sexual abuse. *Psychosomatic Medicine, 54*(6), 658–664.

Wolff, N., Blitz, C. L., & Shi, J. (2007). Rates of sexual victimization in prison for inmates with and without mental disorders. *Psychiatric Services, 58*(8), 1087–1094.

Yaeger, D., Smith, H. G., & Altshuler, L. L. (2006). Atypical antipsychotics in the treatment of schizophrenia during pregnancy and the postpartum. *The American Journal of Psychiatry, 163*(12), 2064–2070.

Yandow, V. (1989). Alcoholism in women. *Psychiatric Annals, 19,* 243–247.

Zavala, S. K., & French, M. T. (2003). Dangerous to your health: The role of chronic drug use in serious injuries and trauma. *Medical Care, 41*(2), 309–322.

Zierler, S., Feingold, L., Laufer, D., Velentgas, P., Kantrowitz-Gordon, I., & Mayer, K. (1991). Adult survivors of childhood sexual abuse and subsequent risk of HIV infection. *American Journal of Public Health, 81*(5), 572–575.

Part II
Selected Disorders

Chapter 6
Depression and Postpartum Disorders

Heather A. Flynn

Depression in Women

In the first part of this chapter, an overview of prevalence and burden of depression in women across the lifespan will be presented, as well as biopsychosocial etiological theories and a brief review of service use and treatment issues. The second part of the chapter will focus specifically on prevalence, clinical, and health care use issues related to depression occurring around the time of childbearing. Pregnant and postpartum women with depression represent an underserved group that, because of the healthcare service use issues, holds promise for improved detection, prevention, and treatment efforts that may improve health and functioning outcomes for women and their families.

Prevalence and Etiology

Depression is both a common and a debilitating disorder, demonstrated by the World Health Organization to have the largest effect on worsening health worldwide compared with the other chronic medical conditions (Moussavi et al. 2007). Epidemiological studies have consistently shown that the prevalence of unipolar major depression in women worldwide is nearly twice that of men (15–25%; Kessler et al. 1998; Weissman et al. 1996). One in five women will experience a major depressive disorder (MDD) at some point in her lifetime, and over a 12-month period, an estimated 6% of women will experience a major depressive episode (Kessler et al. 1998). Interpersonal discord, marital conflict, and poor parent–child relationships have been consistently linked to problems associated with depression in women (Bradbury et al. 1996; Rudolph et al. 2000; Zuckerman et al. 1990). Until puberty,

H. A. Flynn (✉)
Department of Psychiatry, University of Michigan Medical School,
4250 Plymouth Road, Ann Arbor, MI 48109-5766, USA

B. L. Levin, M. A. Becker (eds.), *A Public Health Perspective of Women's Mental Health*,
DOI 10.1007/978-1-4419-1526-9_6, © Springer Science+Business Media LLC 2010

boys and girls experience similar prevalence rates of depression, at which time rates begin to increase in girls.

Developmental etiological theories regarding the emergence of gender differences in depression have received some empirical support and may provide a guide for prevention and intervention opportunities. Because these multifactorial theories have been well-outlined elsewhere (Nolen-Hoeksema and Girgus 1994; Nolen-Hoeksema 1995), they are briefly presented here in terms of health services implications. Biological differences in sex hormones between men and women have been implicated based on evidence of vulnerability to increased depressive symptoms associated temporally with changes in gonadal hormones during the premenstrual, perinatal, and perimenopausal periods. Research studies have found evidence for links between shifts in the hypothylamic-pituitary-adrenal (HPA) axis, ovarian axis functioning (estrogen and progesterin), and testosterone to changes in depression. More recent studies have supported the likelihood of an interaction of biological with social and psychological factors in the development of depression in women. Genetic vulnerabilities, particularly involving serotonin transporter genes, have been found to interact with childhood stress and maltreatment in the development of depression in large cohort prospective studies (Caspi et al. 2003; Kendler et al. 2005). Women experience greater stress over the lifespan, including greater exposure to sexual trauma, multiple social roles, earlier socialization demands based on the development of secondary sex characteristics, discrimination, and poverty (see Le et al. (2003) for a review). Oxytocin, linked in human and animal models to affiliation and caretaking needs, may predispose women to increased vulnerability to interpersonal strife. Psychological theories have implicated both interpersonal and cognitive styles, such as rumination, that are more common in women and have been found to increase depressive symptoms, and to be associated with longer and more severe episodes of depression (Nolen-Hoeksema et al. 1999).

Taken together, the evidence for the importance of the timing of hormonal changes, heightened exposure to stress and trauma, and the interplay of psychological vulnerabilities for the development of depression in women has implications for intervention. Prevention and intervention efforts should be aimed at key developmental periods (such as puberty and the periconceptual and perimenopausal periods) and implemented in settings and agencies where girls and young women encountering stress and trauma may present (such as shelters and crisis centers), as well as in health care settings where women present for physical health issues and around hormonal and life transitions.

Phenomenology of Depression in Women

Although there is some debate regarding differential lifecourse severity of depression in women as compared to men, a study by Kornstein and colleagues of 235 male and 400 female outpatients with chronic MDD found that women showed an earlier age of onset, greater family history of affective disorders, and greater severity based on poorer social adjustment and quality of life as compared to men (Kornstein et al. 2000). Depression in women as compared to men may also have differential somatic and comorbid characteristics. For example, women have been found to experience higher rates of somatic symptoms such as sleep, fatigue, and appetite disturbances (Silverstein 1994). Women with chronic pain have also been found to be more likely to experience depression (Haley et al. 1985). Women with depression are also more likely to suffer from comorbid anxiety and eating disorders. The National Co-morbidity Study found relatively high rates of posttraumatic stress disorder (PTSD) comorbid with depression (Kessler et al. 1995) and also found that pretrauma exposure to an affective disorder was associated with increased rates of PTSD in women (Bromet et al. 1998).

Treatment and Health Service Issues

Gender differences in the phenomenology of depression have not been adequately incorporated into clinical interventions. Generally, efficacious treatments for unipolar depression include antidepressant medications, depression-specific psychotherapies such as cognitive-behavioral therapy (CBT) and interpersonal psychotherapy (IPT), light therapy, exercise, and other biological treatments such as electroconvulsive therapy (ECT). Meta-analyses of clinical trials for the treatment of unipolar depression generally show comparable acute phase symptom response and remission rates for both men and women, particularly for medication and psychotherapy, with overall symptom response rates ranging from 45 to 65% (Hollon et al. 2002). However, emerging research suggests that premenopausal women may show a more favorable response to the selective serotonin reuptake inhibitors (SSRIs) and men to the tricyclic antidepressants. Possible mechanisms of differential response have been linked to sex differences in endogenous central nervous system (CNS) serotonin levels (Nishizawa et al. 1997).

Despite the effectiveness of antidepressant medications for the treatment of depression, many studies have shown that women, particularly minorities, prefer counseling or psychotherapy to medications (Givens et al. 2007). Both IPT and CBT have been found to be effective psychological treatments for depression in women (Frank et al. 2000). IPT typically involves 12–16 sessions and maintains a focus on 1–2 key interpersonal issues that are determined, based on a clinical assessment, to be most closely related to the depression (i.e. interpersonal role disputes/conflicts, interpersonal role transitions, complicated grief, interpersonal deficits/sensitivity). IPT was developed to address the fact that, regardless of etiology, depression commonly occurs in an interpersonal context and is reciprocally affected by interpersonal issues (Weissman et al. 2000).

CBT, also a short-term, structured psychotherapy for depression, has been shown to be efficacious in treating depression across age-ranges and genders in numerous national randomized controlled trials (Butler et al. 2005). Growing evidence suggests that CBT is more effective than antidepressant medication in reducing depression relapse (Hollon et al. 2005; Paykel et al. 2005).

Despite preferences for psychotherapy in general, most women with depression do not present for care in specialty mental health settings. Unfortunately, evidence-based psychotherapies for depression are not commonly available outside of specialty mental health settings. The majority of women receive mental health treatment in general medical settings, such as obstetrics/gynecology (Ob/Gyn) clinics (Scholle et al. 2003), where medication treatments are more readily available than psychological treatments. Following delivery of a child, a time when health care coverage (i.e. Medicaid) may end, women may be less likely to use outpatient healthcare services at all for themselves (Kahn et al. 1999). Therefore, some research and clinical programs have explored depression detection and treatment strategies within the context of pediatric outpatient and emergency care settings (Flynn et al. 2004). Health care regulatory bodies such as the American College of Obstetrics and Gynecology and the American Pediatric Association have both recommended physician screening for depression and associated behavioral health issues in women presenting for care in Ob/Gyn and Pediatric settings, respectively.

According to depression research in primary care settings, depression detection, coupled with delivery of acute phase evidence based treatment and clinical monitoring, has been found to effectively treat depression in the acute phase (Wells et al. 2002a). However, little research has focused on prevention and treatment delivery specifically in Ob/Gyn settings where most women present for care. The sections that follow will provide an overview of depression occurring around the time of pregnancy, as well as the health care service use and policy implications that may provide a model for future directions in reducing the burden of unipolar depression in women.

Perinatal Depression

Depression occurring around the time of childbearing, referred to as perinatal depression, represents a prime opportunity for prevention and treatment for a number of reasons. First, childbearing age is a period of high prevalence for depression in a woman's life. Second, over 80% of women present for prenatal care at some point during their pregnancy (U.S. Department of Health and Human Services (USDHHS) 2004), therefore providing a point of healthcare contact. Third, there are identifiable risk factors for perinatal depression, including a history of perinatal depression, lifetime and family history of depression, and high levels of economic and family stress (see Battle and Zlotnick (2005) for a review). Finally, depression prevention and treatment in women around the time of pregnancy has the potential to prospectively prevent risk to children.

Prevalence and Features of Perinatal Depression

Prevalence rates for depression occurring around the time of childbearing differ depending on the method and timing of assessment. Higher prevalence rates are found using self-report instruments and longer assessment periods, and lower rates are found using diagnostic instruments and shorter time frames (O'Hara and Swain 1996). A meta-analysis of 30 studies of perinatal depression by the Agency for Healthcare Research and Quality (Gaynes et al. 2005) found the point prevalence of minor or major depression to range from 5.5 to 12.9%. Period prevalence estimates through 1 year postpartum were found to be as high as 54% for major or minor depression, with higher rates found in samples composed primarily of economically disadvantaged women (Gaynes et al. 2005).

Although most studies have not found differential rates of depression in childbearing women as compared to age matched nonchildbearing women, there is some evidence of different features of perinatal depression. For example, co-occurring anxiety symptoms may include intrusive thoughts or excessive worry about infant safety issues and maternal caretaking abilities (Miller 2002). The primary way in which perinatal depression is distinct from depression occurring at other developmental periods in women is the impact on pregnancy, fetal, and infant outcomes.

Depression in the antenatal period is correlated with shorter length of gestation and lower birth weight (Hoffman and Hatch 2000), and it results in greater cortisol reactivity in the newborn, an effect that persists into early childhood, placing the child at risk for developing depression (Lundy et al. 1999). Depressed mothers breastfeed less often and stop breastfeeding earlier in infancy (Field et al. 2002). Mothers with depression may have greater difficulty accurately perceiving infant emotional expressions (Broth et al. 2004) and may perceive their children as more difficult and themselves as having poorer competence as a parent (Teti and Gelfand 1991). Behaviorally, infants of depressed mothers are more likely to be withdrawn, less excitable, and less oriented than those of nondepressed mothers (Lundy et al. 1999). They are also more likely to exhibit eating or sleeping difficulties and are less likely to engage with visual or vocal stimuli (Righetti-Veltema et al. 2002).

Importantly, many of these and other studies have shown that elevated depressive symptomatology (and not necessarily diagnosis of MDD) has been linked to low birth weight, preterm delivery, small-sized infants (Field et al. 2004; Hoffman and Hatch 2000; Kelly et al. 2002; Steer et al. 1992), increased fetal activity (Dieter et al. 2001), and infant neurobehavioral dysregulation (see review by Field et al. 2006), suggesting the importance of detecting and addressing subclinical symptoms as well as MDD.

Perinatal Depression: Treatment and Health Services Issues

Given the well-documented extent and risks of maternal depression, it is critical to treat mothers suffering from depression. Persons appropriately treated for depression have shorter periods of illness, are less likely to relapse, and have longer periods of interdepression wellness than those who are not treated, or who are undertreated (Frank et al. 1990; Segal et al. 2002).

Preliminary research suggests that effective treatment for maternal depression may have a positive impact on both maternal and child functioning. Efficacious treatments have been shown in some studies to improve or restore overall maternal functioning, prevent the negative infant neurobehavioral outcomes associated with maternal depression, and improve mother–infant relations immediately postpartum and at 18-month and 5-year follow-up (Logsdon et al. 2003; Moses-Kolko and Roth 2004; Murray et al. 2003; Verduyn et al. 2003). However, a recent study by Forman et al. (2007) showed improvements in maternal depression and functioning outcomes, but not in maternal–infant attachment outcomes following maternal depression treatment with IPT.

Results from the National Institutes of Mental Health STAR*D study showed that mothers whose depression remitted after 3 months of treatment had children with significantly lower rates of psychiatric symptoms and diagnoses than children of mothers who remained depressed (Weissman et al. 2006). Because provision of effective treatment for women has the potential to positively impact maternal and certain child outcomes, it is imperative to reach women in need.

Despite the existence of efficacious treatments, few women with perinatal depression receive adequate treatment (Flynn et al. 2006a; Spitzer et al. 2000). Several recent research studies converge on a rate of approximately 75% of depressed childbearing-aged women in Ob/Gyn settings who are not detected or treated (Kelly et al. 2001; Marcus et al. 2003; Smith et al. 2004; Spitzer et al. 2000). These rates are notably lower than national rates of depression treatment, which range between 30 and 50%, suggesting that this risk group may be accessing treatment at a lower rate than the general population (Young et al. 2001). Although most obstetricians do report having a positive attitude toward screening for depression and performing some form of screening, most do not use validated screening tools, which have been shown to improve accuracy of screening (Evins et al. 2000).

Screening tools generally measure levels of symptoms experienced by women over the course of a specified recent time frame and should not substitute for a diagnosis of depression. The accuracy of prediction of a disorder, based on a screening tool using a specified cut point, is evaluated by comparing screening results to a "gold standard" method of diagnosing depression, usually a validated diagnostic interview. Three indices of accuracy of a screen are considered to be most useful. Sensitivity is the ability of the measure to correctly identify women with postpartum depression (PPD; or true positive rate), specificity is the ability of the screen to correctly identify women without PPD (or true negative rate), and positive predictive value (PPV) is the probability that a woman who scores positive on the screen is truly depressed.

The recent AHQR Evidence Report (Gaynes et al. 2005) reviewed the performance of the most commonly used perinatal depression screening instruments. The Edinburgh Postnatal Depression Scale (EPDS) is the most commonly employed screening tool in research studies and has been translated into several different languages. The EPDS (Cox et al. 1987) is a 10-item measure originally designed to eliminate reliance on somatic symptom items that may be confounded by pregnancy and to be easily scored by health care workers. Items assessing ability to laugh and enjoy oneself, sad and anxious mood, self blame, sleep difficulties not due to childbirth, as well as coping and suicidal thinking are scored on a 4-point likert scale and cover the past 7-day time frame. The most commonly used cut point of 13 to detect MDD in studies using the EPDS show a sensitivity of 0.91 and a specificity of 0.95 (see Gaynes et al. (2005) for a review).

The Beck Depression Inventory (BDI) is another commonly used depression screening measure for perinatal depression. Scores on 21 symptom items are scored from 0 to 3 based on intensity of the symptoms (including somatic symptoms such as sleep and appetite disturbance) over the past week. Using a cut point of 21, sensitivity of the BDI in detecting MDD has been found to range from 0.36 to 0.52, with specificities ranging from 0.99 to 1.0. Lower cut points of 11–13 have yielded higher sensitivities (0.68) and slightly lower specificities (0.88; Gaynes et al. 2005).

The Postpartum Depression Screening Scale (PDSS) was developed (Beck and Gable 2001) to assess mood symptoms commonly reported by women in the first postpartum year, conceptualized along seven dimensions. The performance of the EPDS, the BDI, and the PDSS as initial screening tools has been found to be comparable overall.

Despite the availability of screening tools, barriers to screening within obstetrics include time constraints, discomfort with adequacy of training to address psychosocial issues, and concern that screening will not impact depression outcomes (Janssen et al. 2003; LaRocco-Cockburn et al. 2003). Moreover, screening alone has not been found to improve depression care or to significantly impact depression outcomes based on several primary care setting studies (Carter et al. 2005; Kroenke 2001; Wells et al. 2002a, b). Several large-scale depression management studies in primary care have shown that acute phase depression treatment and outcomes may be improved by systematic screening follow-up, linkage to guideline concordant treatment protocols, and routine monitoring and follow-up (Dickinson et al. 2005; Rost et al. 2001; Wells et al. 2000).

Unfortunately, pregnant and postpartum women who do connect with mental health services commonly receive treatments below depression treatment guidelines (Flynn et al. 2006a; Marcus et al. 2005). Studies by the University of Michigan Women's Mood Disorder research group showed that less than half of women with antenatal MDD received any treatment for depression, and that the majority of those treated were using treatments below recommended guidelines (Flynn et al. 2006a). These studies also found that even in clinic sites where transportation, childcare, access, and payment barriers were absent, less than one-third of depressed women followed through with a mental health appointment (Flynn et al. 2006b).

Despite a preference among perinatal women and minorities for nonpharmacological treatments (Cohen et al. 2004; Van Schaik et al. 2004), evidence-based psychological treatments such as CBT are rarely available in obstetrics settings (Williamson and McCutcheon 2004). The perinatal phase is one filled with physical and emotional changes, such as nausea and mobility limitations, that may interfere with a woman's abilities to seek out and adhere to traditional weekly face-to-face psychotherapy (Buist 2003). Time and childcare demands also present barriers for postpartum women. Given these barriers to traditional face-to-face treatment contact, it is important to consider alternative delivery modalities (such as telephone or obstetrics clinic-based) in an effort to improve engagement and adherence.

Implications for Women's Mental Health

Although routine screening for depression in obstetrics is not necessarily usual care nationwide, it is commonly recommended (Wisner et al. 2006) and likely represents an important first step in impacting depression outcomes. In Britain, the National Institute for Health and Clinical Excellence (National Institute for Health and Clinical Excellence (NICE) 2004) recommends routine, brief screening for depression in primary and prenatal care.

In the USA, the state of New Jersey recently passed a law requiring doctors and nurses to educate and screen expectant mothers about PPD. Subsequently, legislation was introduced in Congress (the Mothers Act S. 3529) that calls for "providing important education and screening on PPD that can lead to early identification and treatment" (June 15, 2006).

Despite these large-scale recommendations and mandates, the effectiveness of screening coupled with provision of information and education has not been adequately studied in obstetrics settings. Much more research is needed on effective strategies to link women identified as depressed to acceptable, accessible, and effective treatments. Research must also consider not only improvement of maternal depression outcomes, but also broader health, social, and child functioning outcomes. Capitalizing on health care settings where women present for care during high risk developmental periods holds great promise for reducing the overall burden of depression in women.

References

Battle, C. L., & Zlotnick, C. (2005). Prevention of postpartum depression. *Psychiatric Annals, 35*(7), 590–598.

Beck, C. T., & Gable, R. K. (2001). Comparative analysis of the performance of the Postpartum Depression Screening Scale with two other depression instruments. *Nursing Research, 50*(4), 242–250.

Bradbury, T. N., Beach, S. R., Fincham, F. D., & Nelson, G. M. (1996). Attributions and behavior in functional and dysfunctional marriages. *Journal of Consulting and Clinical Psychology, 64*(3), 569–576.

Bromet, E., Sonnega, A., & Kessler, R.C. (1998). Risk factors for DSM-III-R Posttraumatic stress disorder: Findings from the National Comorbidity Study, *American Journal of Epidemiology, 147*(4), 353–361.

Broth, M. R., Goodman, S. H., Hall, C., & Raynor, L. C. (2004). Depressed and well mothers' emotional interpretation accuracy and the quality of mother-infant interaction. *Infancy, 6*(1), 37–55.

Buist, A. (2003). Promoting positive parenthood: Emotional health in pregnancy. *Australian Journal of Midwifery, 16*(1), 10–14.

Butler, S. S., Turner, W., Kaye, L. W., Ruffin, L., & Downey, R. (2005). Depression and caregiver burden among rural elder caregivers. *Journal of Gerontological Social Work, 46*(1), 47–63.

Carter, F. A., Carter, J. D., Luty, S. E., Wilson, D. A., Frampton, C. M., & Joyce, P. R. (2005). Screening and treatment for depression during pregnancy: A cautionary note. *The Australian and New Zealand Journal of Psychiatry, 39*(4), 255–261.

Caspi, A., Sugden, K., Moffitt, T. E., Taylor, A., Craig, I. W., Harrington, H., et al. (2003). Influence of life stress on depression: Moderation by a polymorphism in the 5-HTT gene. *Science, 301*(5631), 386–389.

Cohen, L. S., Nonacs, R. M., Bailey, J. W., Viguera, A. C., Reminick, A. M., Altshuler, L. L., et al. (2004). Relapse of depression during pregnancy following antidepressant discontinuation: A preliminary prospective study. *Archives of Women's Mental Health, 7*(4), 217–221.

Cox, J. L., Holden, J. M., & Sagovsky, R. (1987). Detection of postnatal depression. Development of the 10-item Edinburgh Postnatal Depression Scale. *The British Journal of Psychiatry, 150,* 782–786.

Dickinson, L. M., Rost, K., Nutting, P. A., Elliott, C. E., Keeley, R. D., & Pincus, H. (2005). RCT of a care manager intervention for major depression in primary care: 2-year costs for patients with physical vs psychological complaints. *Annals of Family Medicine, 3*(1), 15–22.

Dieter, J. N., Field, T., Hernandez-Reif, M., Jones, N. A., Lecanuet, J. P., Salman, F. A., et al. (2001). Maternal depression and increased fetal activity. *Journal of Obstetrics and Gynaecology, 21*(5), 468–473.

Evins, G. G., Theofrastous, J. P., & Galvin, S. L. (2000). Postpartum depression: A comparison of screening and routine clinical evaluation. *American Journal of Obstetrics and Gynecology, 182*(5), 1080–1082.

Field, T., Diego, M., & Hernandez-Reif, M. (2006). Prenatal depression effects on the fetus and newborn: A review. *Infant Behavior and Development, 29,* 445–455.

Field, T., Diego, M., Hernandez-Reif, M., Vera, Y., Gil, K., Schanberg, S., et al. (2004). Prenatal maternal biochemistry predicts neonatal biochemistry. *The International Journal of Neuroscience, 114*(8), 933–945.

Field, T., Hernandez-Reif, M., & Larissa, F. (2002). Breastfeeding in depressed mother-infant dyads. *Early Child Development and Care, 172*(6), 539–545.

Flynn, H. A., Blow, F. C., & Marcus, S. M. (2006a). Rates and predictors of depression treatment among pregnant women in hospital-affiliated obstetrics practices. *General Hospital Psychiatry, 28*(4), 289–295.

Flynn, H. A., Davis, M., Marcus, S. M., Cunningham, R., & Blow, F. C. (2004). Rates of maternal depression in pediatric emergency department and relationship to child service utilization. *General Hospital Psychiatry, 26*(4), 316–322.

Flynn, H. A., O'Mahen, H. A., Massey, L., & Marcus, S. (2006b). The impact of a brief obstetrics clinic-based intervention on treatment use for perinatal depression. *Journal of Women's Health, 15*(10), 1195–1204.

Forman, D. R., O'Hara, M. W., Stuart, S., Gorman, L. L., Larsen, K. E., & Coy, K. C. (2007, Spring). Effective treatment for postpartum depression is not sufficient to improve the developing mother-child relationship. *Development and Psychopathology, 19*(2), 585–602.

Frank, E., Grochocinski, V. J., Spanier, C. A., Buysse, D. J., Cherry, C. R., Houck, P. R., et al. (2000). Interpersonal psychotherapy and antidepressant medication: Evaluation of a sequential treatment strategy in women with recurrent major depression. *The Journal of Clinical Psychiatry, 61*(1), 51–57.

Frank, E., Kupfer, D. J., Perel, J. M., Cornes, C., Jarrett, D. B., Mallinger, A. G., et al. (1990). Three-year outcomes for maintenance therapies in recurrent depression. *Archives of General Psychiatry, 47*(12), 1093–1099.

Gaynes, B. N., Gavin, N., Meltzer-Brody, S., Lohr, K. N., Swinson, T., Gartlehner, G., et al. (2005). Perinatal depression: Prevalence, screening accuracy, and screening outcomes. *Evidence Report/Technology Assessment (Summary), 119,* 1–8.

Givens, J. L., Houston, T. K., Van Voorhees, B. W., Ford, D. E., & Cooper, L. A. (2007, May–June). Ethnicity and preferences for depression treatment. *General Hospital Psychiatry, 29*(3), 182–191.

Haley, W. E., Turner, J. A., & Romano, J. M. (1985). Depression in chronic pain patients: Relation to pain, activity, and sex differences. *Pain, 23*(4), 337–343.

Hoffman, S., & Hatch, M. C. (2000). Depressive symptomatology during pregnancy: Evidence for an association with decreased fetal growth in pregnancies of lower social class women. *Health Psychology, 19*(6), 535–543.

Hollon, S. D., Jarrett, R. B., Nierenberg, A. A., Thase, M. E., Trivedi, M., & Rush, A. J. (2005). Psychotherapy and medication in the treatment of adult and geriatric depression: Which monotherapy or combined treatment? *The Journal of Clinical Psychiatry, 66*(4), 455–468.

Hollon, S., Thase, M. E., & Markowtiz, J. C. (2002). Treatment and prevention of depression. *Psychological Science in the Public Interest, 3*(2), 39–77.

Janssen, P. A., Holt, V. L., Sugg, N. K., Emanuel, I., Critchlow, C. M., & Henderson, A. D. (2003). Intimate partner violence and adverse pregnancy outcomes: A population-based study. *American Journal of Obstetrics and Gynecology, 188*(5), 1341–1347.

Kahn, R. S., Wise, P. H., Finkelstein, J. A., Bernstein, H. H., Lowe, J. A., & Homer, C. J. (1999). The scope of unmet maternal health needs in pediatric settings. *Pediatrics, 103*(3), 576–581.

Kelly, R. H., Russo, J., Holt, V. L., Danielsen, B. H., Zatzick, D. F., Walker, E., et al. (2002). Psychiatric and substance use disorders as risk factors for low birth weight and preterm delivery. *Obstetrics and Gynecology, 100*(2), 297–304.

Kelly, R., Zatzick, D., & Anders, T. (2001). The detection and treatment of psychiatric disorders and substance use among pregnant women cared for in obstetrics. *The American Journal of Psychiatry, 158*(2), 213–219.

Kendler, K. S., Kuhn, J.W., Vittum, J., Prescott, C. A., & Riley, B. (2005). The interaction of stressful life events and a serotonin transporter polymorphism in the prediction of episodes of major depression: A replication. *Archives of General Psychiatry. 62*(5), 529–535.

Kessler, R. C., Sonnega, A., Bromet, E., & Nelson, C. B. (1995). Posttraumatic stress disorder in the National Comorbidity Survey, *Archives of General Psychiatry, 52*(12), 1048–1060.

Kessler, R. C., Stang, P. E., Wittchen, H. U., Ustun, T. B., Roy-Burne, P. P., & Walters, E. E. (1998). Lifetime manic-depression comorbidity in the National Comorbidity Survey. *Archives of General Psychiatry, 55*(9), 801–808.

Kornstein, S. G., Schatzberg, A. F., Thase, M. E., Yonkers, K. A., McCullough, J. P., Keitner, G. I., et al. (2000). Gender differences in chronic major and double depression. *Journal of Affective Disorders, 60*(1), 1–11.

Kroenke, K. (2001). Depression screening is not enough. *Annals of Internal Medicine, 134*(5), 418–420.

LaRocco-Cockburn, A., Melville, J., Bell, M., & Katon, W. (2003). Depression screening attitudes and practices among obstetrician-gynecologists. *Obstetrics and Gynecology, 101*(5 Pt 1), 892–898.

Le, H., Munoz, R. F., Ippen, C. G., & Stoddard, J. L. (2003). Treatment is not enough: We must prevent major depression in women. *Prevention & Treatment, 6*(10).

Logsdon, M. C., Wisner, K., Hanusa, B. H., & Phillips, A. (2003). Role functioning and symptom remission in women with postpartum depression after antidepressant treatment. *Archives of Psychiatric Nursing, 17*(6), 276–283.

Lundy, B. L., Jones, N. A., Field, T., Nearing, G., Davalos, M., Pietro, P., et al. (1999). Prenatal depression effects on neonates. *Infant Behavior & Development, 22,* 119–129.

Marcus, S. M., Flynn, H. A., Blow, F. C., & Barry, K. L. (2003). Depressive symptoms among pregnant women screened in obstetrics settings. *Journal of Women's Health, 12*(4), 373–380.

Marcus, S. M., Flynn, H. A., Blow, F., & Barry, K. (2005). A screening study of antidepressant treatment rates and mood symptoms in pregnancy. *Archives of Women's Mental Health, 8*(1), 25.

Miller, L. J. (2002). Postpartum depression. *Journal of the American Medical Association, 287*(6), 762–765.

Moses-Kolko, E. L., & Roth, E. K. (2004). Antepartum and postpartum depression: Healthy mom, healthy baby. *Journal of the American Medical Women's Association, 59*(3), 181–191.

Moussavi, S., Chatterji, S., Verdes, E., Tandon, A., Patel, V., & Ustun, B. (2007). Depression, chronic diseases, and decrements in health: Results from the World Health Surveys. *Lancet, 370*(9590), 851–858.

Murray, L., Woolgar, M., Murray, J., & Cooper, P. (2003). Self-exclusion from health care in women at high risk for postpartum depression. *Journal of Public Health Medicine, 25*(2), 131–137.

National Institute for Health and Clinical Excellence (NICE). (2004). Depression: Management of depression in primary and secondary care. *Clinical guideline 23*. London: NICE.

Nishizawa, S., Benkelfat, C., Young, S. N., Leyton, M., Mzengeza, S., de Montigny, C., et al. (1997). Differences between males and females in rates of serotonin synthesis in human brain. *Proceedings of the National Academy of Sciences of the United States of America, 94*(10), 5308–5313.

Nolen-Hoeksema, S. (1995). Epidemiology and theories of gender differences in depression. In M. V. Seeman (Ed.), *Gender and pychopathology*. Washington, DC: American Psychiatric Press.

Nolen-Hoeksema, S., & Girgus, J. S. (1994). The emergence of gender differences in depression during adolescence. *Psychological Bulletin, 115*(3), 424–443.

Nolen-Hoeksema, S., Larson, J., & Grayson, C. (1999). Explaining the gender differences in depressive symptoms. *Journal of Personality and Social Psychology, 77*(5), 1061–1072.

O'Hara, M. W., & Swain, A. M. (1996). Rates and risk of postpartum depression: A meta-analysis. *International Review of Psychiatry, 8*, 37–54.

Paykel, E. S., Scott, J., Cornwall, P. L., Abbott, R., Crane, C., Pope, M., et al. (2005). Duration of relapse prevention after cognitive therapy in residual depression: Follow-up of controlled trial. *Psychological Medicine, 35*(1), 59–68.

Righetti-Veltema, M., Conne-Perreard, E., Bousquet, A., & Manzano, J. (2002). Postpartum depression and mother-infant relationship at 3 months old. *Journal of Affective Disorders, 70*(3), 291–306.

Rost, K., Nutting, P., Smith, J., Werner, J., & Duan, N. (2001). Improving depression outcomes in community primary care practice: A randomized trial of the quEST intervention. Quality enhancement by strategic teaming. *Journal of General Internal Medicine, 16*(3), 143–149.

Rudolph, K. D., Hammen, C., Burge, D., Lindberg, N., Herzberg, D., & Daley, S. E. (2000). Toward an interpersonal life-stress model of depression: The developmental context of stress generation. *Development and Psychopathology, 12*, 215–234.

Scholle, S. H., Haskett, R. F., Hanusa, B. H., Pincus, H. A., & Kupfer, D. J. (2003). Addressing depression in obstetrics/gynecology practice. *General Hospital Psychiatry, 25*(2), 83–90.

Segal, Z. V., Williams, J. M. G., & Teasdale, J. D. (2002). *Mindfulness-based cognitive therapy for depression*. New York, NY: Guilford Press.

Silverstein, B. (1994). Gender difference in the prevalence of clinical depression: The role played by depression associated with somatic symptoms. *American Journal of Psychiatry, 156*, 480–482.

Smith, M. V., Rosenheck, R. A., Cavaleri, M. A., Howell, H. B., Poschman, K., & Yonkers, K. A. (2004). Screening for and detection of depression, panic disorder, and PTSD in public-sector obstetric clinics. *Psychiatric Services, 55*(4), 407–414.

Spitzer, R. L., Williams, J. B., Kroenke, K., Hornyak, R., & McMurray, J. (2000). Validity and utility of the PRIME-MD patient health questionnaire in assessment of 3000 obstetric-gynecologic patients: The PRIME-MD patient health questionnaire obstetrics-gynecology study. *American Journal of Obstetrics and Gynecology, 183*(3), 759–769.

Steer, R. A., Scholl, T. O., Hediger, M. L., & Fischer, R. L. (1992). Self-reported depression and negative pregnancy outcomes. *Journal of Clinical Epidemiology, 45*(10), 1093–1099.

Teti, D. M., & Gelfand, D. M. (1991). Behavioral competence among mothers of infants in the first year: The mediational role of maternal self-efficacy. *Child Development, 62*(5), 918–929.

U.S. Department of Health and Human Services, Health Resources and Services Administration, Maternal and Child Health Bureau. (2004). *Child health USA 2004*. Rockville, MD: U.S. Department of Health and Human Services.

Van Schaik, D. J., Klijn, A. F., van Hout, H. P., van Marwijk, H. W., Beekman, A. T., de Haan, M., et al. (2004). Patients' preferences in the treatment of depressive disorder in primary care. *General Hospital Psychiatry, 26*(3), 184–189.

Verduyn, C., Barrowclough, C., Roberts, J., Tarrier, T., & Harrington, R. (2003). Maternal depression and child behaviour problems. Randomised placebo-controlled trial of a cognitive-behavioural group intervention. *The British Journal of Psychiatry, 183*, 342–348.

Weissman, M. M., Bland, R. C., Canino, G. J., Faravelli, C., Greenwald, S., Hwu, H. G., et al. (1996). Cross-national epidemiology of major depression and bipolar disorder. *Journal of the American Medical Association, 276*(4), 293–299.

Weissman, M. M., Markowitz, J. C., & Klerman, G. I. (2000). *Comprehensive guide to interpersonal psychotherapy*. New York, NY: Basic Books.

Weissman, M. M., Pilowsky, D. J., Wickramaratne, P. J., Talati, A., Wisniewski, S. R., Fava, M., et al. (2006). Remissions in maternal depression and child psychopathology: A STAR*D-child report. *Journal of the American Medical Association, 295*(12), 1389–1398.

Wells, K. B., Miranda, J., Bauer, M. S., Bruce, M. L., Durham, M., Escobar, J., et al. (2002a). Overcoming barriers to reducing the burden of affective disorders. *Biological Psychiatry, 52*(6), 655–675.

Wells, K. B., Sherbourne, C. D., Schoenbaum, M., Duan, N., Meredith, L., Unutzer, J., et al. (2000). Impact of disseminating quality improvement programs for depression in managed primary care: A randomized controlled trial. *Journal of the American Medical Association, 283*(2), 212–220.

Wells, K. B., Sherbourne, C. D., Sturm, R., Young, A. S., & Burnam, M. A. (2002b). Alcohol, drug abuse, and mental health care for uninsured and insured adults. *Health Services Research, 37*(4), 1055–1066.

Williamson, V., & McCutcheon, H. (2004). Postnatal depression: A review of current literature. *Australian Journal of Midwifery, 17*(4), 11–16.

Wisner, K. L., Chambers, C., & Sit, D. K. (2006, December 6). Postpartum depression: A major public health problem. *Journal of the American Medical Association, 296*(21), 2616–2618.

Young, A. S., Klap, R., Sherbourne, C. D., & Wells, K. B. (2001). The quality of care for depressive and anxiety disorders in the United States. *Archives of General Psychiatry, 58*(1), 55–61.

Zuckerman, B., Bauchner, H., Parker, S., & Cabral, H. (1990). Maternal depressive symptoms during pregnancy, and newborn irritability. *Journal of Developmental and Behavioral Pediatrics, 11*(4), 190–194.

Chapter 7
Eating Disorders

Rita DeBate, Heather Blunt and Marion Ann Becker

Introduction

Eating disorders are serious mental health conditions that are more common among women and present with well-documented physical manifestations and psychiatric comorbidities. An estimated 5–10 million females are affected with some form of eating disorder (Gordon 1990; Crowther et al. 1992; Fairburn et al. 1995; Hoek 2002). The American College of Physicians lists eating disorders as one of the nine most serious problems affecting adolescents and young adults, and anorexia nervosa (AN) as the third most common chronic illness (Snyder 1989). Individuals with eating disorders have the highest mortality rate among any groups afflicted with mental illness as 20% of people suffering from eating disorders die prematurely from complications related to their eating disorder, including suicide and heart problems. More specifically, AN has the highest mortality rate of any psychiatric illness (Sullivan 1995). The mortality rate for individuals with AN is 12 times higher than the all-cause death rate for females 15–24 years old (National Eating Disorders Association 2002; Cavanaugh and Lemberg 1999), and 200 times higher than the mortality rate for suicides among women (Cavanaugh and Lemberg 1999). Despite the seriousness of these disorders, many insurance companies continue to deny coverage for treatment (National Eating Disorders Association 2006) even though the outcome of treatment has been found to be better than for obesity or breast cancer (National Eating Disorders Association 2005a). This chapter will provide an overview of eating disorders including classification, epidemiology, comorbidities, health consequences, and treatment. In addition, mental health policy implications will be presented.

R. DeBate (✉)
Department of Community & Family Health, College of Public Health,
University of South Florida, 13201 Bruce B. Downs Blvd. MDC 56,
Tampa, FL 33612, USA

B. L. Levin, M. A. Becker (eds.), *A Public Health Perspective of Women's Mental Health*,
DOI 10.1007/978-1-4419-1526-9_7, © Springer Science+Business Media LLC 2010

Epidemiology of Eating Disorders

Epidemiology is described as the assessment and understanding of the distribution and determinants of death, disease, and disability in a population (Rossignol 2007). The measures of disease frequency in epidemiology are defined as incidence and prevalence (Rossignol 2007). Incidence can be defined as the number of new cases in the population over a specified period of time (typically 1 year) and is expressed per 100,000 of the population per year. Prevalence pertains to the proportion of the population that has the particular disease at a specific point in time (Rossignol 2007). Epidemiological studies of eating disorders have many limitations due to the methodological differences with regard to the selection of populations, assessment criteria, and participant bias due to the highly secretive nature of these disorders (Hoek and van Hoeken 2003). The most widely used and accepted method for assessing the prevalence of eating disorders is the two-stage screening strategy (Hoek 2002; Hoek and van Hoeken 2003). With this strategy, the first stage consists of screening a large number of individuals using a questionnaire. The second stage involves interviews with persons who screened positive for an eating disorder in addition to a random selection of persons who did not screen positive (Hoek 2002).

Generally speaking, epidemiological studies of eating disorders suggest a significant increase in AN and binge eating disorder (BED) in the mid- to late twentieth century, and a leveling off of bulimia nervosa (BN) in recent years (Hudson et al. 2007; Hoek and van Hoeken 2003). As part of the National Comorbidity Survey Replication (NCS-R) study, a subsample (n = 2,980) of US respondents was randomly assigned to have an assessment of eating disorders using DSM-VI criteria (Hudson et al. 2007). Results indicate a lifetime prevalence of eating disorders among women to be 1.75–3 times higher than men. This population-based study found lifetime prevalence estimates of AN, BN, and BED among women to be 0.9%, 1.5%, and 3.5% respectively. These prevalence estimates are similar to those observed in population-based studies in Austria which revealed prevalence estimates of 1.2% for BN and 3.3% for BED (Kinzl et al. 1999). In a population-based study in the USA, estimates of lifetime risk of developing an eating disorder by the age of 80 were revealed as 0.6% for AN, 1.1% for BN, and 3.9% for BED (Hudson et al. 2007).

Classification and Diagnostic Criteria

Classification of eating disorders as mental disorders began with AN in the 1970s followed by BN in the early 1980s and the classification of atypical eating disorders (e.g., eating disorders not otherwise specified (EDNOS)). Although diagnostic criteria for these disorders have not been firmly established, BED and night eating syndrome (NES) have also recently been identified as EDNOS subtypes.

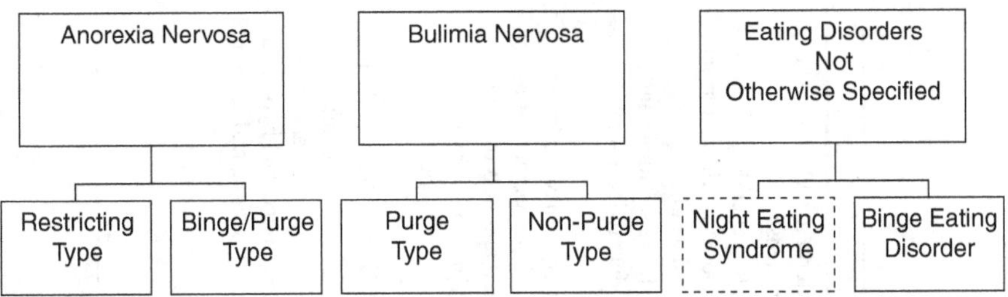

Fig. 7.1 Classification of eating disorders

The following section describes the classification of eating disorders based on the Diagnostic and Statistical Manual for Mental Disorders, 4th edition (DSM-IV; American Psychiatric Association 1994). As depicted in Fig. 7.1, the DSM-IV includes three main classifications for eating disorders. These include AN, BN, and EDNOS.

Anorexia Nervosa

Diagnostic criteria for AN include core physical and psychological criteria including (a) refusal to maintain a body weight at or above 85% of what is expected for the individual's height and age; (b) amenorrhea; (c) intense fear of gaining weight; and (d) body image distortion including an undue influence of body weight on self-evaluation. As per Fig. 7.1, two AN subtypes have been identified. AN subtypes can be classified via the absence or presence of binge–purge behaviors (see Table 7.1).

Although the diagnostic criteria for AN are well established, concerns and controversy among researchers and clinicians exist regarding the inclusion of amenorrhea and the weight threshold as diagnostic criteria. For example, community studies have found that women who indicate all criteria for AN but continue to menstruate are as ill as those who meet all diagnostic criteria. Additionally, individuals who take oral contraceptives may regulate their menstrual cycles, thereby running the risk of being misdiagnosed.

Bulimia Nervosa

As with AN, diagnostic criteria for BN includes aspects of body image as an influencing factor on overall self-image. However, different from AN, diagnostic criteria for BN mainly comprise recurrent episodes of binging (eating large amounts of food in a discrete period of time with an associated feeling of loss of control) and purging behaviors. Diagnosis of BN requires that the individual engage in these binge/purge

Table 7.1 Diagnostic criteria. (Adapted from American Psychiatric Association (1994))

Anorexia nervosa		Bulimia nervosa		EDNOS	
Refusal to maintain body weight at or above normal weight for age and height		Recurrent episodes of binge eating		For females, meets all criteria for AN, however individual has regular menses	
Intense fear of gaining weight although markedly underweight		Recurrent inappropriate compensatory behaviors to prevent weight gain		Meets all criteria for AN, however despite significant weight loss, individual is within normal weight range for age and height	
The absence of at least 3 consecutive periods (or periods only occur when given hormones)		The binge eating and purging behaviors occur at least twice a week for 3 months		Meets all criteria for BN, however, binge and purge behaviors occurs less than twice a week for less than 3 months	
Abnormal body perception shown by undue emphasis on weight or shape, denial of seriousness of low weight, distorted body shape or weight		Self-evaluation influenced by body shape and weight		Regular use of compensatory behaviors by an individual with normal body weight for age and height after eating small amounts of food	
		Does not occur exclusively during episodes of anorexia nervosa		Repeatedly chewing and spitting out by not swallowing large amounts of food	
Restricting type	Binge/Purge type	Purging type	Nonpurging type	Binge eating disorder	Night eating syndrome
Not regularly engaged in binge eating and purging behaviors	Regularly engaged in binge eating and purging behaviors	Regularly engaged in purging behaviors such as self-induced vomiting, or the misuse of laxatives, diuretics, or enema	Engaged in the use of inappropriate compensatory behaviors such as fasting, excessive exercise, but not regularly engaged in purging behaviors	Regular episodes of binge eating without the regular use of purging or inappropriate compensatory behaviors	Combination of: morning anorexia, nocturnal hyperphagia, and insomnia

behaviors at least two times per week for a period of 3 months. Concerns exist regarding the optimum threshold for number of binge/purge episodes required for diagnosis. BN subtypes are further categorized by the types of purging behaviors. Whereas the BN purging type is engaged with self-induced vomiting, laxative, diuretic, and/or enema misuse, the nonpurging subtype compensates for calories ingested from a binge by fasting and/or engaging in excessive exercise (Fig. 7.1).

Eating Disorders Not Otherwise Specified (EDNOS)

Generally speaking, diagnostic criteria for individuals who meet some, but not all, criteria for AN or BN are considered EDNOS. Identified EDNOS subtypes include BED and NES. Table 7.1 describes the criteria for BED as presented in the DSM-IV. Although currently not a separate classification, BED is considered a specific EDNOS subtype. BED can be described as regular episodes of binge eating without the regular use of purging or inappropriate compensatory behaviors indicated in the two BN subtypes. More specifically, BED consists of the following characteristics: (a) recurrent episodes of binge eating; (b) the binge episodes are associated with three or more of the following: eating more rapidly than normal, eating until feeling uncomfortably full, eating large amounts of food when not physically hungry, eating alone due to embarrassment regarding amount of food eaten, feeling disgusted, depressed or guilty after overeating; (c) distress over binge eating; (d) on average binge eating episodes occur at least 2 days per week for 6 months; and (e) binge eating is not associated with inappropriate purging or compensatory behaviors. Although these characteristics have been described in the DSM-IV, they are considered areas for further research. Most noteworthy are the 2 day and 6 month threshold for binge eating episodes.

Another EDNOS subtype is NES. First described in 1955, NES is considered an atypical eating disorder as it seems to be a unique combination of morning anorexia, evening or nocturnal overeating, and insomnia (Townsend 2007). NES has not been classified in the DSM-IV; however, there is a renewed interest in the relationship between eating disorders and obesity. Further research is needed regarding characteristics pertaining to diagnostic criteria for NES.

Incidence and Prevalence of AN

Incidences of AN have largely been based on records from hospitals and primary care facilities in addition to inpatient and outpatient mental health treatment facilities (Hoek 2002). Using medical records to calculate incidence of AN may underestimate the problem, because not all persons with AN seek treatment. Epidemiological studies implemented from 1931 to 1995 using hospital records indicate an increase in the incidence of eating disorders from 0.10/100,000 in 1931 to 1.17/100,000 in 1995 (Hoek and van Hoeken 2003). Studies using case registers from 1965 to 1989 vary greatly with incidence rates ranging from 0.37/100,000 to 5.0/100,000. Incidence rates based on large representative samples from primary care facilities reveal incidence rates of 4.2/100,000 in the UK and 8.1/100,000 in the Netherlands (Hoek 2002). Similarly, studies conducted in the USA using medical records report an overall incidence rate of 8.3/100,000.

Epidemiological studies using the two-stage approach reveal prevalence rates for AN to be approximately 0–0.9% among young females. For partial syndrome AN (meeting some but not all of the clinical criteria for AN) prevalence rates are reported to be approximately 0.29% (Hoek and van Hoeken 2003). In a large community study of 4,285 females in Canada, 0.56% met clinical criteria for AN (Garfinkel et al. 1996). Another community-based study found a lifetime prevalence of 2.2% of DSM-IV criteria for AN, and 4.2% for broad case (Keski-Rahkonen et al. 2007).

With regard to age, the highest incidence of AN occurs among 15–19-year-old women (73.9 per 100,000 person-years) followed by incidence rates of 9.5 per 100,000 person-years for 30–39 year olds, 5.9 per 100,000 person-years for 40–49 year olds, and 1.8 per 100,000 person-years for 50–59 year olds (Lucas et al. 1999). According to a more recent study, the incidence for DSM-IV AN in 15–19-year-old women was 270 per 100,000 person-years (Keski-Rahkonen et al. 2007).

Incidence and Prevalence of BN

Generally speaking, incidence studies pertaining to BN are lacking. The reasons for the lack of research investigating incidence rates include the following: (1) BN was first distinguished as an eating disorder by the American Psychological Association in 1980; (2) the taboo surrounding BN and accompanying behaviors (Hoek and van Hoeken 2003). Although few epidemiological studies assessing incidence of BN have been conducted in the USA (Soundy et al. 1995), the Netherlands (Hoek et al. 1995), and the UK (Turnbull et al. 1996), observed incidence rates from these studies were 13.5, 11.5, and 12.2 respectively, with an average incidence rate of 12/100,000. The highest incidence rates of BN occur among 20–27-year-old females with incidence rates of approximately 88/100,000 (Soundy et al. 1995; Hoek et al. 1995). Determining prevalence of BN using the two-stage approach reveals the prevalence rate of BN as 1% among young females (Fairburn and Beglin 1990) with the lifetime prevalence of 1.1% among women (0.1% among 15–65-year-old men; Garfinkel et al. 1995).

Incidence and Prevalence of BED and NES

In a community sample of 910 individuals in the USA, prevalence estimates of BED among women were 6.4% (Grucza et al. 2006). The prevalence of NES has been estimated around 1.5% in the general population; however, it is much higher among obese individuals. Prevalence estimates in obesity clinics can run as high as 9–15% (Marshall et al. 2004).

Risk Factors and Correlates

Factors associated with the development and perpetuation of eating disorders are multifaceted and may occur in various life stages. Conceptualization of these multiple factors requires an understanding of the differences between correlates and risk factors that predispose, precipitate, and/or perpetuate these disorders. A correlate can be described as a characteristic, experience, or event that has been found to be associated with eating disorders, but without any empirical evidence of temporal sequence (Kazdin et al. 1997). In other words, a factor would be considered a correlate if it has not been shown via longitudinal studies that the characteristic, experience, or event occurred *prior* to the development of the eating disorder. On the other hand, a risk factor can be described as a characteristic, exposure, or event that has been identified as preceding the eating disorder. As such, when present, a risk factor is associated with an increased risk of the development of an eating disorder (Kazdin et al. 1997). Risk factors can be further characterized into fixed or variable markers. Fixed markers are risk factors that cannot be changed (e.g., race, year of birth, genotype), whereas variable markers can change (e.g., age) or can be changed (e.g., attitudes, beliefs, skill, etc.). Understanding the differences between the various types of risk factors and correlates is crucial for effective prevention and policy efforts to decrease the development of eating disorders. Table 7.2 depicts the multiple risk factors and correlates of AN, BN, and BED. The risk factors and correlates presented are based largely on a current review of risk factors presented by Jacobi (2005), and Schmidt (2005) describes the multifactorial risk factors and correlates associated with the development of AN, BN, and BED. Table 7.2 depicts these risk factors and correlates as they occur over various life stages.

Common Risk Factors and Correlates for AN, BN, and BED

As depicted in Table 7.2, genetic factors, gender, and race/ethnicity are fixed markers associated with AN, BN, and BED. As described previously, epidemiological studies have found AN and BN to occur predominately among females, with lower rates among Asians. With regard to BED, gender is described as a nonspecific fixed risk factor (2:5 female to male ratio) and race/ethnicity as a fixed marker of unknown specificity as epidemiological studies found similar distributions among Caucasians and African-Americans (Jacobi 2005).

Additionally, concerns about weight, dieting, and body image disturbances have all been classified as variable risk factors for AN, BN, and BED. Findings from numerous

Table 7.2 Etiology of anorexia nervosa, bulimia nervosa, and binge eating disorder

		Anorexia nervosa	Bulimia nervosa	Binge eating disorder
Life-stage	Risk factors and retrospective correlates			
Birth	Genetic factors	**FM**	**FM**	**FM**
	Gender	**FM**	**FM**	**FM**
	Ethnicity	**FM**	**FM**	**FM**
	Pregnancy complications	X	◄	
	Preterm birth, birth trauma	X		
	Season of birth	**FM**		
Childhood	Early childhood eating health problems	X	X	
	Gastrointestinal problems	◄		
	Infant sleep difficulties	◄		
	High concern over parenting	◄		
	Anxiety	◄	◄	
	Depression		X	
	Acculturation	◄	◄	
	Obsessive-compulsive personality disorder and traits	◄		
	Sexual abuse	◄	X	X
	Physical abuse/neglect		X	X
	Perceived paternal neglect and rejection			◄
	Higher level of loneliness, shyness and inferiority	◄		
	Childhood obesity		◄	◄
Adolescence	Adolescent age	X	X	
	Age of menarche	**FM**	**FM**	
	Weight concerns/dieting/negative body image	X	X	X
	High level of exercise	◄		
	Body dysmorphic disorder	◄		
	Greater level of exposure to dieting risk	◄	◄	◄
	Low self-esteem/ineffectiveness		X	X
	General psychiatric illness/negative emotions		X	
	Prodromal symptoms		◄	
	Higher level of shyness		◄	
	High use of escape-avoidance coping			X
	Low perceived social support			X
	Bullying			◄
	Critical comments about shape, weight, or eating		◄	◄

FM = fixed marker, X = variable marker, ◄ = correlate

longitudinal studies revealed "fear of gaining weight," dieting behaviors, and negative body image as predictors for the development of eating disorders (Jacobi 2005).

Shared Risk Factors and Correlates

Adolescent age, early childhood eating and health problems, age of menarche, and pregnancy complications are shared risk factors for AN and BN. As described previously, the peak incidence of AN and BN occurs within the range between adolescence to early adulthood. As such, one can classify age as a variable risk factor. With regard to early childhood eating and health problems, picky eating, digestive problems, eating conflicts, struggles, and unpleasant meals have all been identified as variable markers for AN, whereas longitudinal studies have identified early health problems in infancy and toddlerhood as variable risk factors for BN. Inconsistent evidence exists for age of menarche as a fixed risk factor. Cross-sectional studies have identified early menarche as associated with both AN and BN. However, no association was found in longitudinal studies.

Retrospective correlates of AN/BN include childhood anxiety disorders and acculturation. Current studies with various ethnicities, including Cuban-Americans and Mexican-Americans, have supported the paradigm that highly acculturated women are more vulnerable to eating disorders (Jane et al. 1999; Chamorro and Flores-Ortiz 2000). However, it is important to note that the level of acculturation may not always be predictive of eating disorders as more research is needed to discern how acculturation will affect individuals based on their ethnicity (Kempa and Thonas 2000; French et al. 1997).

Sexual abuse, physical neglect, and low self-esteem are shared risk factors for BN and BED. Although cross-sectional studies have consistently found an association between sexual abuse and physical neglect among those with BN, one longitudinal study in a large community-based sample found an increased risk of BN and BED among those who had experienced sexual abuse and/or physical neglect during childhood. Longitudinal studies have also consistently identified low self-esteem and negative self-concept as variable risk factors for both BN and BED. In addition, various case–control and cohort studies have revealed that family and personal history of obesity and family comments made to the individual regarding weight, shape, and eating have been identified as important correlates of both BN and BED.

Specific to AN

Season of birth and preterm birth are risk factors specific to AN. Epidemiological studies have found a significant number of births among those with AN between April and June (Watkins et al. 2002). As such, season of birth has been classified as a fixed marker for AN. Additionally, women with AN may not gain enough weight during pregnancy, risking perinatal complications, premature birth, and low birth weight. These perinatal complications have been associated with an increased risk of developing AN (Schmidt 2005).

Other retrospective correlates found to be associated with eating disorders include sleep difficulties as an infant, parenting concerns, obsessive-compulsive disorder (OCD), sexual abuse, shyness, excessive exercise, and body dysmorphic disorder.

Specific to BN

Psychiatric morbidity, depression, and substance abuse have been identified via longitudinal studies as variable risk factors for BN. However, because anxiety disorders and negative affectivity have been identified as risk factors for other psychiatric conditions and substance abuse, these risk factors should be considered nonspecific risk factors (Jacobi 2005).

Specific to BED and NES

High use of escape–avoidance coping and low perceived social support have both been identified as variable risk factors specific to BED. In addition, retrospective studies have described individuals with BED reporting low parental contact, perceived neglect from the father, and higher rates of bullying by peers. With regard to NES, overweight or obesity is a risk factor for NES, in addition to sleep disturbances including a circadian pattern delay (Townsend 2007).

Eating Disorders and Comorbidities

Many of the results discussed here are based on a large nationally representative study of the US population, the NCS-R, conducted from 2001 to 2003 (Hudson et al. 2007; also see Chap. 5 in this volume for additional information on multiple morbidities). Participants were English-speaking residents over the age of 18, sampled through a multistage clustered design. This study addressed the comorbidities of many DSM-IV disorders, including eating disorders, specifically AN, BN, and BED.

In general, women with eating disorders may have an increased likelihood of having a first degree relative with a history of alcoholism. Again, causality cannot be determined for the co-occurrence of eating disorders and a family member with alcoholism. Overall, women with eating disorders and a family member with alcoholism tend to suffer more from binge eating, vomiting, laxative use, and diet pills than women with eating disorders but no alcoholism in relatives (Redgrave et al. 2007).

Anorexia Nervosa

Anxiety

The comorbidity of anxiety and AN has important implications for both the pathology and treatment of AN. Anxiety disorders include panic disorder, agoraphobia, social phobia, OCD, generalized anxiety disorder, and posttraumatic stress disorder. The most common comorbidities of anorexia and anxiety are generalized anxiety disorder, social phobia, and OCD (Godart et al. 2003). Childhood separation anxiety is also associated with both subtypes of anorexia (Godart et al. 2003). However, in the NCS-R, AN was only found to be significantly correlated with specific phobia (Hudson et al. 2007).

The exact relationship between anxiety and AN is still uncertain. Studies have reported cases of anxiety disorders preceding the onset of anorexia, in particular OCD and social phobia (Kaye et al. 2004). However, occurrence of anorexia preceding anxiety disorders has also been noted, as well as simultaneous occurrences of both disorders (Godart et al. 2003). Part of the difficulty in determining causation among disorders is the different ages of onset of these disorders.

Mood Disorders

Mood disorders are also frequently comorbid with AN. Anorexia nervosa has been found to be comorbid with two types of depression: major depressive disorder and dysthymia (Hudson et al. 2007). Some studies have found major depressive disorder to be 2.6–4 times higher in women suffering from anorexia than in community residents without anorexia (Godart et al. 2007). Most frequently major depressive disorder is found at relatively similar rates between anorexia nervosa restricting type (AN-R) and anorexia nervosa binge–purge type AN-BP. However, it is also important to note that malnutrition, which is frequent with anorexia, is also a major factor in depressive symptoms, and therefore may be a confounder in these studies. Some evidence has been reported on twin studies that found genetic contributions to anorexia with comorbid major depression (Wade et al. 2000). Bipolar disorder is rarely found to be comorbid with AN, but likely to co-occur with BN (Hudson et al. 2007). For additional information on depression, see Chap. 6 in this volume.

Substance Use/Abuse

AN is frequently comorbid with substance abuse, and in the NCS-R study, was found to be significantly correlated with all types of substance use, with the exception of illicit drug dependence (Hudson et al. 2007; also see Chap. 9 in this volume for additional information on substance abuse).

Bulimia Nervosa

Anxiety

Like anorexia, BN has two subtypes: binge eating/purging type (BN-P) and nonpurging type (BN-NP). Both subtypes of bulimia also have a high comorbidity with anxiety disorders. In the NCS-R, BN was significantly comorbid with all of the anxiety disorders, with the exception of generalized anxiety disorder (Hudson et al. 2007).

Mood Disorders

Mood disorders are also frequently comorbid with BN, including bipolar disorder, which has been found to be more likely in bulimia inpatients than outpatients (Godart et al. 2007). Bipolar II in particular seems to be significantly correlated with BN. BN has also been found to be significantly correlated with major depression and dysthymia (Hudson et al. 2007).

Substance Use/Abuse

Women with BN may be more likely to engage in substance use and/or abuse, particularly alcohol. Some studies have suggested that women with BN may be more likely to drink excessively and have comorbid alcohol use disorder than those without (Redgrave et al. 2007; Luce et al. 2007). BN has been found to be significantly correlated with any type of substance abuse, including alcohol and illicit drugs (Hudson et al. 2007).

Impulse Control Disorders

In the NCS-R, BN was also found to be comorbid with all impulse disorders except intermittent explosive disorder (Hudson et al. 2007).

Binge Eating Disorder

Perhaps surprisingly, due to the fact that BED has only recently received a DSM diagnosis as an eating disorder, in the NCS-R study it was found to be correlated with all anxiety, mood, impulse-control, and substance use disorders (Hudson et al. 2007).

Substance Use/Abuse

Based on self-report, women with BED reported significantly more weekend drinking than others, based on typical number of drinks (Luce et al. 2007). Women with

BED are more likely to binge drink and engage in increased drinking partially as a coping mechanism. This commonality of both binge eating and binge drinking may be indicative of a maladaptive coping mechanism.

Night Eating Syndrome

Although NES in specific was not included in the NCS-R study, other studies have reported on some of the comorbidities found with NES.

Substance Use/Abuse

Within psychiatric outpatient populations, NES was found in 12.9% of the sample. Higher rates of substance use disorders were found in patients with NES than those without (Lundgren et al. 2006).

Mood Disorders

NES is frequently associated with depression (Marshall et al. 2004) and low self-esteem (Gluck et al. 2001).

Other Eating Disorders

It is worth noting that literature on NES has frequently pointed out that NES has a low comorbidity with other eating disorders including AN and BN, therefore suggesting that NES may be fundamentally different than the other eating disorders typically studied.

Medical Complications

Table 7.3 depicts the medical complications for AN, BN, and BED. Generally speaking, health consequences of eating disorders are resultant of the associated disordered eating behaviors (e.g., food restriction, binging, purging).

Medical complications associated with AN and BN include electrolyte abnormalities due to potassium loss, cardiovascular abnormalities, gastrointestinal complications, osteopenia, reproductive function complications, pregnancy complications, dermatological issues, and dental complications (Abraham and Llewellyn-Jones 1995; Pomeroy and Mitchell 2002). Among female athletes, the combination of long-term restriction of caloric and fat intake, amenorrhea, and osteopenia is referred to as the "female athlete triad."

Table 7.3 Medical complications of eating disorders

Anorexia nervosa (AN)	Bulimia nervosa (BN)	Binge eating disorder (BED)
• Electrolyte complications • Cardiovascular complications – Low blood pressure – Slow heart rate – Dizziness – Fainting – Heart failure • Gastrointestinal complications – Enlarged parotid gland – Esophageal problems including rupture – Gastric rupture – Ulcers – Chronic irregular bowel movements and constipation from overuse and misuse of laxatives • Osteopenia • Reproductive and pregnancy complications – Infertility – Higher rates of miscarriage, complications during delivery, and postpartum depression – Low-birth weight baby • Skin complications – Growth of Lanugo (fine downy white hair growth on face) – Loss of hair on head – Dry skin – Brittle nails – Finger calluses • Dental complications	• Electrolyte complications • Cardiovascular complications – Low blood pressure – Slow heart rate – Dizziness – Fainting – Heart failure • Gastrointestinal complications – Enlarged parotid gland – Esophageal problems including rupture – Gastric rupture – Ulcers – Chronic irregular bowel movements and constipation from overuse and misuse of laxatives • Osteopenia • Reproductive and pregnancy complications – Infertility – Higher rates of miscarriage, complications during delivery, and postpartum depression – Low-birth weight baby • Skin complications – Loss of hair on head – Dry skin – Brittle nails – Finger calluses • Dental complications	• Cardiovascular complications – High blood pressure – Heart disease • Metabolic complications – High cholesterol • Endocrine complications – Type II diabetes – Gall bladder disease

With regard to BED, medical complications primarily are resultant of consistent binging behaviors which lead to obesity. As with obesity, medical complications include cardiovascular, hypercholesterolemia, Type II diabetes, and gallbladder disease (National Eating Disorders Association 2005b).

Treatment

Due to the multifaceted etiology of eating disorders, the most effective treatment involves a treatment team involving a mental health specialist, physician, and nutritionist. Under this approach, individual treatment plans will ultimately vary according to the severity of the disorder and the individual problems, needs, and strengths.

Anorexia Nervosa

The primary goal for treatment of AN is weight gain. Other goals also include increasing body satisfaction and decreasing the drive for thinness, decreasing over-exercising and bingeing/purging behaviors, and restoring menstruation. Several methods have been used in treating AN, including psychotherapy, medication, hormone treatment, and combination treatments, each with varying success. The 5-year recovery rate for AN has been reported to be 66.8% for DSM-IV criteria, and 69.1% for broad criteria (Keski-Rahkonen et al. 2007).

The inclusion of zinc supplements with other therapy has also shown success in helping to restore a more appropriate body mass index. Zinc may have a positive impact on the neurotransmitters in the brain, and thus help normalize the activity of the amygdala, which is frequently abnormal in anorexia patients (Birmingham and Gritzner 2006). To be comprehensive, treatment of AN should be multidimensional, including mental health treatment, dietary supervision and education, and medical attention for complications of weight loss.

A systematic review of treatments for AN conducted by Bulik et al. (2007) reported the following results. Treatment of AN with medication only is not well advised, particularly based on the significant need for increased weight in anorexia patients, which medication does not address. Cognitive-behavioral therapy (CBT) shows positive results for reducing relapse into AN for adult patients after restoring weight. Family therapy has shown some positive results for younger patients with AN including weight gain and psychological improvements.

Bulimia Nervosa

Main goals of BN treatment include reducing both binge eating and compensatory behavior. Compensatory behaviors may include vomiting, inappropriate use of laxatives or diuretics, fasting, and overexercising. In addition to these, goals of treatment include increases in body satisfaction and decreases in anxiety and depressive symptoms. Frequent side effects of BN include dental destruction; therefore, dental attention should also be included as part of a treatment plan.

Methods for treating BN have primarily included medication, psychotherapy, and combination treatments, although light therapy has been tested as well. The success rates of each of these treatments have been inconclusive to a best or most effective treatment.

A systematic review of treatment studies for BN by Shapiro et al. (2007) reported that medication treatment has most frequently included fluoxetine, an antidepressant which has shown positive results for decreasing binge eating, purging, and depressive mood, and improvements in weight concern, food preoccupation, drive for thinness, and body satisfaction. These results have generally been found to sustain over up to 16 weeks. Fluoxetine in combination with CBT was superior to medication alone at reducing vomiting frequency and weekly objective and subjective binge and vomit episodes. Fluoxetine, both alone and in combination with a self-help book, showed decreased objective bingeing, vomiting, restrained eating, and depression.

In addition to CBT, family therapy has received some attention in the BN treatment literature (Shapiro et al. 2007). However, in a direct comparison of CBT-guided self-care and family therapy, CBT showed an advantage in reducing binge eating faster and at lower cost. In addition, adolescents were more accepting of CBT-guided self-care, as family involvement in treatment was not always supported by young participants. Both therapies showed improvements in bingeing and vomiting over 6 and 12 months.

Binge Eating Disorder

BED shares the binge eating component of bulimia, but lacks the compensatory behaviors. Thus, women with BED rarely suffer from the same low body weight problems associated with AN and BN, but frequently struggle with obesity. Therefore, in addition to eliminating binge eating, other goals of treatment for BED include weight loss, rather than weight gain, and reduction in dietary restraint, depression, and anxiety. Typical treatments for BED have included medication, behavioral therapy, combination treatment, and infrequently, virtual reality. However, it should be noted that currently none of these treatments has been approved by the FDA for treatment of BED (McElroy et al. 2007).

One of the newer drug treatments for BED is Topiramate. This has been shown to have positive impacts on reducing frequency of binge eating, illness severity, obsessive eating-related thoughts, and weight (Brownley et al. 2007). Another study found that both reduced binge eating and weight loss were sustained at a 42-week follow-up (McElroy et al. 2004).

Systematic reviews of BED treatments by Brownley et al. (2007) found the following results. Similar to its effects on bulimia, fluoxetine decreased weekly bingeing frequency, illness severity and depression, and was also associated with less weight gain. Combinations of CBT and fluoxetine revealed combination therapy was superior at decreasing hunger and weight concerns, and depressive mood. Studies using fluvoxamine, another antidepressant, have shown reductions in binge eating frequency and BMI, and improvements in illness severity. Combination therapy and medication studies were not reported with fluvoxamine.

In general, the review by Brownley et al. (2007) found that selective serotonin reuptake inhibitors (SSRIs) indicated some reduction in binge eating and weight symptoms, and that sibutramine and topiramate specifically showed good results for weight reduction. CBT was also effective in reducing binge eating episodes and reported binge eating days. This appears to lead to a greater rate of abstinence from binge eating at 4-month follow-ups. In addition, CBT is superior at also reducing the psychological components including hunger and disinhibition, but not self-rated depressive symptoms.

Night Eating Syndrome

Although NES has not been as widely studied as the other eating disorders discussed in this chapter, the recent primary treatment for NES has included in particular an SSRI (Sertraline). Like BED, NES is associated with obesity, and therefore goals include weight loss.

One study of Sertraline for NES resulted in significant decreases in number of night awakenings, number of nocturnal ingestions, and percentage of calories ingested after dinner (O'Reardon et al. 2004). Stress reduction has also been implicated as an additional treatment for NES, with some studies suggesting that night eating is related to increased stress and depression (Pawlow et al. 2003).

Cost of Treatment

The cost of treatment for eating disorders has been researched and compared to other mental disorders.

The cost of AN treatment has been found to be similar to the cost of treatment for schizophrenia, but higher than the treatment cost for OCD; the cost of treatment for BN was found to be significantly lower than for schizophrenia but higher than the OCD treatment cost; and the cost of treatment for EDNOS was found to be significantly lower than the treatment cost for schizophrenia, but similar to that for OCD (Striegel-Moore et al. 2000). These results were found through an analysis of private insurance claims, which likely had a significant impact on the number of cases that were included, since many insurance companies do not cover eating disorders. Inpatient and outpatient services were collapsed, which may have also had an impact on the comparison in costs of treatment.

Insurance Parity

As mentioned previously, despite the serious health implications presented by eating disorders, many insurance companies continue to deny coverage for treatment (National Eating Disorders Association 2006) even though research has demonstrated the cost effectiveness of early treatment (National Eating Disorders Association 2005a). As of 2008, only 17 states in the US mandate coverage for treatment of anorexia and bulimia (Rubin and Wiehle 2008). However, it is also important to ensure that the coverage provided is adequate to cover appropriate treatment.

It is theorized that one of the reasons that anorexia has such a high mortality rate is because eating disorders do not receive the appropriate long-term treatment (DeAngelis 2002). The average number of sessions that a health insurer will cover is 10–15 sessions for eating disorders, which is much lower than the recommendations of the American Psychiatric Association (Stein 2004).

Implications for Women's Mental Health

Despite low lifetime and 12-month prevalence estimates, eating disorders represent a serious public health concern because they are frequently associated with other mental disorders, increased morbidity, role impairment, and are often underdiagnosed and undertreated. For mothers with eating disorders, there is added impact on child development and family functioning. As mentioned previously, despite the serious health implications presented by eating disorders, many insurance companies continue to deny coverage for treatment (National Eating Disorders Association 2006) even though significant advances have been made in the development of psychological therapies for eating disorders and research has demonstrated the cost effectiveness of psychological treatments. Finding treatment for eating disorders remains a challenge because treatment is expensive, trained providers are scarce, and professional training in psychological treatment of eating disorders remains very limited (Wilson et al. 2007).

Further research aimed at the identification of risk and protective factors for eating disorders is needed for the development of prevention programs and the refinement of current therapies. In addition to continuing research to improve current prevention and therapy, researchers should continue to explore possible psychobiological mechanisms that impact and sustain eating disorders and identify mechanisms of therapeutic change. Such research holds the potential to improve treatment outcomes and women's prospects for improved mental health. At a societal level, wide-ranging messages from the media about acceptance of a variety of body shapes and sizes could also have a positive impact. Finally, every effort should be made to expand insurance coverage for the treatment of eating disorders and ensure the delivery of needed training for service providers.

References

Abraham, S., & Llewellyn-Jones, D. (1995). Sexual and reproductive function in eating disorders and obesity. In K. Brownell & C. Fairburn (Ed.), *Eating disorders and obesity: A comprehensive handbook* (pp. 281–288). New York, NY: The Guilford Press.

American Psychiatric Association. (1994). *Diagnostic and statistical manual of mental disorders* (4th ed.). Washington, DC: American Association Press.

Birmingham, C., & Gritzner, S. (2006). How does zinc supplementation benefit anorexia nervosa? *Eating and Weight Disorders, 11*(4), 109–111.

Brownley, K., Berkman, N. D., Sedway, J. A., Lohr, K. N., & Bulik, C. M. (2007). Binge eating disorder treatment: A systematic review of randomized controlled trials. *International Journal of Eating Disorders, 40,* 337–348.

Bulik, C., Berkman, N. D., Brownley, K. A., Sedway, J. A., & Lohr, K. N. (2007). Anorexia nervosa treatment: A systematic review of randomized controlled trials. *International Journal of Eating Disorders, 40,* 310–320.

Cavanaugh, C., & Lemberg, R. (1999). What we know about eating disorders: Facts and statistics. In R. Lemberg & L. Cohn (Eds.), *Eating disorders: A reference sourcebook* (pp. 7–11). Phoenix, AZ: The Oryx Press.

Chamorro, R., & Flores-Ortiz, Y. (2000). Acculturation and disordered eating patterns among Mexican American women. *International Journal of Eating Disorders, 25*(1), 65–70.

Crowther, J. H., Wolf, E. M., & Sherwood, N. (1992). Epidemiology of bulimia nervosa. In M. Crowther, D. L. Tennenbaum, S. E. Hobfoll, & M. A. P. Stephens (Eds.), *The etiology of bulimia nervosa: The individual and familial context* (pp. 1–26). Washington, DC: Taylor & Francis.

DeAngelis, T. (2002). Pressing for better insurance coverage for eating disorders. *Monitor on Psychology, 33*(3).

Fairburn, C., & Beglin, S. (1990). Studies of the epidemiology of bulimia nervosa. *American Journal of Psychiatry, 147,* 401–408.

Fairburn, C. G., Hay, P. J., & Welch, S. L. (1995). Binge eating and bulimia nervosa: Distribution and determinants. In C. G. Fairburn & G. T. Wilson (Eds.), *Binge eating: Nature, assessment, and treatment* (pp. 123–143). New York, NY: The Guilford Press.

French, S. A., Story, M., Neumark-Sztainer, D., Downes, B., Resnik, M. & Blum, R. (1997). Ethnic differences in psychosocial and health behavior correlates of dieting, purging, and binge eating in a population-based sample of adolescent females. *International Journal of Eating Disorders, 22*(3), 315–322.

Garfinkel, P. E., Lin, E., Goering, P., Spegg, C., Goldbloom, D., Kennedy, S., et al. (1995). Bulimia nervosa in a Canadian community sample: Prevalence and comparison subgroups. *American Journal of Psychiatry, 152,* 1052–1058.

Garfinkel, P. E., Lin, E., Goering, P., Spegg, C., Goldbloom, D., Kennedy, S., et al. (1996). Should amenorrhoea be necessary for the diagnosis of anorexia nervosa? Evidence from a Canadian community sample. *British Journal of Psychiatry, 168,* 500–506.

Gluck, M. E., Geliebter, A., & Satov, T. (2001). Night eating syndrome is associated with depression, low self-esteem, reduced daytime hunger, and less weight loss in obese outpatients. *Obesity Research, 9,* 264–267.

Godart, N., Flament, M. F., Curt, F., Perdereau, F., Lang, F., Venisse, J. L., et al. (2003). Anxiety disorders in subjects seeking treatment for eating disorders: A DSM-IV controlled study. *Psychiatry Research, 117*(3), 245–258.

Godart, N., Perdereau, F., Rein, Z., Berthoz, S., Wallier, J., Jeammet, P. H., et al. (2007). Comorbidity studies of eating disorders and mood disorders. Critical review of the literature. *Journal of Affective Disorders, 97,* 37–49.

Gordon, R. (1990). *Anorexia and bulimia: Anatomy of a social epidemic.* New York, NY: Blackwell.

Grucza, R. A., Przybeck, T. R., & Cloninger, C. R. (2006). Prevalence and correlates of binge eating disorder in a community sample. *Comprehensive Psychiatry, 48*(2), 124–131.

Hoek, H. W. (2002). Distribution of eating disorders. In C. G. Fairburn & K. D. Brownell (Eds.), *Eating disorders and obesity: A comprehensive handbook* (2nd ed., pp. 233–237). New York, NY: The Guilford Press.

Hoek, H. W., Bartelds, A. I., Bosveld, J. J., van der Graaf, Y., Limpens, V. E., Maiwald, M., et al. (1995). Impact of urbanization on detection rates of eating disorders. *American Journal of Psychiatry, 152,* 1272–1278.

Hoek, H., & van Hoeken, D. (2003). Review of the prevalence and incidence of eating disorders. *International Journal of Eating Disorders, 34,* 383–396.

Hudson, J. I., Hiripi, E., Pope, H. G. Jr., & Kessler, R. C. (2007). The prevalence and correlates of eating disorders in the National Comorbidity Survey Replication. *Biological Psychiatry, 61,* 348–358.

Jacobi, C. (2005). Psychosocial risk factors for eating disorders. In S. Wonderlich, J. Mitchell, M. de Zwann, & H. Steiger (Eds.), *Eating disorders review: Part 1* (pp. 59–86). Seattle, WA: Radcliffe Publishing.

Jane, D. M., Hunter, G. C., & Lozzi, B. M. (1999). Do Cuban American women suffer from eating disorders? Effects of media exposure and acculturation. *Hispanic Journal of Behavioral Sciences, 21*(2), 212–218.

Kaye, W., Bulik, C. M., Thorton, L., Barbarich, N., & Masters, K. (2004). Comorbidity of anxiety disorders with anorexia and bulimia nervosa. *American Journal of Psychiatry, 161,* 2215–2221.

Kazdin, A. E., Kraemer, H. C., Kessler, R. C., Kupfer, D. J., & Offord, D. R. (1997). Contributions of risk-factor research to developmental psychopathology. *Clinical Psychology Review, 17*(4), 375–406.

Kempa, M., & Thonas, A. (2000). Adolescent weight management and perceptions: An analysis of the National Longitudinal study of Adolescent Health. *Eating Disorders, 8,* 17–30.

Keski-Rahkonen, A., Hoek, H. W., Susser, E. S., Linna, M. S., Sihvola, E., Raevuori, A., et al. (2007). Epidemiology and course of anorexia nervosa in the community. *American Journal of Psychiatry, 164*(8), 1259–1265.

Kinzl, J. F., Traweger, C., Trefalt, E., Mangweth, B., & Biebl, W. (1999). Binge eating disorder in females: A population based investigation. *International Journal of Eating Disorders, 25,* 287–292.

Lucas, A. R., Crowson, C. S., O'Fallon, W. M., & Melton, L. J. III. (1999). The ups and downs of anorexia nervosa. *International Journal of Eating Disorders, 26,* 397–405.

Luce, K., Engler, P. A., & Crowther, J. H. (2007). Eating disorders and alcohol use: Group differences in consumption rates and drinking motives. *Eating Behaviors, 8,* 177–184.

Lundgren, J., Allison, K. C., Crow, S., O'Reardon, J. P., Berg, K. C., Galbraith, J., et al. (2006). Prevalence of the night eating syndrome in a psychiatric population. *American Journal of Psychiatry, 163,* 156–158.

Marshall, H. M., Allison, K. C., O'Reardon, J. P., Birketvedt, G., & Skunkard, A. J. (2004). Night eating syndrome among nonobese persons. *International Journal of Eating Disorders, 35,* 217–222.

McElroy, S., Hudson, J. I., Capece, J. A., Beyers, K., Fisher, A. C., & Rosenthal, N. R. (2007). Topiramate for the treatment of binge eating disorder associated with obesity: A placebo-controlled study. *Biological Psychiatry, 61,* 1039–1048.

McElroy, S., Shapira, N. A., Arnold, L. M., Keck, P. E., Rosenthal, N. R., Wu, S. C., et al. (2004). Topiramate in the long-term treatment of binge-eating disorder associated with obesity. *Journal of Clinical Psychiatry, 65,* 1463–1469.

National Eating Disorders Association. (2002). *Statistics: Eating disorders and their precursors.* http://www.nationaleatingdisorders.org

National Eating Disorders Association. (2005a). *Facts for activists.* Retrieved January 13, 2009, from http://www.nationaleatingdisorders.org

National Eating Disorders Association. (2005b). *Health consequences of eating disorders.* Retrieved January 13, 2009, from http://www.nationaleatingdisorders.org

National Eating Disorders Association. (2006). *Insurance issues.* Retrieved January 13, 2009, from http://www.nationaleatingdisorders.org

O'Reardon, J., Stunkard, A. J., & Allison, K. C. (2004). Clinical trial of sertraline in the treatment of night eating syndrome. *International Journal of Eating Disorders, 35,* 16–26.

Pawlow, L., O'Neil, P. M., & Malcolm, R. J. (2003). Night eating syndrome: Effects of brief relaxation training on stress, mood, hunger, and eating patterns. *International Journal of Obesity, 27*(8), 970–978.

Pomeroy, C., & Mitchell, J. (2002). Medical complications of anorexia nervosa and bulimia nervosa. In C. Fairburn & K. Brownell (Eds.), *Eating disorders and obesity: A comprehensive handbook* (pp. 278–285). New York, NY: The Guilford Press.

Redgrave, G., Coughlin, J. W., Heinberg, L. J., & Guarda, A. S. (2007). First-degree relative history of alcoholism in eating disorder patients: Relationship to eating and substance use psychopathology. *Eating Behaviors, 8,* 15–22.

Rossignol, A. (2007). *Principles and practice of epidemiology: An engaged approach.* New York, NY: McGraw Hill.

Rubin, B. M., & Wiehle, A. (2008, June 23). Anorexia, bulimia may soon become part of mandatory health insurance in Illinois. *Chicago Tribune.* Retrieved May 15, 2009, from http://www.timberlineknolls.com/news-20080623.asp

Schmidt, U. (2005). Epidemiology and aetiology of eating disorders. *Diagnosis, Epidemiology and Aetiology, 4*(4), 5–9.

Shapiro, J., Berkman, N. D., Brownley, K. A., Sedway, J. A., Lohr, K. N., & Bulik, C. M. (2007). Bulimia nervosa treatment: A systematic review of randomized controlled trials. *International Journal of Eating Disorders, 40,* 321–336.

Snyder, L. (1989). Health care needs of the adolescent: Position paper. *Annals of Internal Medicine.*

Soundy, T. J., Lucas, A. R., Suman, V. J., & Melton, L. J. (1995). Bulimia nervosa in Rochester, Minnesota from 1980–1990. *Psychological Medicine, 25*(5), 1065–1071.

Stein, M. K. (2004) National conference aims to increase awareness of eating disorders. *Eating Disorders Review, 15*(1), 6–7.

Striegel-Moore, R. H., Lesie, D., Petrill, S. A., Garvin, V., & Rosenheck, R. A. (2000). One-year use and cost of inpatient and outpatient services among female and male patients with an eating disorder: Evidence from a national database of health insurance claims. *International Journal of Eating Disorders, 27,* 381–389.

Sullivan, P. F. (1995). Mortality in anorexia nervosa. *American Journal of Psychiatry, 152,* 1073–1074.

Townsend, A. B. (2007). Night eating syndrome. *Holistic Nursing Practice, 21*(5), 217–221.

Turnbull, S., Ward, A., Treasure, J., Jick, H., & Derby, L. (1996). The demand for eating disorder care. An epidemiological study using the General Practice Research Database. *British Journal of Psychiatry, 169,* 705–712.

Wade, T., Bulik, C. M., Neale, M., & Kendler, K. S. (2000). Anorexia nervosa and major depression: Shared genetic and environmental risk factors. *American Journal of Psychiatry, 157,* 469–471.

Watkins, B., Willoughby, K., Waller, G., Serpell, L., & Lask, B. (2002). Pattern of birth in anorexia nervosa: Early-onset cases in the United Kingdom. *International Journal of Eating Disorders, 32,* 11–17.

Wilson, G. T., Grilo, C. M., & Vitousek, K. M. (2007). Psychological treatment of eating disorders. *American Psychologist, 62*(3), 199–216.

Chapter 8
Menopause

Tonita Wroolie and Megan Holcomb

Introduction

Menopause transition is an experience all women undergo either naturally or surgically. This chapter defines the stages of menopause including mental health conditions that have been studied in various populations during these life transition periods. Symptomatology including hot flashes, night sweats, insomnia, and psychiatric symptoms is outlined and examined. Theories about the relationship between menopause and depression such as hormonal fluctuations, psychosocial, and neurobiological factors are discussed along with evidence for and against such theories. Use of hormone/estrogen therapy and its effect on depression in perimenopausal and postmenopausal women is also discussed in this chapter. Surgical versus natural menopause is outlined with evidence suggesting many factors interplay with regard to depression and surgical menopause. Implications for treatment of various psychiatric disorders including anxiety, bipolar disorder, and schizophrenia are discussed. Finally, evidence is presented that shows an increase in sexual dysfunction during menopause transition due to multiple factors including no partner, depressed mood, or living with a child. Treatment implications are included to guide care providers working with women who are undergoing this stage of life change.

Menopause is defined as the permanent cessation of menstrual periods. It occurs naturally as part of the normal aging process or can be induced by surgery, chemotherapy, or radiation. According to the National Institutes of Health (NIH 2005), "natural menopause is recognized after 12 consecutive months without menstrual periods that are not associated with a physiologic (i.e., lactation or pregnancy) or pathologic cause." Perimenopause is the period of transition from regular menstrual cycles to amenorrhea (Rapkin et al. 2002). During this transition, intermittent ovula-

---

T. Wroolie (✉)
Department of Psychiatry and Behavioral Sciences,
Center for Neuroscience in Women's Health,
Stanford University, School of Medicine,
401 Quarry Road, Stanford, CA 94305-5723, USA

B. L. Levin, M. A. Becker (eds.), *A Public Health Perspective of Women's Mental Health*,
DOI 10.1007/978-1-4419-1526-9_8, © Springer Science+Business Media LLC 2010

tion causes hormone levels to fluctuate erratically and menses to become irregular. The World Health Organization and the Stages of Reproductive Aging Workshop (Soules et al. 2001) define menopause transition as "the time of an increase in follicle-stimulating hormone and increased variability in cycle length, two skipped menstrual cycles with 60 or more days of amenorrhea (absence of menstruation), or both. The menopausal transition concludes with the final menstrual period (FMP) and the beginning of postmenopause." However, postmenopause is not recognized until 12 months of amenorrhea.

Natural menopause (i.e., time of the FMP) typically occurs between the ages of 48 and 52 years with a median age of 51.4 years, but can range from 35 to 58 years (Avis and McKinlay 1991, 1995; Burt et al. 1998; McKinlay 1996). The median age for onset of perimenopause is 47.5 years (McKinlay 1996) and this transitional period usually lasts around 4 or 5 years (Burger et al. 2007; McKinlay 1996), but can last up to 10–15 years (Morrison et al. 2006). Menopause prior to age 45 is classified as early (Burger et al. 2007). Factors shown to be associated with early menopause include cigarette smoking, chronic disease, hysterectomy, and adverse socioeconomic conditions (Chang et al. 2007; Harlow and Signorello 2000; Wise et al. 2002). Approximately 1% of women experience menopause very early (prior to age 40) and these women are defined as having premature ovarian failure (Coulam et al. 1986).

Symptoms

Symptom profiles of women transitioning into menopause range from little or no symptoms to severe or even disabling symptoms (NIH 2005), and more than 80% of women experience some degree of menopausal symptoms (McKinlay and Jefferys 1974). Vasomotor symptoms (VMS), including hot flashes/flushes and night sweats, are the most commonly reported menopause transition symptoms. Hot flashes are experienced as a spontaneous sensation of warmth sometimes preceded or accompanied by palpitations, perspiration, nausea, dizziness, anxiety, headache, weakness, or a feeling of suffocation. Other commonly reported symptoms include sleep disturbance, vaginal dryness and painful intercourse, urinary problems, cognitive complaints, sexual dysfunction, and uterine bleeding (Nelson et al. 2006). Psychiatric symptoms such as feeling blue are also prevalent among women going through menopause transition.

The Menopause Epidemiology Study found that amongst women in the US, VMS prevalence was 79% during perimenopause and 65% during postmenopause (Williams et al. 2008). VMS, such as hot flashes and night sweats, tend to occur intermittently and often decrease in frequency during postmenopause but may continue for decades; however, their intensity typically declines over time (Rödström et al. 2002). Some women experience severe VMS during menopause transition, and thus may seek medical advice for the management of symptoms.

Women transitioning into menopause are more likely to report difficulty sleeping compared to premenopausal women (Bromberger et al. 2003; Kuh et al. 1997).

Previous research has established numerous factors associated with poor sleep including ethnicity, VMS, psychological symptoms, self-perceived health, health behaviors, arthritis pain, and educational level (Kravitz et al. 2003).

A factor analytic evaluation of self-reported perimenopausal symptoms in the longitudinal Seattle Midlife Women's Health Study found that menopause symptoms could be classified into five separate categories including vasomotor, somatic, neuromuscular, insomnia, and dysphoric mood (Mitchell and Woods 1996). However, many symptoms in perimenopause are not unique to the transition, suggesting a considerable overlap with medical and psychiatric problems. Mitchell and Woods (1996) evidenced persistent dysphoric mood across a 3-year time period, suggesting that these symptoms may result from chronic high levels of stress and/or longstanding emotional illness. Similarly, neuromuscular and insomnia symptoms were stable across time and associated with underlying chronic physical conditions. In contrast, vasomotor and somatic symptoms varied over time and are likely due to hormonal fluctuations and acute episodic illness.

Menopause involves not only biological and reproductive changes, but psychological and social changes as well. Biological changes, within the context of the psychosocial and cultural environment, influence the extent to which a woman is affected by the end of her reproductive life. For example, North American women tend to report twice as many menopausal symptoms as Japanese women (Avis et al. 1993). In Western cultures, particularly in Europe and the USA, women in lower socioeconomic classes report a higher frequency and severity of symptoms. However, in Asia, the reverse is true as increased reports of symptom frequency and severity occur in women in higher socioeconomic classes (Dennerstein 1996). This suggests that factors other than just physical symptoms affect how women experience and interpret menopause. In fact, in the large community-based Study of Women's Health Across the Nation (SWAN) longitudinal study in the USA, African-American, Chinese, and Japanese middle-aged women reported less mood symptoms than Caucasian women (Bromberger et al. 2003).

Ethnic background often precludes how women adjust to and interpret the end of their reproductive life. For instance, one community-based study in a sample of African-American and Caucasian women found that African-American women reported significantly more positive attitudes regarding well-being, sexuality, and physical changes (Pham et al. 1997). This group was also more apt to view menopause as a relief from worry about becoming pregnant. Caucasian women on the other hand were more apt to view menopause as a medical problem that may require treatment.

Menopause Transition and Depression

Most of the literature that pertains to psychiatric symptoms during the menopause transition focuses on mood symptoms, particularly depression. Although most women going through menopause transition do not develop clinical depression

(Schmidt and Rubinow 2006), studies do suggest a greater incidence of depressive mood disturbances during menopause transition when compared to the premenopausal (Cohen et al. 2006; Freeman et al. 2004; Schmidt et al. 2004a) and postmenopausal periods (Schmidt and Rubinow 2006). In a subset of their original population-based sample, Freeman et al. (2006) found a fourfold increase in significant depressive symptoms (CES-D scores >16) and a 2.5-fold increase in the diagnosis of depression in women during perimenopause compared to premenopause. Women appear to be even more vulnerable to depression during the late perimenopause period. In a prospective evaluation of 29 asymptomatic, regularly cycling premenopausal women monitored for an average of 5 years until at least 6 months of amenorrhea, Schmidt et al. (2004a) found a 14-fold increase in depression onset in the 24 months surrounding the last menstrual period.

In addition, community-based longitudinal studies confirm that up to 10% of women report mood fluctuations and an increase in mild depressive symptoms (Hunter 1992; Matthews 1992; Martens et al. 2001; Woods et al. 2002). The largest community-based study to date (SWAN) examined the association between menopausal status and persistent mood symptoms. Women during early perimenopause were found to have higher rates (14.9–18.4%) of irritability, nervousness, and frequent mood changes as compared to the rates of mood symptoms in premenopausal women (8–12%); additionally, these symptoms were particularly prominent in women with lower educational attainment (Bromberger et al. 2003).

There are several risk factors associated with an increased vulnerability to depression onset during perimenopause, the most significant being a prior history of depression (Amore et al. 2004; Dennerstein 1996). Other risk factors include a personal or family history of a psychiatric disorder, social stress, impaired health (Rapkin et al. 2002), a history of distress during other hormonal events (Stewart and Boydell 1993), and VMS (Avis et al. 2001; Cohen et al. 2006). There is also evidence suggesting that during this time, the vulnerability to depression is increased in women without a history of depression (Freeman et al. 2004; Harlow et al. 2003), particularly when transition into menopause occurs at an early age (<40 years) (Harlow et al. 1995; Liao et al. 2000) or has a longer (>27 months) duration (Avis et al. 1994).

Several theories have been posited to explain why vulnerability to depression increases during perimenopause. The psychosocial theory suggests that depression is the result of a reaction to the numerous life changes that commonly occur during the same time as menopause transition. This theory postulates that the subjective experiences regarding the changes in role relationships interact and trigger mood symptoms, which consequently spiral into depression (Rapkin et al. 2002). Changes in estrogen levels that occur during perimenopause also give rise to physical symptoms such as hot flashes/flushes, night sweats, insomnia, and emotional lability. The "domino" theory posits that these emotional and physical changes from hormonal instability, in conjunction with poor understanding of their cause, trigger the symptoms of depression (Campbell and Whitehead 1977). More recently, it has been hypothesized that depression and VMS share physiological mechanisms that are both influenced by the hormonal changes seen during menopause transition (Cohen et al. 2006). The neurobiological theory of perimenopausal depression relates to the biochemical changes occurring during this transitional period. This theory proposes that declining estrogen levels influence neurotransmitters (i.e., dopamine, serotonin, and others) in the brain, causing a significant increase in depressive symptoms.

Psychosocial Factors

Stressful life events are associated with the onset of depression in women (Maciejewski et al. 2001), and both perceived stress and exposure to more stressful events are associated with mood complaints in women during the menopause transition (Kaufert et al. 1992; Schmidt et al. 2004b). Women with histories of early stressful life events (e.g., maltreatment, poverty, chronic illness) are particularly vulnerable to depression that may be exacerbated during perimenopause (see Alexander et al. (2007) for a review).

Women in perimenopause often undergo numerous psychosocial transitions that may cause distress and provoke symptoms of depression. Potential stressors at midlife include undesired childlessness, relationship difficulties, divorce or widowhood, changes in physical appearance, adjusting to adolescent or adult children, onset of personal or familial medical problems, and responsibility for both children and elders at the same time in addition to career and educational pressures (Kaufert et al. 1992). Many women transition through these life changes without developing depression; however, difficulties arise as a consequence of negative attitudes toward aging and menopause and when life changes associated with menopause transition are interpreted as negative stressors (Avis and McKinlay 1991; Dennerstein et al. 2004). As concerns and worries about commonly encountered psychosocial disruptions heighten, clinical manifestations of anxiety and depression may develop (McKinlay et al. 1987; Kaufert et al. 1992; Avis and McKinlay 1991).

The "empty nest" syndrome, related to children becoming adults and leaving home, often triggers feelings of loss. When maladjustment to the empty nest is present, marital conflict may ensue as spouses withdraw from one another (El-Guebaly et al. 1984). Physical changes associated with menopause may also impact libido with resultant sexual withdrawal, further negatively influencing a woman's marital relationship and self-concept/esteem (El-Guebaly et al. 1984). Marital stress can also be related to, or the result of, adolescent children rebelling against parental figures, an increase in physical illness in oneself or partner, and adopting the role of caretaker for aging or ailing parents (Dennerstein 1996). Women also face greater choices in terms of career opportunities and daily schedules, and they may feel overwhelmed by decisions and possibilities (El-Guebaly et al. 1984).

There is some support to show that factors other than life changes are responsible for the development of depression during menopause transition. One longitudinal study found no difference in frequency of real or perceived losses (e.g., death of a loved one, divorce, child leaving home) at 6 months prior to a depressive episode or at any other time during the study; however, these events significantly amplified the negative impact on mood for women during menopause transition (Schmidt et al. 2004b). Although psychosocial variables may not fully account for depression during menopause transition, many studies do show a relationship. For example, women having to adjust to significant role changes in the context of children, spouses, and parents report feeling less satisfied with the meaning of their role than women in earlier stages of development (Deeks and McCabe 2004).

Several studies also demonstrate that psychosocial variables affect symptom reporting and subjective well-being during menopause transition. In a sample of nearly 2,000 Australian women, Dennerstein et al. (1994) found that menopausal status did not affect perceived well-being, whereas psychological and lifestyle characteristics did. Lower levels of reported symptomatology were associated with more education, better health and less medication use, less interpersonal stress, not currently smoking, regular exercise, and positive attitudes toward aging and menopause. Various social parameters including low perceived stress, living with a partner, and daily exercise were similarly positively associated with well-being (Dennerstein et al. 1999).

Conversely, negative mood and negative attitudes toward aging and menopause, as well as currently being a smoker, were associated with increased interpersonal stress. Psychosocial variables also appear to affect self-rated health. Smith et al. (1994) found that positive self-reported health was correlated with older age, full-time employment, being separated or divorced, and regular exercise. On the other hand, women who worried about job and income, and/or experienced the recent death of a loved one, reported more ill health-related symptoms. Women who report poor health are shown to be four times more likely to become depressed than women who report good heath (Kaufert et al. 1992). These studies demonstrate that symptom reporting is not merely due to the physical symptoms associated with hormone changes, but that lifestyle, stressors, and personal interpretation also have a significant impact on a woman's perceived health.

Problems relating to life changes during menopause are often a focus in research; however, these same changes can be positively interpreted by some women. Rather than eliciting a negative response, children leaving home may result in a feeling of relief, newfound freedom, increased creativity, and career opportunities (El-Guebaly et al. 1984; Deeks and McCabe 2004). Deeks and McCabe (2004) studied 304 women in their 40s who were in pre-, peri-, or postmenopausal status. They consistently found that women appeared to experience more positive ratings of purpose in life compared to the prior 10 years. These women also reported that they experienced higher levels of self-acceptance and had greater confidence in the future than in the past. While some women find it difficult to cope and adapt to the life changes that occur during menopause transition, others utilize this phase as an opportunity for personal growth and positive transformation (El-Guebaly et al. 1984), thus challenging the notion that menopause is only associated with feelings of loss and negative change.

Hormonal Changes

Menopausal transition is marked by intermittent ovulation, causing hormone levels to fluctuate erratically and menses to become irregular. This changing hormonal milieu is thought to contribute to an increased susceptibility to depression, at least for some women (Freeman et al. 2004, 2006; Rasgon et al. 2005). Women with histories of mood symptoms during times of other hormonal events appear to have increased risk of depression during the menopause transition, supporting the theory that psychiatrically vulnerable women have an increased sensitivity to reproductive hormones. Psychological distress in perimenopause is also shown to be associated with a history of oral contraception dysphoria, premenstrual dysphoria, postnatal blues, and postpartum depression (Freeman et al. 2004; Stewart and Boydell 1993). In fact, 47.9% of women with histories of premenstrual complaints, attending a menopause outpatient clinic, were found to have psychiatric symptoms during peir-menopause (Novaes et al. 1998).

The interaction between estrogen levels and depression is complex, and there is no consistent evidence that demonstrates clear differences between women with and without perimenopausal depression. A variety of confounding factors are likely involved in the relationship between depression and estrogen status. For example, low serum estrogen levels are associated with decreased vigilance and abnormal frontal brain activation, which, in turn, is associated with increased depression (Saletu et al. 1996).

Some studies show that declining estrogen levels are associated with greater vulnerability to major depressive episodes (Almeida et al. 2005; Halbreich et al. 1995; Rehman and Masson 2005), whereas other studies have found that increasing estrogen levels, particularly in early menopause, are related to depressed moods (Freeman et al. 2004). On the other hand, one cross-sectional study compared women with first onset of depression during perimenopause to a nondepressed control group and found no differences between groups on measures of basal ovarian estrogens, testosterone, or gonadotropins, suggesting that estrogen is not the only factor associated with depression in perimenopause. The only difference found between these groups was lower levels of morning dehydroepiandrosterone (DHEA) in the depressed group (Schmidt et al. 2002).

These inconsistencies are clarified by findings from a longitudinal study that followed premenopausal women aged 35–47 years with normal menstrual cycles and without a history of depression for 8 years. The results revealed an increase in depression with (within-woman) estradiol variability, rather than absolute levels, during menopause transition when compared to premenopausal levels (Freeman et al. 2006). This study also found that overall increased (within-woman) levels and variability of FSH and LH were associated with higher rates of depression. Almeida et al. (2005) also evidenced that depression in older postmenopausal women was associated with decreased serum estradiol, but only when estradiol levels fell below a certain threshold.

Animal studies suggest that VMS are due to hormonal instability (Simpkins 1984). Women, who are anxious and/or depressed, are shown to have more prevalent VMS (Freeman et al. 2005; Joffe et al. 2002) with or without a prior history of depression (Avis et al. 1994). Cohen et al. (2006) also found that women who reported greater VMS had higher risks of developing depression during menopause transition than those without reported vasomotor complaints. Hot flashes and night sweats are also related to symptoms of mild depression including depressed mood, irritability, poor concentration, and fatigue due to sleep deprivation, as a result of VMS. Although physical symptoms are associated with perimenopausal depression, there is clear evidence that they do not solely account for the depression (Schmidt et al. 2004b).

Depressed mood is shown to be associated with menopausal stage (Cohen et al. 2006; Freeman et al. 2007; Schmidt et al. 2004a). Estrogen levels are declining and most unstable from late perimenopause to early postmenopause, and at this time there is a greater vulnerability to depression (Schmidt et al. 2004a). These researchers found that women who were depressed during this late transition period became less depressed when the transition was completed, presumably when estrogen levels stabilized.

A lengthier perimenopause also contributes to higher rates of depression. Data obtained from the Massachusetts Women's Health Study found that women who experienced a long perimenopausal period (at least 27 months) had an increased risk of depression (Avis et al. 1994). However, this association appeared to be transitory and the result of increased menopausal symptoms. Another study found that women with a rapidly increasing follicle-stimulating hormone profile, resulting in a shorter duration of perimenopause, were less likely to have depressive symptoms as well (Freeman et al. 2006).

A history of depression may, in turn, shorten overall reproductive life due to early decline in ovarian function. In a longitudinal study, Harlow et al. (2003) investigated the impact of lifetime history of major depression and evidenced that women aged 36–45 years with a history of depression had 1.2 times the rate of perimenopause compared to nondepressed women of the same age with no history of depression. Symptom severity was also associated with earlier menopause such that women with more marked depressive symptoms at study enrollment were twice as likely to enter into menopause earlier compared to women without a history of depression. Furthermore, women with greater depressive symptoms and reported antidepressant use had nearly three times the risk of early transition into menopause. Additionally, the group with depression histories had lower estradiol levels as well as higher levels of follicle-stimulating hormone and luteinizing hormone at study enrollment and follow-up. For additional information on depression, see Chap. 6 in this volume.

Neurobiological Factors

Neurobiological mechanisms may account for the most basic explanation of perimenopausal depression. Research has shown that estrogen impacts brain levels and metabolism of various neurotransmitters known to have a role in regulating emotion pathways, namely dopamine (Gordon1980), beta-endorphin (Kumar et al. 1979), norepinephrine (Ball et al. 1972) and serotonin (5-HT; Guicheney et al. 1988; Sherwin and Suranyi-Cadotte 1990). Estrogen appears to have a particular effect on multiple levels of the serotonergic system (Cone et al. 1981; Biegon

1990), increasing sites for transport of serotonin into neurons and producing a greater number of binding sites (Sherwin and Suranyi-Cadotte 1990), therefore leading to a higher overall level of serotonin in the brain (Guicheney et al. 1988). The role of serotonin in mood disorders has been well documented, especially in women, who seem to be more likely to develop depressive symptoms as a result of lower levels of 5-HT when compared to men (Booij et al. 2002; Moreno et al. 2006). The findings taken together suggest that lower levels of estrogen during perimenopause could increase the likelihood of developing depressive symptoms during this period.

It is also thought that the changing hormonal environment directly affects neurobiological mechanisms and increases the risk of depression during the menopause transition independent of previous history, physiological difficulties, or psychosocial stressors. During perimenopause, menstrual cycles occur more frequently due to extreme fluctuations in estradiol and progesterone levels (Santoro et al. 1996), and this instability may have a direct impact on brain function and increased susceptibility to depressive disorders. Another possible underlying etiology of the higher rates of mood disorders in women during the menopausal stages is that, unlike the male brain, the female brain must adjust to and function in response to fluctuating hormone levels (Deecher et al. 2008). This requires a certain development of flexibility during puberty and throughout the reproductive years in response to cyclical and timed changes in the neuroendocrine system. Even greater flexibility is required during the menopausal transition in response to disruption of the normal cycle and unpredictable ovarian hormone levels (Santoro et al. 1996). It is possible that the brain's inability to rapidly adjust to these changes in estradiol and progesterone levels increases the risk for mood disorders and depressive symptoms (Deecher et al. 2008).

It has been hypothesized that mood disorders and VMS share an underlying etiology related to hormonal changes and associated pathways (Cohen et al. 2006). Not only is adaptation to changing hormone levels required for mood stabilization, it is also required for maintaining normal temperature regulation. During postmenopause, in the absence of cyclical levels of ovarian hormones, a new baseline level of homeostasis is established and VMS are reduced. Since the risk for mood disorders is greatest during perimenopause and declines during postmenopause (Freeman et al. 2004, 2006), it has been hypothesized that an analogous hormonal adaptation process takes place. Thus, as postmenopausal women adapt to changing hormonal environments and "reset" their brain functions, their risk for developing depressive disorders decreases.

Estrogen/Hormone Therapy and Depression

The use of estrogen/hormone therapy (E/HT) in treatment of depression remains controversial, and few studies have examined its role in antidepressant response. Studies regarding the use of adjunctive E/HT in postmenopausal depression have yielded conflicting results (Amsterdam et al. 1999; Klaiber et al. 1979; Shapira et al. 1985), often due to differences in study design (retrospective versus prospective), differences in HT preparations (e.g., estrogen or estrogen plus progesterone, type of estrogen), heterogeneity of clinical populations with respect to severity of depressive illness, phase of menopause, and type of antidepressants used (e.g., tricyclics versus selective serotonin reuptake inhibitors (SSRIs)). For instance, no benefits were seen with the addition of ET in early investigations with tricyclic antidepressants or a more recent retrospective study of SSRIs in depressed women (Amsterdam et al. 1999; Prange et al. 1972; Shapira et al. 1985). In contrast, clinical placebo-controlled trials have demonstrated augmentation of antidepressant response in women on ET compared to women taking placebo (Klaiber et al. 1979; Schneider et al. 1997). In fact, some studies provide evidence that ET may even accelerate the response to antidepressants (Rasgon et al. 2007).

Menopause status (i.e. age and time since menopause) may also affect the antidepressant response to E/HT in the treatment of depression in women in midlife. In a review by Schmidt (2005), estrogen use was considered effective as an antidepressant agent in perimenopausal women with depressive symptoms but not for women who were 5–10 years postmenopause. Antidepressant response may be delayed in these older women due to normal age-related changes to the 5-HT (serotonin) as this system is known to contribute to the regulation of behavior and mood, particularly in affective disorders (Meltzer 1990; Schneider et al. 1997). ET may help to reduce depressive symptoms by enhancing serotonin synthesis, decreasing serotonin reuptake (Shors and Leuner 2003), augmenting serotonergic activity (Halbreich et al. 1995), and/or inhibiting of monoaminoxidase (MAO; Luine et al. 1975). ET has also been shown to increase the number of sites available for active transport of 5-HT into brain cells (Sherwin and Suranyi-Cadotte 1990). However, E/HT may not be adequate as a primary treatment for those with major depressive disorder, as established by severe symptomatology (Morrison et al. 2004; Schneider et al. 1997).

In contrast, the antidepressant effects of estrogen may be mitigated by HT preparations that contain progesterone (Soares et al. 2003). Progesterone may increase monoamine oxidase activity and GABA-inhibitory action resulting in mood-destabilization (Sherwin and Suranyi-Cadotte 1990). Progesterone is commonly prescribed in addition to estrogen for prevention of uterine cancer and most, if not all, studies use hormone preparations that contain progesterone.

Surgical Menopause

Although early clinical studies had reported that a hysterectomy often led to increased psychiatric and psychological difficulties, more recent research has found that this effect often depends on multiple variables, including premorbid level of functioning and mental health, reasons for surgery, and type of surgery (Shifren and Avis 2007).

One study compared a sample of women undergoing hysterectomy, before and after surgery, to gynecological outpatients and women in the general population (Davies and Doyle 2002). Although these women undergoing surgery had significantly elevated rates of depression, 6 months after surgery the prevalence of depression in this group was similar to the other populations, suggesting that hysterectomy did not lead to increased psychiatric morbidity. Another recent, large-scale study examined 1,100 women undergoing hysterectomy, assessing the participants before and after surgery (Kjerulff et al. 2000). Results suggested that for women with no history of psychiatric disorders, surgical menopause often led to improvements in mood, whereas mood symptoms were not alleviated in women with presurgical depression or emotional difficulties (Kjerulff et al. 2000). Two other studies found that there were no differences in depression or mood symptoms after surgery between women who had ovaries preserved, and women who had full hysterectomies (Aziz et al. 2005; Farquhar et al. 2006). However, one study examined hysterectomy and mental health with regard to loss of fertility and found that women who had desired a child presurgery exhibited significantly higher levels of depression and anxiety after surgery than women who had not wanted a child (Leppert et al. 2007). Therefore, there are numerous variables affecting postoperative mental health among women undergoing surgical menopause.

Implications for Treatment

The importance of establishing which women are at risk for perimenopausal depression is essential, since both major and minor depressions are associated with significant disability and morbidity (Schmidt and Rubinow 2006). Most women present to their primary care clinicians with symptoms of psychological problems before they consult a mental health professional (Landau and Milan 1996). Therefore, it is the responsibility of the primary care clinician to be aware of various difficulties women experience in midlife. Women may experience beginning or worsening of premenstrual syndrome or onset of other numerous physical and psychological symptoms as early as 35 without recognizing that they are associated with perimenopause (NAMS 2000), and education and anticipatory guidance from healthcare providers, especially with women in their 30s, can often help to alleviate the distress related to these symptoms.

Because prior history of depression is a strong predictive risk factor for perimenopausal depression (for a review, see Burt et al. (1998)), primary care clinicians should conduct careful psychosocial assessments with women reporting mood disturbances. These assessments should cover changes in mood, appetite, sleep, energy, sexual functioning, concentration, memory, and suicidal thoughts, as well as mood disturbances particularly related to other periods of hormonal fluctuations (e.g., premenstrual, pregnancy, postpartum, or during use of oral contraceptives). Additionally, because some medications and substances are related to depression, documentation of dose and frequency should be included in the assessment.

There are various options available for perimenopausal women with depression. Nonpharmocalogical methods often target coping with stress and include relaxation, daily exercise (yoga may be particularly beneficial), healthy diet, and self-care in addition to enjoyable activities, creative outlets, and psychological support/therapy. If nonpharmocalogical methods do not alleviate vasomotor and psychological disturbances, HT may be beneficial, especially for women whose mood is affected by hormonal fluctuations (Soares et al. 2003). Additionally, clinical depression may require psychopharmacological treatments.

In summation, women at midlife experience various physical and psychosocial transitions that may be related to symptoms of depression, which are often presented first to primary care clinicians (NAMS 2000). By increasing awareness, education, and guidance related to this phase of transition, clinicians may decrease the distress associated with symptoms of perimenopause.

Other Psychiatric Disorders and Menopause Transition

Although most research on the menopausal transition has focused on unipolar depression and depressive symptoms, a few studies have examined the relationship between menopause and other psychiatric disorders such as anxiety, schizophrenia, and bipolar disorder. The relationship between menopause and these disorders remains unclear and further research is certainly warranted.

Sajatovic et al. (2006) examined expectations and concerns regarding menopause in women with schizophrenia/schizoaffective disorder, bipolar disorder, or major depressive disorder. Slightly more than half of the total sample believed they felt more stressed due to menopause or approaching menopause and that menopause negatively affected their emotional state. Nearly 80% of the total sample reported feeling depressed, anxious, tired or worn out and lacking energy. Additionally, these women showed deficits in knowledge regarding menopause. In a similar sample of severely chronically mentally ill women, frequent vasomotor, psychosocial, physical, and sexual symptoms were reported; however, the women with major depression reported these symptoms more often (Friedman et al. 2005).

Anxiety

The relationship between anxiety symptoms and menopause has been examined in several studies, although it is often difficult to separate anxiety symptoms from the experience of depression. Almeida et al. (2005) found that lower levels of serum estradiol and estrone were associated with increased anxiety symptoms in a sample of older postmenopausal women (mean age of 74.6 years). In a longitudinal study that followed 238 women over a 6-year period, a strong association was shown between anxiety symptoms and hot flashes, even after controlling for menopausal stage, smoking status, BMI, race, age, time, estradiol levels, and depressive symptoms (Nelson et al. 2004). The same study noted that anxiety symptoms often preceded hot flashes.

Bipolar Disorder

Freeman et al. (2002) documented new onset and/or worsening of bipolar disorder during perimenopause. These researchers interviewed 50 women with a diagnosis of bipolar disorder and found three cases of new onset and 12 women reporting a worsening mood during the menopausal transition. These women reported an increase in depressive symptoms, and the majority also complained of increased irritability, hypomania or mania, and more rapid cycling. Women not on HT were more likely to report intensifying mood symptoms during perimenopause than women on HT, suggesting that HT may have a positive effect on mood stabilization and affect regulation. Other studies have similarly suggested that bipolar women cycle more rapidly during the perimenopausal period (Kukopulos et al. 1980) and that a significant percentage of postmenopausal women with bipolar disorder reported severe emotional distress during the menopausal transition (Blehar et al. 1998).

Schizophrenia

The course of schizophrenia also seems to be affected by the menopausal transition. A review by Lindamer et al. (1997) evidenced that a significantly higher percentage of women (37%) than men (16.4%) tend to develop schizophrenia after the age of 45, suggesting that late onset of schizophrenia for women seems to overlap with the beginning stages of menopause. Furthermore, in direct contrast to men, who experience predominantly negative symptoms, women experience more positive symptoms, such as hallucinations and delusions (Aloysi et al. 2006). Lindamer et al. (1997) examined a community sample of postmenopausal women diagnosed with schizophrenia and found that women with a history of HT were also receiving significantly lower doses of daily antipsychotic medications. These findings support earlier studies that suggested higher serum levels of estradiol may be related to decreased symptoms of thought disturbances (Riecher-Rossler et al. 1994; Hallonquist et al. 1993).

Implications for Treatment

Women with serious mental illness may be particularly vulnerable to the symptoms of menopause. Psychiatrists and other physicians should be aware of the overlap and increased frequency of both physical and emotional symptoms when planning treatment for this population of women during midlife (Friedman et al. 2005). Treating physicians should also address the deficits in knowledge regarding menopause seen in this population.

Sexuality and Menopause

The literature on sexual functioning in women in midlife is sparse and limited by factors such as study design, lack of validated measures, reliance on retrospective data and consideration of confounding variables such as hormone status. In addition, the effects of aging and menopause on sexual functioning are difficult to separate since they occur simultaneously. Both advancing age and menopause are associated with a decline in sexual functioning, particularly in sexual responsivity (Dennerstein et al. 2005b; Gracia et al. 2007). Decline in sexual functioning, however, does not necessarily denote sexual dysfunction since there may not be distress associated with functional decline. For instance, distress associated with loss of sexual desire has been shown to be inversely related to age (Graziottin 2007).

Sexual dysfunction is not uncommon in midlife, and population-based studies estimate 27–33% of middle-aged women may meet diagnostic criteria (Dennerstein et al. 2001; Gracia et al. 2007; Osborn et al. 1988). Sexual dysfunction appears to increase over the menopause transition with positive correlations between menopause status and ratings of sexual complaints in the domains of desire, arousal, lubrication, orgasm, satisfaction, and pain. Rates of sexual dysfunction are shown to be 2.4 and 2.3 times higher in women in late transition and postmenopause, respectively, compared to premenopausal women (Gracia et al. 2007). Common risk factors associated with sexual dysfunction include the absence of a sexual partner, negative feelings toward a partner, prior level of sexual function, decreased mood and/or increased anxiety, and living with a child under the age of 18 years (Dennerstein et al. 2005b; Gracia et al. 2007).

The role of hormones in sexual functioning in midlife has not been fully elucidated. However, a 3-year longitudinal study has shed some light on the role of hormones and sexuality in women transitioning into menopause. As part of the larger Penn Ovarian Aging Study, researchers found that after controlling for numerous covariates, low dehydroepiandrosterone sulfate (DHEAS) serum concentrations were associated with greater sexual dysfunction. Although FSH and LH increased over the study period, these hormones did not differentiate between women with and without sexual dysfunction. Findings regarding changes in estrogen or androgen levels in sexual dysfunction are inconclusive (Gracia et al. 2007), although Dennerstein et al. (2005a) found that declines in estradiol were related to sexual response and dyspareunia (pain during intercourse) although not to the extent of prior sexual functioning and relationship factors. On the other hand, common symptoms associated with hormonal changes in menopause transition are associated with decreased libido. Sleep disturbance, night sweats, and depressive symptoms are higher in women reporting decreased libido (Reed et al. 2007).

Sexuality in midlife is heterogeneous, and there are numerous emotional, psychological, and physiological factors that influence sexual desire and activity (as cited in Gracia et al. (2007)). However, decline in sexual interest appears to be related more to life circumstances and well-being than hormone and menopause status. Cross-sectional studies show that women seeking help for low sexual desire differ in terms of mental health (e.g., depression), personality factors (e.g., poor self-esteem), relationship quality, past sexual experiences, and physical health (Hartmann et al. 2004). Sexual functioning prior to menopause and variables related to sexual partners also appear to have a higher impact on sexuality than hormonal changes (Dennerstein et al. 2005a, b).

Shifren and Avis (2007) reviewed the literature regarding the effects of hysterectomy on psychological well-being and sexuality. They concluded that sexual functioning and well-being varied depending on preoperative problems and surgical procedure. Improvements were seen in well-being and sexual functioning following hysterectomy for benign disease. This is likely due to remediation of the problems related to the need for surgery. Libido tended to worsen, however, for women who underwent bilateral salpingo-oophorectomy (removal of both ovaries). Finally, existence of depression or sexual problems prior to hysterectomy was associated with postoperative worsening of mood and libido.

Hartmann et al. (2004) found that older women were more satisfied in their relationships albeit less physically connected to their partners compared to younger women. Women in older cohorts tend to have more restrictive ideas of sexuality and greater negative associations with sex due to the conservative societal norms present during their upbringing (Hartmann et al. 2004). Conformance to the social modeling to which they were exposed may lead to difficulty openly discussing sexual experiences as well as actively pursuing their own sexual satisfaction (Wood et al. 2007). This learned lack of "social agency" has sizeable health implications for women since it may prevent them from seeking out assistance for lowered sex drives, vaginal dryness, and other problems that may occur during middle and older age (Wood et al. 2007).

Implications for Treatment

Since problems with sexual functioning in the various stages of menopause are due to multiple etiologies, multifactorial assessment is warranted. Treatment teams that address biological, psychological, and relational issues produce the most favorable outcomes (Wylie et al. 2007). Evaluation of sexuality in menopausal women should include a thorough history of sexual experiences, trauma, and partner-related feelings of intimacy. Use of validated measures such as the Female Sexual Function Index (Rosen et al. 2000) are useful in determining problems related to desire, arousal, lubrication, orgasm, satisfaction, and pain. Cutoff scores of 20 are thought to provide a conservative estimate of sexual dysfunction in menopausal and perimenopausal woman (Wiegel et al. 2005).

Implications for Women's Mental Health

Previous medical and mental health conditions may negatively affect women transitioning through menopause. Caucasian women are shown to have more difficulty with this transition and therefore may seek mental health treatment in greater numbers. In particular, women are more vulnerable to depression during the late perimenopausal period and/or when they experience a longer transition into menopause. It is important for medical and mental health providers to understand mental health symptoms in relation to the status of menopause transition status. Health providers need to thoroughly assess for difficulties in current life circumstances (e.g., depressed mood, empty nest, marital difficulty, work stressors), past medical and mental health backgrounds (previous history of mood disorder, history of cigarette smoking) in order to address the increased vulnerability of mood disturbance during this period of life. Because women typically seek relief from menopause symptoms from primary care providers, standard practice should involve thorough assessment of mood and physical symptoms. Sexual dysfunction is also often associated with various stages of menopause; therefore practitioners should be sensitive to these changes as well. Educating clinicians about the development and/or exacerbation of mental health issues will serve to improve treatment outcomes.

References

Alexander, J. L., Dennerstein, L., Woods, N. F., McEwen, B. S., Halbreich, U., Kotz, K., et al. (2007). Role of stressful life events and menopausal stage in wellbeing and health. *Expert Review of Neurotherapies, 7*(Suppl. 11), 93–113.

Almeida, O. P., Lautenschlager, N., Vasikaram, S., Leedman, P., & Flicker, L. (2005). Association between physiological serum concentration of estrogen and the mental health of community-dwelling postmenopausal women age 70 years and over. *American Journal of Geriatric Psychiatry, 13*(2), 142–149.

Aloysi, A., Van Dyk, K., & Sano, M. (2006). Women's cognitive and affective health and neuropsychiatry. *Mount Sinai Journal of Medicine, 73*(7), 967–975.

Amore, M., Di Donato, P., Papalini, A., Berti, A., Palareti, A., Ferrari, G., et al. (2004). Psychological status at the menopausal transition: An Italian epidemiological study. *Maturitas, 48*(2), 115–124.

Amsterdam, J., Garcia-España, F., Fawcett, J., Quitkin, F., Reimherr, F., Rosenbaum, J., et al. (1999). Fluoxetine efficacy in menopausal women with and without estrogen replacement. *Journal of Affective Disorders, 55,* 11–17.

Avis, N. E., Brambilla, D., McKinlay, S. M., & Vass, K. (1994). A longitudinal analysis of the association between menopause and depression: Results from the Massachusetts Women's Health Study. *Annals of Epidemiology, 4*(3), 214–220.

Avis, N. E., Crawford, S., Stellato, R., & Longcope, C. (2001). Longitudinal study of hormone levels and depression among women transitioning through menopause. *Climacteric, 4*(3), 243–249.

Avis, N. E., Kaufert, P. A., Lock, M., McKinlay, S. M., & Vass, K. (1993). The evolution of menopausal symptoms. *Baillieres Clinical Endocrinology and Metabolism, 7*(1), 17–32.

Avis, N. E., & McKinlay, S. M. (1991). A longitudinal analysis of women's attitudes toward the menopause: Results from the Massachusetts Women's Health Study. *Maturitas, 13*(1), 65–79.

Avis, N. E., & McKinlay, S. M. (1995). The Massachusetts Women's Health Study: An epidemiologic investigation of the menopause. *Journal of American Medical Women's Association, 50*(2), 45–49.

Aziz, A., Brannstrom, M., Berquist, C., & Silfverstolpe, G. (2005). Perimenopausal androgen decline after oophorectomy does not influence sexuality or psychological well-being. *Fertility and Sterility, 83,* 1021–1028.

Ball, P., Knuppen, R., Haupt, M., & Breuer, H. (1972). Interactions between estrogens and catechol amines. 3. Studies on the methylation of catechol estrogens, catechol amines and other catechols by the ctechol-O-methyltransferases of human liver. *Journal of Clinical Endocrinology Metabolism, 34*(4), 736–746.

Biegon, A. (1990). Effects of steroid hormones on the serotonergic system. *Annals of the New York Academy of Sciences, 600,* 426–432.

Blehar, M. C., DePaulo, J. R. Jr., Gershon, E. S., Reich, T., Simpson, S. G., & Nurnberger, J. I. Jr. (1998). Women with bipolar disorder: Findings from the NIMH Genetics Initiative sample. *Psychopharmacology Bulletin, 34*(3), 239–243.

Booij, L., Van Der Does, W., Benkelfat, C., Bremner, J. D., Cowen, P. J., Fava, M., et al. (2002). Predictors of mood response to acute tryptophan depletion. A reanalysis. *Neuropsychopharmacology, 27*(5), 852–861.

Bromberger, J. T., Assmann, S. F., Avis, N. E., Schocken, M., Kravitz, H. M., & Cordal, A. (2003). Persistent mood symptoms in a multiethnic community cohort of pre- and perimenopausal women. *American Journal of Epidemiology, 158*(4), 347–356.

Burger, H., Woods, N. F., Dennerstein, L., Alexander, J. L., Kotz, K., & Richardson, G. (2007). Nomenclature and endocrinology of menopause and perimenopause. *Expert Review of Neurotherapies, 7*(Suppl. 11), 35–43.

Burt, V. K., Alshuler, L. L., & Rasgon, N. (1998). Depressive symptoms in the perimenopause: Prevalence, assessment, and guidelines for treatment. *Harvard Review of Psychiatry, 6,* 121–132.

Campbell, S., & Whitehead, M. (1977). Oestrogen therapy and the menopausal syndrome. *Clinics in Obstetrics and Gynaecology, 4,* 31–47.

Chang, S. H., Kim, C. S., Lee, K. S., Kim, H., Yim, S. V., Lim, Y. J., et al. (2007). Premenopausal factors influencing premature ovarian failure and early menopause. *Maturitas, 58*(1), 19–30.

Cohen, L. S., Soares, C. N., Vitonis, A. F., Otto, M. W., & Harlow, B. L. (2006). Risk for new onset of depression during the menopausal transition: The Harvard study of moods and cycles. *Archives of General Psychiatry, 63*(4), 385–390.

Cone, R. I., Davis, G. A., & Goy, R. W. (1981). Effects of ovarian steroids on serotonin metabolism within grossly dissected and microdissected brain regions of the ovariectomized rat. *Brain Research Bulletin, 7,* 639–644.

Coulam, C. B., Adamson, S. C., & Annegers, J. F. (1986). Incidence of premature ovarian failure. *Obstetrics and Gynecology, 67*(4), 604–606.

Davies, J., & Doyle, P. (2002). Quality of life studies in unselected gynecological outpatients and inpatients before and after hysterectomy. *Journal of Obstetrics and Gynecology, 22,* 523–526.

Deecher, D., Andree, T. H., Sloan, D., & Schechter, L. E. (2008). From menarche to menopause: Exploring the underlying biology of depression in women experiencing hormonal changes. *Psychoneuroendocrinology, 33,* 3–17.

Deeks, A. A., & McCabe, M. P. (2004). Well-being and menopause: An investigation of purpose in life, self-acceptance and social role in premenopausal, perimenopausal and postmenopausal women. *Quality of Life Research, 13*(2), 389–398.

Dennerstein, L. (1996). Well-being, symptoms and the menopausal transition. *Maturitas, 23*(2), 147–157.

Dennerstein, L., Dudly, E., & Burger, H. (2001). Are changes in sexual functioning during midlife due to aging or menopause? *Fertility and Sterility, 76,* 456–460.

Dennerstein, L., Guthrie, J. R., Clark, M., Lehert, P., & Henderson V. W. (2004). A population-based study of depressed mood in middle-aged, Australian-born women. *Menopause, 11*(5), 563–568.

Dennerstein, L., Lehert, P., & Burger, H. (2005a). The relative effects of hormones and relationship factors on sexual function of women through the natural menopausal transition. *Fertility and Sterility, 84,* 174–180.

Dennerstein, L., Lehert, P., Burger, H., & Dudley, E. (1999). Mood and the menopausal transition. *Journal of Nervous Mental Disease, 187*(11), 685–691.

Dennerstein, L., Lehert, P., Burger, H., & Guthrie, J. (2005b). Sexuality. *The American Journal of Medicine, 118*(12B), 59S–63S.

Dennerstein, L., Smith, A. M., & Morse, C. (1994). Psychological well-being, mid-life and the menopause. *Maturitas, 20*(1), 1–11.

El-Guebaly, N., Atchison, B., & Hay, W. (1984). The menopause: Stressors and facilitators. *Canadian Medical Association Journal, 131*(8), 865–869.

Farquhar, C., Harvey, S., Yu, Y., Sadler, L., & Stewart, A. (2006). A prospective study of 3 years of outcomes after hysterectomy with and without oophorectomy. *American Journal of Obstetrics and Gynecology, 194,* 711–717.

Freeman, E. W., Sammel, M. D., Lin, H., Gracia, C. R., Kapoor, S., & Ferdousi, T. (2005). The role of anxiety and hormonal changes in menopausal hot flashes. *Menopause, 12,* 258.

Freeman, E. W., Sammel, M. D., Liu, L., Gracia, C. R., Nelson, D. B., & Hollander, L. (2004). Hormones and menopausal status as predictors of depression in women in transition to menopause. *Archives of General Psychiatry, 61*(1), 62–70.

Freeman, E. W., Sammel, M. D., Lin, H., Gracia, C. R., Pien, G. W., Nelson, D. B., et al. (2007). Symptoms associated with menopausal transition and reproductive hormones in midlife women. *Obstetrics and Gynecology, 110*(2), 230–240.

Freeman, E. W., Sammel, M. D., Lin, H., & Nelson, D. B. (2006). Associations of hormones and menopausal status with depressed mood in women with no history of depression. *Archives of General Psychiatry, 63*(4), 375–382.

Freeman, M. P., Smith, K. W., Freeman, S. A., McElroy, S. L., Kmetz, G. E., Wright, R., et al. (2002). The impact of reproductive events on the course of bipolar disorder in women. *Journal of Clinical Psychiatry, 63*(4), 284–287.

Friedman, S. H., Sajatovic, M., Schuermeyer, I. N., Safavi, R., Hays, R. W., West, J., et al. (2005). Menopause-related quality of life in chronically mentally ill women. *International Journal of Psychiatry in Medicine, 35*(3), 259–271.

Gordon, J. H. (1980). Modulation of apomorphine-induced stereotypy by estrogen: Time course and dose response. *Brain Research Bulletin, 5*(6), 679–682.

Gracia, C. R., Freeman, E. W., Sammel, M. D., Lin, H., & Mogul, M. (2007). Hormones and sexuality during transition to menopause. *Obstetrics and Gynecology, 109*(4), 831–840.

Graziottin, A. (2007). Prevalence and evaluation of sexual health problems—HSDD in Europe. *Journal of Sexual Medicine, 4*(Suppl. 3), 211–219.

Guicheney, P., Leger, D., Barrat, J., Trevoux, R., De Lignieres, B., Roques, P., et al. (1988). Platelet serotonin content and plasma tryptophan in peri- and postmenopausal women: Variations with plasma oestrogen levels and depressive symptoms. *European Journal of Clinical Investigation, 18*(3), 297–304.

Halbreich, U., Rojansky, N., Palter, S., Tworek, H., Hissin, P., & Wang, K. (1995). Estrogen augments serotonergic activity in postmenopausal women. *Biological Psychiatry, 37,* 434–341.

Hallonquist, J. D., Seeman, M. V., Lang, M., & Rector, N. A. (1993). Variation in symptom severity over the menstrual cycle of schizophrenics. *Biological Psychiatry, 33*(3), 207–209.

Harlow, B. L., Cramer, D. W., & Annis, K. M. (1995). Association of medically treated depression and age at natural menopause. *American Journal of Epidemiology, 141*(12), 1170–1176.

Harlow, B. L., & Signorello, L. B. (2000). Factors associated with early menopause. *Maturitas, 35*(1), 3–9.

Harlow, B. L., Wise, L. A., Otto, M. W., Soares, C. N., & Cohen, L. S. (2003). Depression and its influence on reproductive endocrine and menstrual cycle markers associated with menopausal transition: The Harvard Study of Moods and Cycles. *Journal of Women's Health and Gender Based Medicine, 60,* 29–36.

Hartmann, U., Philippsohn, S., Heiser, K., & Ruffer-Hesse, C. (2004). Low sexual desire in midlife and older women: Personality factors, psychosocial development, present sexuality. *Menopause, 11*(6), 726–740.

Hunter, M. (1992). The south-east England longitudinal study of the climacteric and postmenopause. *Maturitas, 14*(2), 117–26.

Joffe, H., Hall, J. E., Soares, C. N., Hennen, J., Reilly, C. J., Carlson, K., et al. (2002). Vasomotor symptoms are associated with depression in perimenopausal women seeking primary care. *Menopause, 9,* 392.

Kaufert, P. A., Gilbert, P., & Tate, R. (1992). The Manitoba Project: A re-examination of the link between menopause and depression. *Maturitas, 14*(2), 143–155.

Kjerulff, K., Langenberg, P., Rhodes, J., Harvey, L. A., Guzinski, G. M., & Stolley, P. D. (2000). Effectiveness of hysterectomy. *Obstetrics and Gynecology, 95*(3), 319–326.

Klaiber, E. L., Broverman, D. M., Vogel, W., & Kobayashi, Y. (1979). Estrogen therapy for severe persistent depressions in women. *Archives of General Psychiatry, 36,* 550–554.

Kravitz, H. M., Ganz, P. A., Bromberger, J., Powell, L. H., Sutton-Tyrrel, K., & Meyer, P. M. (2003). Sleep difficulty in women at midlife: A community survey of sleep and the menopausal transition. *Menopause, 10,* 19–28.

Kuh, D. L., Wadsworth, M., & Hardy, R. (1997). Women's health in midlife: The influence of the menopause, social factors and health in earlier life. *British Journal of Obstetrics and Gynaecolgy, 104,* 923–933.

Kukopulos, A., Reginaldi, D., Laddomada, P., Floris, G., Serra, G., & Tondo, L. (1980). Course of the manic-depressive cycle and changes caused by treatment. *Pharmakopsychiatrie Neuropsychopharmakologie, 13*(4), 156–167.

Kumar, M. S., Chen, C. L., & Muther, T. F. (1979). Changes in the pituitary and hypothalamic content of methionine-enkephalin during the estrous cycle of rats. *Life Sciences, 25*(19), 1687–1696.

Landau, S., & Milan, F. B. (1996). Assessment and treatment of depression during the menopause: A preliminary report. *Menopause, 3,* 201–207.

Leppert, P. C., Legro, R. S., & Kjerulff, K. H. (2007). Hysterectomy and loss of fertility: Implications for women's mental health. *Journal of Psychosomatic Research, 63,* 269–274.

Liao, K. L., Wood, N., & Conway, G. S. (2000). Premature menopause and psychological well-being. *Journal of Psychosomatic Obstetrics and Gynecology, 21*(3), 167–174.

Lindamer, L. A., Lohr, J. B., Harris, M. J., & Jeste, D. V. (1997). Gender, estrogen, and schizophrenia. *Psychopharmacology Bulletin, 33*(2), 221–228.

Luine, V. N., Khylchevskaya, R. I., & McEwen, B. (1975). Effect of gonadal steroids on activities of monoaminooxidase and choline acetylase in rat brain. *Brain Research, 86,* 293–306.

Maciejewski, P. K., Prigerson, H. G., & Mazure, C. M. (2001). Sex differences in event-related risk for major depression. *Psychological Medicine, 31*(4), 593–604.

Martens, L. W., Leusink, G. L., Knottnerus, J. A., Smeets, C. G., & Pop, V. J. (2001). Climacteric complaints in the community. *Family Practice, 18,* 189–194.

Matthews, K. A. (1992). Myths and realities of the menopause. *Psychosomatic Medicine, 54,* 1–9.

McKinlay, S. M. (1996). The normal menopause transition: An overview. *Maturitas, 23,* 137–145.

McKinlay, S. M., & Jefferys, M. (1974). The menopausal syndrome. *British Journal of Preventive and Social Medicine, 28,* 108–115.

McKinlay, J. B., McKinlay, S. M., & Brambilla, D. (1987). The relative contributions of endocrine changes and social circumstances to depression in mid-aged women. *Journal of Health and Social Behavior, 28*(4), 345–363.

Meltzer, H. Y. (1990). Role of serotonin in depression. *Annals of the New York Academy of Sciences, 600,* 486–500.

Mitchell, E. S., & Woods, N. F. (1996). Symptom experiences of midlife women: Observations from the Seattle Midlife Women's Health Study. *Maturitas, 25*(1), 1–10.

Moreno, F. A., McGahuey, C. A., Freeman, M. P., & Delgado, P. L. (2006). Sex differences in depressive response during monoamine depletions in remitted depressive subjects. *Journal of Clinical Psychiatry, 67*(10), 1618–1623.

Morrison, J. H., Brinton, R. D., Schmidt, P. J., & Gore, A. C. (2006). Estrogen, menopause, and the aging brain: How basic neuroscience can inform hormone therapy in women. *Journal of Neuroscience, 26*(41), 10332–10348.

Morrison, M. F., Kallan, M. J., Have, T. T., Katz, I., Tweedy, K., & Battistini, M. (2004). Lack of efficacy of estadiol for depression in postmenpausal women: A randomized, controlled trial. *Biological Psychiatry, 55,* 406–412.

National Institutes of Health. (2005, March 21–23). NIH State-of-the-Science Conference Statement on Management of Menopause-Related Symptoms. State-of-the-Science Conference Statement.

Nelson, D. B., Sammel, M. D., Freeman, E. W., Liu, L., Langan, E., & Gracia, C. R. (2004). Predicting participation in prospective studies of ovarian aging. *Menopause, 11*(5), 543–548.

Nelson, H. D., Vesco, K. K., Haney, E., Fu, R., Nedrow, A., Miller, J., et al. (2006). Nonhormonal therapies for menopausal hot flashes: systematic review and meta-analysis. *Journal of the American Medical Association, 295*(17), 2057–2071.

North American Menopause Society. (2000). Clinical challenges of perimenopause: Consensus opinion of the North American Menopause Society. *Menopause, 7,* 5–13.

Novaes, C., Almeida, O. P., & de Melo, N. R. (1998). Mental health among perimenopausal women attending a menopause clinic: Possible association with premenstrual syndrome? *Climacteric, 1*(4), 264–270.

Osborn, M., Hawton, K., & Gath, D. (1988). Sexual dysfunction among middle-aged women in the community. *British Medical Journal, 296,* 959–962.

Pham, K. C., Grisso, J. A., & Freeman, E. W. (1997). Ovarian Aging and Hormone Replacement Therapy Hormonal Levels, Symptoms, and Attitudes of African-American and White Women. *Journal of General Internal Medicine, 12,* 230–236.

Prange, A. J., Wilson, I. C., & Alltop, L. B. (1972). Estrogen may well affect response to antidepressants. *Journal of the American Medical Association, 219,* 143–144.

Rapkin, A. J., Mikacich, J. A., Moatakef-Imani, B., & Rasgon, N. (2002). The clinical nature and formal diagnosis of premenstrual, postpartum, and perimenopausal affective disorders. *Current Psychiatry Reports, 4*(6), 419–428.

Rasgon, N. L., Dunkin, J., Fairbanks, L., Altshuler, L. L., Troung, C., Elman, S., et al. (2007). Estrogen and response to sertraline in postmenopausal women with major depressive disorder: A pilot study. *Journal of Psychiatric Research, 41*(3–4), 338–343.

Rasgon, N., Shelton, S., & Halbreich, U. (2005). Perimenopausal mental disorders: Epidemiology and phenomenology. *CNS Spectrums, 10*(6), 471–478.

Reed, S. D., Newton, K. M., LaCroix, A. Z., Grothaus, L. C., & Ehrlich, K. (2007). Night sweats, sleep disturbance, and depression associated with diminished libido in late menopausal transition and early postmenopause: Baseline data from the Herbal Alternative for Menopause Trial (HALT). *American Journal of Obstetrics and Gynecology, 196,* 593.e1–593.e7.

Rehman, H. U., & Masson, E. A. (2005). Neuroendocrinology of female aging. *Gender Medicine, 2*(1), 41–56.

Riecher-Rössler, A., Häfner, H., Dütsch-Strobel, A., Oster, M., Stumbaum, M., van Gülick-Bailer, M., et al. (1994). Further evidence for a specific role of estradiol in schizophrenia? *Biological Psychiatry, 36*(7), 492–494.

Rödström, K., Bengtsson, C., Lissner, L., Milsom, I., Sundh, V., & Björkelund, C. (2002). A longitudinal study of the treatment of hot flushes: The population study of women in Gothenburg during a quarter of a century. *Menopause, 9*(3), 156–161.

Rosen, R., Brown, C., Heiman, J., Leiblum, S., Meston, C., Shabsigh, R., et al. (2000). The Female Sexual Function Index (FSFI): A multidimensional self-report instrument for the assessment of female sexual function. *Journal of Sex & Marital Therapy, 26*(2), 191–208.

Sajatovic, M., Friedman, S. H., Schuermeyer, I. N., Safavi, R., Ignacio, R. V., Hays, R. W., et al. (2006). Menopause knowledge and subjective experience among peri- and postmenopausal women with bipolar disorder, schizophrenia and major depression. *Journal of Nervous Mental Disease, 194*(3), 173–178.

Saletu, B., Brandstatter, N., Metka, M., Stamenkovic, M., Anderer, P., Semlitsch, H. V., et al. (1996). Hormonal syndromal and EEG mapping studies in menopausal syndrome patients with and without depression compared with controls. *Maturitas, 23,* 91–105.

Santoro, N., Brown, J. R., Adel, T., & Skurnick, J. H. (1996). Characterization of reproductive hormonal dynamics in the perimenopause. *Journal of Clinical Endocrinology & Metabolism, 81*(4), 1495–1501.

Schmidt, P. J. (2005). Mood, depression, and reproductive hormones in the menopausal transition. *American Journal of Medicine, 118*(Suppl. 12B), 54–58.

Schmidt, P. J., Haq, N., & Rubinow, D. R. (2004a). A longitudinal evaluation of the relationship between reproductive status and mood in perimenopausal women. *American Journal of Psychiatry, 161*(12), 2238–2244.

Schmidt, P. J., Murphy, J. H., Haq, N., Danaceau, M. A., & St. Clair, L. (2002). Basal plasma hormone levels in depressed perimenopausal women. *Psychoneuroendocrinology, 27*(8), 907–920.

Schmidt, P. J., Murphy, J. H., Haq, N., Rubinow, D. R., & Danaceau, M. A. (2004b). Stressful life events, personal losses, and perimenopause-related depression. *Archives of Women's Mental Health, 7*(1), 19–26.

Schmidt, P. J., & Rubinow, D. R. (2006). Reproductive ageing, sex steroids and depression. *The Journal of the British Menopause Society, 12*(4), 178–185.

Schneider, L. S, Small, G. W., Hamilton, S. H., Bystritsky, A., Nemeroff, C. B., & Meyers, B. S. (1997). Estrogen replacement and response to fluoxetine in a multicenter geriatric depression trial. Fluoxetine Collaborative Study Group. *American Journal of Geriatric Psychiatry, 5*(2), 97–106.

Shapira, B., Oppenheim, G., Zohar, J., Segal, M., Malach, D., & Belmaker, R. H (1985). Lack of efficacy of estrogen supplementation to imipramine in resistant female depressives. *Biological Psychiatry, 20,* 576–579.

Sherwin, B. B., & Suranyi-Cadotte, B. E. (1990). Up-regulatory effect of estrogen on platelet 3H-imipramine binding sites in surgically postmenopausal women. *Biological Psychiatry, 28,* 339–348.

Shifren, J. L., & Avis, N. E. (2007). Surgical menopause: Effects on psychological well-being and sexuality. *Menopause, 14*(3), 586–591.

Shors, T. J., & Leuner, B. (2003). Estrogen-mediated effects on depression and memory formation in females. *Journal of Affective Disorders, 74,* 85–96.

Simpkins, J. W. (1984). Spontaneous skin flushing episodes in the aging female rat. *Maturitas, 6*(3), 269–278.

Smith, A. M., Shelley, J. M., & Dennerstein, L. (1994). Self-rated health: Biological continuum or social discontinuity? *Social Science and Medicine, 39*(1), 77–83.

Soares, C. N., Poitras, J. R., & Prouty, J. (2003). Effect of reproductive hormones and selective estrogen receptor modulators on mood during menopause. *Drugs and Aging, 20,* 85–100.

Soules, M. R., Sherman, S., Parrott, E., Rebar, R., Santoro, N., Utian, W., et al. (2001). Stages of reproductive aging workshop (STRAW). *Journal of Women's Health & Gender-Based Medicine, 10*(9), 843–848.

Stewart, D. E., & Boydell, K. M. (1993). Psychologic distress during menopause: Associations across the reproductive life cycle. *International Journal of Psychiatry in Medicine, 23,* 157–162.

Wiegel, M., Meston, C., & Rosen, R. (2005). The female sexual function index (FSFI): Cross-validation and development of clinical cutoff scores. *Journal of Sex and Marital Therapy, 32,* 1–20.

Williams, R. E., Kalilani, L., Dibenedetti, D. B., Zhou, X., Granger, A. L., Fehnel, S. E., et al. (2008). Frequency and severity of vasomotor symptoms among peri- and postmenopausal women in the United States. *Climacteric, 11*(1), 32–43.

Wise, L. A., Krieger, N., Zierler, S., & Harlow, B. L. (2002). Lifetime socioeconomic position in relation to onset of perimenopause. *Journal of Epidemiology and Community Health, 56*(11), 851–860.

Wood, J. M., Mansfield, P. K., & Koch, P. B. (2007). Negotiating sexual agency: Postmenopausal women's meaning and experience of sexual desire. *Qualitative Health Research, 17,* 189–200.

Woods, N. F., Mariella, A., & Mitchell, E. S. (2002). Patterns of depressed mood across the menopausal transition: Approaches to studying patterns in longitudinal data. *Acta Obstetricia Et Gynecologica Scandinavica, 81*(7), 623–632.

Wylie, K., Daines, B., Jannini, E. A., Hallam-Jones, R., Boul, L., Wilson, L., et al. (2007). Loss of sexual desire in the postmenopausal woman. *Journal of Sexual Medicine, 4*(2), 395–405.

Chapter 9
Substance Abuse

Kristen L. Barry and Frederic C. Blow

Introduction

Recent research has shown that women and men differ in substance abuse etiology, disease progression, and access to treatment for substance abuse. This is particularly important given the recent changes in alcohol and drug use among young women. There is a trend among boys and girls aged 12–17 years toward comparable rates of use and initiation for alcohol, cocaine, heroin, and tobacco (Greenfield et al. 2003). If this trend continues, over time there may be a narrowing of the male-to-female prevalence ratios of substance abuse in the older age groups.

With the aging of the Baby Boom generation, a generation that uses alcohol and drugs at a higher rate than the current older adult cohort, and the longer life expectancy of women compared to men, it is anticipated that society will be faced with the increased need for specialized screening, interventions, and treatment over time (Blow et al. 2002). This possibility is particularly disturbing because women have a heightened vulnerability to medical, physical, mental, and social consequences of substance use across age groups (Barry and Blow 2006; Greenfield et al. 2003).

Women also carry additional unique risks during pregnancy because of the effect on neonates. In addition, they have certain gender-specific cancer risks. Given this and the declining age of initiation of substance use in women, prevention and treatment efforts especially geared toward women (e.g., education of all medical and paramedical staff, screening in primary care clinics, detection of drug use) are exceedingly important to stop and ultimately reverse this growing trend.

This chapter addresses the prevalence, etiology, and comorbid conditions unique to women with substance abuse issues. It also highlights screening, identification, brief intervention, and treatment issues for women in general and for special populations (women of child-bearing age/pregnancy, older adults) who experience increased vulnerability to the effects of alcohol.

K. L. Barry (✉)
Department of Psychiatry, University of Michigan,
Ann Arbor, MI 48109, USA

B. L. Levin, M. A. Becker (eds.), *A Public Health Perspective of Women's Mental Health*,
DOI 10.1007/978-1-4419-1526-9_9, © Springer Science+Business Media LLC 2010

Prevalence

Household surveys find that approximately 60% of American women report alcohol consumption in the past year, with around 44% reporting alcohol use in the past month (National Institute on Alcohol Abuse and Alcoholism (NIAAA) 2004a). The 2003 National Survey on Drug Use and Health (Substance Abuse and Mental Health Services Administration, Office of Applied Studies (SAMHSA, OAS) 2004a) reported that 14.8% of females over the age of 12 reported binge alcohol use (five or more drinks on the same occasion) in the past month and 3.4% reported heavy alcohol use (five or more drinks on the same occasion on each of five or more days in the past 30 days). Additionally, 6.5% of females aged 12 or older reported any illicit drug use, which includes marijuana/hashish, cocaine (including crack), heroin, hallucinogens, inhalants, or any prescription-type psychotherapeutic used nonmedically.

In general, women typically consume less alcohol than men when they drink, drink alcohol less frequently and are less likely than men to use illicit drugs (Fillmore et al. 1997; Greenfield et al. 2003). Some of these patterns, however, may be shifting. Recent research in New Zealand showed adult women's and men's substance use patterns becoming more similar in the past few years (McPherson et al. 2004). Among adolescents, recent rates of substance use also show fewer gender differences. For example, the 2003 National Survey on Drug Use and Health reported an estimated 11.1% of girls and 11.4% of boys had used an illicit drug in the past month (SAMHSA, OAS 2004a).

Slightly over 2% of females aged 12 or older are classified with alcohol dependence (DSM-IV definition) and 1.5% with substance dependence on any illicit drug (SAMHSA, OAS 2004a). This compares to 4.3% of males aged 12 or older with alcohol dependence and 2.2% of males with any illicit drug dependence. Women who use psychotropic drugs, such as sedatives or tranquilizers, are more likely than men to develop dependence on those drugs (Kandel et al. 1998).

Diagnostic Criteria

The American Psychiatric Association, in the *Diagnostic and Statistical Manual, Fourth Edition* (DSM-IV-TR, APA, 2000) provides the criteria for the clinical diagnosis of substance **abuse** (pp. 198–199) and substance **dependence** (pp. 197–198.)

Risk for abuse and dependence can be based on how much and how often the patient consumes alcohol or other substances. Quantity and frequency of substance use, as well as the consequences of substance use and the individual's perceptions of substance use behavior are important to diagnose substance abuse or dependence.

There are recommended levels of alcohol consumption to minimize risky or problematic drinking and to prevent alcohol-related problems. For example, the National Institute for Alcoholism and Alcohol Abuse (NIAAA 2007) defines moderate alcohol use guidelines for most adult women as 3–7 drinks per week or up to one drink per day. Guidelines for most adult men are 4–14 drinks per week/up to two drinks per day. Drinking at these levels is usually not associated with health risks (Dietary Guidelines for Americans 2005). A drink is 12 g of alcohol (e.g., 12 ounces of beer or wine cooler, 5 ounces of wine, or 1.5 ounces of 80-proof distilled spirits).

Typical risk-assessment questions include:

- How many days a week do you drink alcohol?
- On a typical day when you drink, how many drinks do you have?
- What is the maximum number of drinks you had on any given occasion during the past month?

Some individuals, however, should not consume alcohol at all. These include women who are pregnant or trying to become pregnant, individuals taking certain over-the-counter or prescription medications, those with medical conditions that can be made worse by drinking, individuals planning to drive a car or engage in other activities requiring alertness and skill, recovering alcoholics, and people younger than 21 (NIAAA 2007).

Because women differ from men in etiology and progression to substance use problems (see below for more detail), the recommendations for quantity/frequency differ from that for men, and the criteria for substance abuse and dependence are not always appropriate. Women often experience problems related to use at lower levels than typically seen in males referred to treatment.

Etiology

Female substance use is more likely than male substance use to be associated with high rates of mental health problems, such as depression, anxiety, bipolar affective disorder, posttraumatic stress disorder (PTSD), phobias, eating disorders, psychosexual disorders, and suicidal ideation (Brady et al. 1998; Merikangas and Stevens 1998; Saxe and Wolfe 1999). Kessler et al. (1997) found that an onset of affective or anxiety disorder more commonly preceded substance use disorders in women than in men.

The antecedents for substance use for women differ from those for men. Female substance use is often initiated after traumatic or difficult life events, such as sexual or physical violence, an accident, a sudden physical illness, or a disruption in family life (Grella and Joshi 1999; Kilpatrick et al. 1998; Martin et al. 2003; Najavits et al. 1997). Women with substance use problems have been found to be significantly more likely than men to exhibit recent physical, emotional, or sexual abuse (Gentilello et al. 2000). Women may use alcohol or other drugs in an effort to "self-medicate" or relieve the psychological strain of traumatic events, leaving them at risk to develop substance-related problems (Miranda et al. 2002; Teusch 2001;

Young et al. 2002). For example, women victimized by intimate partner violence have increased risk for subsequent heavy drinking years later (Martino et al. 2005). Women with substance abuse problems may also be encouraged to use substances by partners or may have been raised in a family environment of substance abuse (Ramlow et al. 1997; Stein and Cyr 1997).

Women appear to be physiologically more susceptible to the effects of alcohol than men. Female bodies generally have less water than male bodies. Consequently, when a similar amount of alcohol is consumed, it is less diluted and the alcohol level in the bloodstream typically reaches a higher level in women than in men (Bradley et al. 1998; Redgrave et al. 2003). Women often may become more impaired by the effects of alcohol, and they can be more vulnerable to substance-related problems due to differences in the way female bodies absorb, distribute, eliminate, and metabolize alcohol or other substances (Mumenthaler et al. 1999; Wasilow-Mueller and Erickson 2001).

Women generally begin regular patterns of intoxication at an older average age than men (26.6 versus 22.7 years), as well as first experience alcohol-related problems (27.5 versus 25.0 years) and loss of control of drinking at older ages (29.8 versus 27.2 years; Randall et al. 1999). When women develop substance abuse problems, however, they tend to develop more quickly than with men. Women, when compared to men, have a shorter time gap between first getting intoxicated regularly and first encountering drinking problems (0.9 versus 2.3 years), first loss of drinking control and onset of their worst drinking problems (5.5 versus 7.8 years), and a shorter average progression time between first getting intoxicated regularly and seeking treatment for the first time (11.6 versus 15.8 years; Randall et al. 1999).

Negative consequences of substance abuse for women include interpersonal difficulties, negative intrapersonal changes (such as decreased self-esteem or personality changes), physical problems, poor impulse control, and reduced ability to maintain their social roles and responsibilities (Green 2006). Compared to men, women experience substance-related problems that interfere with functioning in more life domains (Fillmore et al. 1997). Testa et al. (2003) found that women's use of hard drugs was associated with increased odds of experiencing intimate partner violence over the next 12 months within an ongoing relationship. Both marijuana and hard drug use were associated with increased likelihood of experiencing violence in new relationships, while women's heavy episodic drinking did not predict subsequent episodes of intimate partner violence. Women in substance abuse treatment report more problems related to physical and sexual abuse and domestic violence victimization than men (Wechsberg et al. 1998).

Women also develop alcohol-related physical problems at lower levels of consumption than men, generally due to physiological differences in the way women's bodies process alcohol. Medical problems related to alcohol consumption among women include hypertension, stroke, alcohol-related organ damage, breast cancer, increased menstrual symptoms, increased infertility, and spontaneous abortion (Bradley et al. 1998; NIAAA 2004b; Gentilello et al. 2000). Grazier (2001) found that women with alcohol abuse or dependence had poorer physical functioning, more impairment, and poorer physical and mental health than men with alcohol abuse or dependence.

Comorbidities

Women suffer from a number of serious physical and mental health comorbidities related to alcohol and drug/medication use, often at lower levels of use than reported for men.

Psychiatric Disorders

Comorbidity between mental health problems, disorders, and substance use disorders is common. In general, people with a substance use disorder have higher comorbid rates of mental disorders than vice versa, and people with illicit drug disorders have the highest rates of comorbid mental disorders (Jane-Llopis and Matytsina 2006). There is a strong direct association between the magnitude of comorbidity and the severity of substance use disorders. There is also evidence that alcohol is a casual factor for depression.

Women have a significantly higher prevalence of comorbid psychiatric disorders, including depression and anxiety, than men (Brady and Randall 1999). Comorbid depression and substance use disorder are more severe than either condition singly. For women, affective disorders are present before the onset of substance abuse disorders more typically than for men (Kessler et al. 1997).

Recent mixed-age research found that both alcohol dependence and major depression posed a significant risk for the development of the other disorder (Gilman and Abraham 2001). Mixed-age research has also shown that when comorbid depression and alcohol use disorders are present, both disorders tend to be more severe than when either one occurs alone (Grant et al. 1996; Hanna and Grant 1997). Patients with this comorbidity can be more difficult to diagnose and treat because each illness may complicate the other (McKenna and Ross 1994). Atkinson (1999) provides an excellent discussion of current research regarding the complex connections between late-life depression and alcohol use disorders.

Subsyndromal depression may be aggravated by drinking, leading to depressive disorder. This is exemplified in grief-associated depressive symptoms or late-life adjustment disorders with depressed mood (Atkinson 1999) that may increase to levels indicative of a major depressive disorder. For example, a recently widowed person may be depressed and use alcohol in an attempt to mitigate these feelings. The reinforcing positive feelings associated with the drinking can then lead to continued alcohol use, which may increase depressive symptoms—those associated with the loss of the partner as well as those brought on by alcohol misuse (e.g., health-related difficulties, rejection by others due to drinking, financial strain). Further drinking episodes can be used to attempt to assuage increasing depressed feelings, and the resultant cycle of alcohol use and depressed feelings can lead to a major depression episode.

Because the rates of co-occurring psychiatric disorders, particularly depression, are high and potential consequences are great, it is clinically important to determine the levels of substance use as well as the presence of depression and/or depressed feelings to be able to adequately treat women suffering from either or both.

Physical Disorders

Compared to men, women develop alcoholic liver diseases such as cirrhosis or hepatitis after a shorter duration and less intensive drinking. Research suggests the female liver is more vulnerable to the effects of chronic alcohol consumption (Colantoni et al. 2003; Mandayam et al. 2004; Mann et al. 2003). Proportionately more women with alcohol dependence die of cirrhosis than men with alcohol dependence (Mann et al. 2003; NIAAA 1999). Women may be more at risk of alcohol-related cardiac difficulties (Blum et al. 1998; Piano 2002). Fernandez-Sola et al. (1997) found that women with alcohol dependence had similar rates of heart disease than their male counterparts despite significantly lower daily alcohol intake, shorter duration of alcohol dependence, and lower total lifetime alcohol intake. The telescoping of alcohol-related symptoms in women requires that providers understand these comorbidities and ask screening questions to determine the impact of alcohol/medication use and misuse on physical health conditions. For additional information on multiple morbidities, see Chap. 5 in this volume.

Special Populations

This section will focus briefly on two special female populations: (1) women of childbearing age, including pregnancy; and (2) older adult women. Both groups pose unique considerations and challenges to be addressed in terms of rates, presentation, intervention, and barriers to help.

Women of Childbearing Age/Pregnancy

Rates of substance use among adolescents and young women who are of childbearing age and/or pregnant are of particular importance. Recent national treatment data estimated 4% of women admitted to substance abuse treatment had known pregnancies at admission (SAMHSA 2004b). The 2002 and 2003 National Surveys on Drug

Use and Health found that 10% of pregnant respondents reported alcohol use, 4% reported binge alcohol use, and nearly 1% reported heavy alcohol use in the past month (SAMHSA 2004c). The additional psychological stress of pregnancy may cause some women to be more at risk of substance use. For example, a study of substance use before and during pregnancy by women who had experienced intimate partner violence found that after the women became pregnant, the links between women's experiences of intimate partner violence and their use of substances became stronger (Martin et al. 2003). The women who experienced intimate partner violence (including psychological aggression, physical abuse, and sexual coercion) were more likely to use both alcohol and illicit drugs. The substance-using women who were psychologically and physically abused had somewhat elevated levels of substance disorder symptoms during pregnancy compared with women who did not suffer such victimization.

Pregnancy or becoming a parent may interfere with treatment seeking and engagement for women with problems related to substance use. For some women, pregnancy and childbearing can be a barrier to treatment seeking due to concerns of prosecution or fear of losing custody of their children (Ayyagari et al. 1999; Chavkin et al. 1998; Figdor and Kaeser 2005). Women seeking treatment have frequently indicated their responsibilities for children and inadequate access to childcare are barriers to treatment entry and completion (Grella and Joshi 1999; Kaltenbach and Finnegan 1998; van Olphen and Freudenberg 2004).

Alcohol consumption and tobacco use by women during pregnancy remain major public health concerns in the USA (Chang et al. 1999). Prenatal exposure to alcohol has been consistently shown to have detrimental effects on the developing fetus (Abel 1995; Jacobson and Jacobson 1999). These harmful consequences on the infant and society in general point to the importance of developing programs to determine rates of use, risk factors associated with use/abuse, and methods to intervene with risk drinking for women during pregnancy and, more generally, with women of childbearing age. Despite increasing public awareness of the risks of alcohol use during pregnancy and the potential to expose infants to detrimental health risks, a substantial number of women still use alcohol during pregnancy (Flynn et al. 2003).

Flynn et al. (2003) found that, among a sample of 1,131 pregnant women screened in obstetrics clinics, 15.1% reported any alcohol use during pregnancy with the majority of those women reporting relatively low levels of use. Studies have also found that 3–9% of pregnant women drink "heavily" (variously defined) throughout pregnancy (Gladstone et al. 1997; Randal 2001; Flynn et al. 2003). One study has suggested that alcohol consumption rates during pregnancy are increasing. There is evidence that a large percentage of women spontaneously stop using alcohol when they learn that they are pregnant. In terms of alcohol consumption, two-thirds of women who drank prior to pregnancy stopped during pregnancy. However, it is clear that a significant proportion remain at risk due to their alcohol use in pregnancy. The following section discusses effective preventive interventions to assist individuals who are risk drinkers, including women who are pregnant and women of childbearing age.

Prevention/Early Brief Intervention Strategies for At-Risk Drinking

The Center for Substance Abuse Treatment's Treatment Improvement Protocol (TIP) Series #34, "Brief Interventions and Brief Therapies for Substance Abuse" (Barry 1999), defined brief alcohol interventions as time limited (5 minutes to five brief sessions) targeting a specific health behavior (at-risk drinking). Brief intervention studies have been successfully conducted in a wide range of healthcare settings, including hospitals and primary healthcare locations (e.g., Wallace et al. 1988; Anderson and Scott 1992; Senft et al. 1997; Fleming et al. 1997, 1999; Ockene et al. 1999; Maisto et al. 2001; Curry et al. 2003). Individuals recruited from such settings are likely to have some contact with a healthcare professional over the course of study participation, and therefore they would have potential alcohol-related professional assistance available if needed. Nonetheless, many or most of these patients would not be identified as having an alcohol problem by their healthcare provider and would not ordinarily receive any alcohol-specific intervention. The results of the many clinical trials have been evaluated and summarized in meta-analyses and reviews by Bien et al. (1993), Kahan et al. (1995), Wilk et al. (1997), Poikolainen (1999), Ballesteros et al. (2004), Whitlock et al. (2004), and Beich et al. (2003).

Many of the brief alcohol intervention clinical trials were conducted in primary care settings. The U.S. Preventive Taskforce (Whitlock et al. 2004) conducted a systematic review of the evidence for the efficacy of behavioral counseling interventions in primary care to reduce at-risk or harmful alcohol use by adults. There were 12 trials that met their quality and relevance inclusion criteria (adequate randomization; maintenance of comparable groups; high follow-up rates; equal, reliable, and valid measurements; clear definitions of the interventions; consideration of important outcomes; and intention-to-treat analysis). The trials that met inclusion criteria included Wallace et al. (1988), Scott and Anderson (1990), Nilssen (1991), Anderson and Scott (1992), Richmond et al. (1995), WHO Brief Intervention Study Group (1996), Senft et al. (1997), Fleming et al. (1997, 1999), Ockene et al. (1999), Maisto et al. (2001), and Curry et al. (2003).

Results across the Task Force studies indicated that participants in the experimental groups reduced their average number of drinks per week by 13–34% more than controls. The proportion of participants in the intervention conditions drinking at moderate or safe levels was 10–19% greater than controls. In terms of health-related outcomes, the WHO Brief Intervention Study Group (1996) and Anderson and Scott (1992) found that both the intervention and control groups improved in morbidity problem scores over 12 months, while one trial (Fleming et al. 1997) found a significant reduction in self-reported hospital days for the intervention group at 12 months. Maisto et al. (2001) found improved quality of life related to alcohol problems for those who decreased consumption by 20% or more in the intervention/control. Few studies followed patients for longer than 12 months. However, Fleming et al. (2002) followed patients for 48 months and found fewer total hospital days at 48 months for the intervention group compared to the control group (429 versus 664 days; $p < .05$). That study also saw significantly greater reductions in alcohol use by the intervention group over 48 months.

One of the brief intervention trials conducted a cost/benefit analysis (Fleming et al. 2002). The analysis found that the total cost per patient for the brief intervention was $205 (both clinic and patient costs). The cost advantage between the intervention and control group was significant for medical ($p = .02$) and motor vehicle ($p = .03$) events. Overall, the analysis suggested a $43,000 reduction in future health costs for every $10,000 invested in early intervention.

From this meta-analysis, the U.S. Prevention Task Force concluded that (1) brief interventions can reduce alcohol use for at least 12 months among younger and older adults, (2) the approach is acceptable to younger and older adults, and (3) results remain mixed on longer-term utilization and the reduction of alcohol-related harm.

Prevention/Early Intervention Strategies with Women of Childbearing Age

In terms of interventions with women aged 18–44, significant time effects were found for women in studies conducted by Scott and Anderson (1990) and Fleming et al. (1997), indicating that for both control and intervention conditions, women more readily reduced their alcohol consumption compared to men. Scott and Anderson (1990) found that women who had received any previous alcohol consultation changed their drinking behavior more than those who had not been counseled previously. In addition, although the reason is unclear, women may be more responsive to nonspecific influences on drinking behavior. Simple discussions of health concerns, such as has been done during screening and assessment for both control and experimental conditions, may in themselves be sufficient to change behavior in a greater proportion of women than men (Fleming et al. 1997).

In the Blow et al. (2006) Emergency Department study, younger adult females (ages 19–22) who received brief advice were the most likely to decrease their heavy episodic drinking. Because binge drinking is a particular risk factor for young women of childbearing age, the effectiveness of brief advice in decreasing binge episodes in this population is important as part of an overall strategy to prevent more serious consequences of risk drinking.

Brief Interventions for Women at Risk for Alcohol-Exposed Pregnancies

Because prenatal alcohol exposure is the leading cause of neurodevelopmental deficits in children, the Centers for Disease Control and Prevention sponsored a multisite single-arm study to test the feasibility and impact of a motivational intervention to reduce alcohol consumption and/or increase the use of effective contraception in women who were at risk. This was the first study to target a group at risk because of both contraceptive and alcohol use patterns. The intervention included four manual-driven brief counseling sessions with a mental health professional and one contraceptive counseling session with a family planning clinician. Of the 230 eligible women, 190 were consented and enrolled, and 143 (75.3%) completed a 6-month follow-up interview. At 6-month follow-up, 68.6% were no longer at risk for an alcohol-exposed pregnancy. Of those, 12.6% reduced drinking only, 23.1% used effective contraception only, and 32.9% reduced drinking and used effective contraception. The results were consistent across the diverse sites. The promising results from the innovative dual-outcome (alcohol use, contraception) approach used in Project CHOICES provides the basis for the development of randomized clinical trials to further test these methods (Ingersoll et al. 2003).

Older Adult Women

As a larger proportion of the US population reaches late life (Adams et al. 1996), there are new challenges to providing quality healthcare services for this group. Record numbers of older adults are seeking health care for acute and chronic conditions. Older women represent the largest single group of healthcare utilizers in this country. Research has shown that 12% of older women regularly drink in excess of recommended guidelines and can be considered hazardous drinkers. Problems related to alcohol use and misuse can seriously affect many of the health concerns common among older women, including chronic illnesses, depression, and health functioning. Because of the seriousness of alcohol misuse in this group, it is imperative that targeted identification and treatment approaches be employed to prevent major health consequences and to maximize outcomes. Older women with alcohol problems, in particular, are underscreened and underdiagnosed, have significant access to care issues, and respond differentially to standard specialized treatment protocols. To date, research on these topics has been limited. Furthermore, there has been a paucity of research focused on treatment outcomes for elderly adults with alcohol problems, with almost no emphasis on older women (Blow, CSAT 1998).

Because most older women who drink at risky levels do not meet DSM criteria for alcohol abuse or dependence, alcohol use disorders are least likely to be detected and treated in this population (Adams et al. 1996). In addition, there are more older women living alone, and their substance abuse can be difficult to identify (Blow 1998). Older women with alcohol problems often conceal their drinking or medication/drug misuse (Ashley et al. 2003).

Compared with men, women have less insurance coverage and supplemental income (such as a pension). There is a lower level of coverage for women, and fewer women have any coverage at all (Estes 1995). Older women are less likely to have worked, more likely to lose insurance coverage with the death of a spouse, and more likely to live in poverty. Women drink less often in public places and are, therefore, less likely to drive while intoxicated or engage in other behaviors that might reveal an alcohol problem. Overall, elderly women are healthier and more independent than men in that age group but are also more isolated. They often drink alone. In addition, older women are prescribed more and consume more psychoactive drugs, particularly benzodiazepines, than are men, and they are more likely to be long-term users of these substances.

Because of increased healthcare needs, older adults are more likely than younger adults to seek services from their primary and specialty care providers, and older women are more likely to seek out healthcare than older men. This provides the opportunity for healthcare "gate-keepers" to identify and refer older women who drink at hazardous levels (Blow 1998). As the larger number of adults in the "Baby Boom" generation reaches older adulthood, the need for new systematized alcohol screening and brief intervention, and treatment techniques targeted at older women will be even more critical to the national health services research agenda.

The introduction of elder-specific alcohol screening instruments such as the Michigan Alcoholism Screening Test-Geriatric version (Blow et al. 1992) and the development of brief alcohol interventions for older adults (Fleming et al. 1999; Blow, CSAT 1998), which are particularly successful in reducing alcohol use in older women, make it possible to focus innovative approaches targeted at this vulnerable underrecognized population. For additional information on older adult women, see Chap. 4 in this volume.

Gender-Related Treatment Research

Gender is an important variable to consider in substance abuse treatment research. The proportion of females among substance abuse treatment clients has increased over the past decade, and female clients currently constitute about one-third of the treatment population. Reports have shown that female substance abusers experience a number of barriers to receiving treatment, including childcare responsibilities, stigmatization, and inability to pay for treatment. Female substance abusers are more vulnerable than male substance abusers to some of the physiological effects of substance use, and substance abuse among females is rooted more often in psychosocial problems and traumatic life events. These important gender differences suggest the need for specialized treatment programming for women.

The proportion of substance abuse treatment clients who are females has increased moderately over the past decade. In 2002, according to the Treatment Episode Data Set (TEDS), about 30% (565,000) of admissions to substance abuse treatment facilities were females, up from 28% in 1992 (SAMHSA 2004b). This report included analyses of retention among a nationally representative sample of substance abuse treatment facilities serving male and female clients. Treatment retention is measured in two ways in this study: (1) as the percentage of clients who successfully completed treatment and (2) as mean length of stay (LOS) in treatment. Both measures are important because they are associated with improved treatment outcomes, such as reduced drug use, criminality, or unemployment (Hser et al. 2004; Hubbard et al. 2003; Satre et al. 2004; TOPPS-II Interstate Cooperative Study Group 2003; Wallace and Weeks 2004). Longer stays in treatment among pregnant substance abusers have been associated with improved pregnancy and neonatal outcomes (Kissin et al. 2004). In a drug treatment program for pregnant and postpartum women in New York City, for example, LOS was associated with less maternal drug use, as well as greater mean birth weight and less intrauterine growth retardation among infants (McMurtrie et al. 1999).

Women's roles in families and intimate partnerships have an influence on their seeking and engaging in substance abuse treatment, as well as treatment completion and relapse. Compared to men, women may more typically have partners or spouses who are not supportive of treatment efforts. Women with substance abuse disorders are more likely than men with substance abuse disorders to have spouses or partners who also abuse substances (Blum et al. 1998; Riehman et al. 2003). Partners may discourage treatment entry by threatening violence or an end to the relationship, or they may undermine efforts by continuing to abuse substances (Riehman et al. 2000).

Negative relationship patterns and stressors that may have contributed to women's substance abuse may continue to have an influence during the treatment process. For example, relationship dynamics (power, control, dependence, insecurity, and decision-making power) have been shown to influence treatment engagement and abstinence among heroin users in methadone treatment (Riehman et al. 2003). In addition, some women enter substance abuse treatment by court mandate, often as required to keep or regain child custody (Clark 2001), making the need for childcare particularly important for the maintenance of family relationships while providing quality treatment.

Finally, given the connection between women's substance abuse and a history of traumatic experiences, some therapeutic approaches to substance abuse treatment, such as confrontational models, may be unpalatable and ineffective with female treatment clients (Copeland 1997). Substance abuse treatment clients' substance use outcomes can be affected negatively by partner interpersonal stressors and the client's belief that the partner has a substance use problem (Tracy et al. 2005).

Ashley et al. (2003) reviewed 38 studies of the effect on treatment outcomes of substance abuse treatment programming for women. The review, which included seven randomized controlled trials and 31 nonrandomized studies, examined six components of substance abuse treatment programming for women: childcare, prenatal care, women-only programs, supplemental services, and workshops that address women-focused topics, mental health programming, and comprehensive programming. Positive associations were found between these components and the following treatment outcomes: treatment completion, LOS, decreased use of substances, reduced mental health symptoms, improved birth outcomes, employment, self-reported health status, and HIV risk reduction.

Anxiety or depressive disorders, which tend to be more prevalent and severe among women, may also prevent women from seeking help with substance abuse problems (Brady and Randall 1999) and may make it more likely that women will relapse. A qualitative in-depth examination of relapse among substance-abusing women identified four major themes that contributed to women's relapse: (1) low self-worth and its connection to intimate relationships with men, (2) interpersonal conflicts and/or negative emotion, (3) less ability to sever the tie with the using network and establish a tie with the nonusing network, and (4) a lack of alcohol or other drug-related knowledge and relapse prevention coping skills (Sun 2007).

A number of studies have shown that males remain in substance abuse treatment longer than females (e.g., Hser et al. 2004; Petry and Bickel 2000; Sayre et al. 2002) even after controlling for other factors and regardless of type of care (Arfken et al. 2001). However, relatively few data are available about retention among female substance abuse treatment clients, and findings are not consistent. Other factors associated with retention include age, race/ethnicity, education, marital status, partner's drug use, presenting substance abuse problem at admission, severity of substance abuse, age at first use, psychiatric symptom severity, referral source, type of care, and intensity or level of service (Ashley et al. 2003; Green et al. 2002; Grella et al. 2000; Haller et al. 2002). However, large, nationally representative studies are lacking, and knowledge gaps still exist about factors influencing retention in substance abuse treatment, particularly among females.

Barriers to Treatment

Women with risky alcohol/drug/medication use face a number of barriers that need to be addressed to ensure positive long-term outcomes. Substance use among females is more highly stigmatized than among males (Grella and Joshi 1999), and for females, social stigma, labeling, and guilt are significant barriers to receiving treatment (Ayyagari et al. 1999). Stigma and guilt may foster denial of problems by females, creating a further barrier to treatment. In addition, females in a variety of treatment settings have been found to be more likely than males to belong to minority racial/ethnic groups (Hser et al. 2003). As such, women in substance abuse treatment may have experienced racism and may harbor mistrust of the medical and substance abuse treatment systems, which may compromise provider–patient relationships and hinder treatment and recovery.

Women are more likely to experience economic barriers to treatment (Brady and Ashley 2005). It has been shown that providing comprehensive services, such as housing, transportation, education, and income support, reduces posttreatment substance use among both men and women, but it has been clear that greater numbers of women need such services (Marsh et al. 2000) and that these services are not always available for the women who need them most. Women are also more likely to have difficulty attending regular treatment sessions because of family responsibilities (Brady and Ashley 2005; Brady and Randall 1999), and even if they can attend treatment sessions, women are more likely to report feeling shame or embarrassment because they are in substance abuse treatment, leading to lower participation. Programming to address these barriers is becoming more of a priority for treatment programs across the country, but funding and resources are limited.

Conclusion

Women differ from men in the presentation and course of problems related to substance use. With the declining age of initiation of substance use in women, the development of prevention and treatment efforts targeting women is of critical importance. There are now brief strategies—including screening, minimal advice, structured brief interventions, and specialized treatment—for use with women whose drinking patterns and drug/medication use put them at risk for more serious problems. While progress has been made in understanding the effectiveness of substance use screening, brief interventions, and treatments with women, it remains to be determined how these protocols will fit into the broad spectrum of healthcare settings as a routine part of clinical care and how to target specific interventions/treatments to appropriate subgroups of women.

Implications for Women's Mental Health

Research in the substance abuse field has led to the development of screening, intervention, and referral techniques that are both clinically and cost-effective. Changes in the healthcare environment in the USA underscore the importance of using these brief cost-effective techniques and technologies for women across the lifespan. The use of alcohol screening and interventions targeted to the unique issues faced by women at various stages in the lifespan can move the field toward providing best practices care to a large segment of the population.

References

Abel, E. L. (1995). An update on incidence of FAS: FAS is not an equal opportunity birth defect. *Neurobehavioral Toxicology, 17,* 437–443.

Adams, W. L., Barry, K. L, & Fleming, M. F. (1996). Screening for problem drinking in older primary care patients. *Journal of the American Medical Association, 276,* 1964–1967.

American Psychiatric Association. (2000). *Diagnostic and statistical manual of mental disorders* (4th ed., Text Revision: DSM-IV-TR). Washington, DC: Author.

Anderson, P., & Scott, E. (1992). The effect of general practitioners' advice to heavy drinking men. *British Journal of Addiction, 87,* 891–900.

Arfken, C. L., Klein, C., di Menza, S., & Schuster, C. R. (2001). Gender differences in problem severity at assessment and treatment retention. *Journal of Substance Abuse Treatment, 20,* 53–57.

Ashley, O. S., Marsden, M. E., & Brady, T. M. (2003). Effectiveness of substance abuse treatment programming for women: A review. *American Journal of Drug and Alcohol Abuse, 29,* 19–35.

Atkinson, R. M. (1999). Depression, alcoholism, and aging: A brief review. *International Journal of Geriatric Psychiatry, 14,* 905–910.

Ayyagari, S., Boles, S., Johnson, P., & Kleber, H. (1999). Difficulties in recruiting pregnant substance abusing women into treatment: Problems encountered during the cocaine alternative treatment study. *Abstract Book Association for Health Services Research, 16,* 80–81.

Ballesteros, J., Gonzalez-Pinto, A., Querejeta, I., & Arino, J. (2004). Brief interventions for hazardous drinkers delivered in primary care are equally effective in men and women. *Addiction, 99,* 103–108.

Barry, K. L. (1999). *Brief Interventions and Brief Therapies for Substance Abuse* (Treatment Improvement Protocol (TIP) Series No. 34). Rockville, MD: U.S. Department of Health and Human Services, Public Health Service, Substance Abuse and Mental Health Services Administration, Center for Substance Abuse Treatment.

Barry, K. L., & Blow, F. C. (2006). Substance safety. In S. S. Gorin & J. Arnold (Eds.), *Health promotion in practice* (pp. 329–360). San Francisco, CA: Jossey-Bass.

Beich, A., Thorsen, T., & Rollnick, S. (2003). Screening in brief intervention trials targeting excessive drinkers in general practice: Systematic review and meta-analysis. *British Medical Journal, 327,* 536–542.

Bien, T. H., Miller, W. R., & Tonigan, J. S. (1993). Brief interventions for alcohol problems: A review. *Addiction, 88,* 315–336.

Blow, F. C. (1998). Treatment Improvement Protocol #26: Substance Abuse Among Older Adults. Center for Substance Abuse Treatment, Substance Abuse and Mental Health Services Administration (DHHS No. (SMA) 98-3179).

Blow, F. C., Barry, K. L., Walton, M. A., Maio, R., Chermack, S. T., Bingham, C. R., et al. (2006) The efficacy of brief tailored alcohol messages among injured at risk drinkers in the emergency department. *Journal of Studies on Alcohol, 6,* 568–578.

Blow, F. C., Barry, K. L., Welsh, D., & Booth, B. M. (2002). National longitudinal alcohol epidemiologic survey (NLAES): Alcohol and drug use across age groups. In S. P. Korper & C. L. Council (Eds.), *Substance use by older adults: Estimates of future impact on the treatment system* (DHHS Publication No. SMA 03-3763, Analytic Series A-21, pp. 105–122). Rockville, MD: Substance Abuse and Mental Health Services Administration, Office of Applied Studies.

Blow, F. C., Brower, K. J., Schulenberg, J. E., Demo-Dananberg, L. M., Young, J. P., & Beresford, T. P. (1992). The Michigan alcoholism screening test – geriatric version (MAST-G): A new elderly-specific screening instrument. *Alcoholism: Clinical and Experimental Research, 16,* 372.

Blum, L. N., Nielsen, N. H., & Riggs, J. A. (1998). Alcoholism and alcohol abuse among women: Report of the council on scientific affairs, American Medical Association. *Journal of Women's Health, 7,* 861–871.

Bradley, K. A., Badrinath, S., Bush, K., Boyd-Wickizer, J., & Anawalt, B. (1998). Medical risks for women who drink alcohol. *Journal of General Internal Medicine, 13,* 627–639.

Brady, T. M., & Ashley, O. S. (Eds.). (2005). *Women in substance abuse treatment: Results from the Alcohol and Drug Services Study (ADSS)* (DHHS Publication No. SMA 04-3968, Analytic Series A-26). Rockville, MD: Substance Abuse and Mental Health Services Administration, Office of Applied Studies.

Brady, K. T., Dansky, B. S., Sonne, S. C., & Saladin, M. E. (1998). Posttraumatic stress disorder and cocaine dependence: Order of onset. *American Journal on Addictions, 7,* 128–135.

Brady, K. T., & Randall, C. L. (1999). Gender differences in substance use disorders. *Psychiatric Clinics of North America, 22,* 241–252.

Chang, G., Wilkins-Haug, L., Berman, S., & Goetz, M. A. (1999). Brief interventions for alcohol use in pregancy: A randomized trial. *Addiction, 94,* 1499–1508.

Chavkin, W., Breitbart, V., Elman, D., & Wise, P. H. (1998). National survey of the states: Policies and practices regarding drug-using pregnant women. *American Journal of Public Health, 88,* 117–119. Erratum in 88, 438, and 88, 820. Comment in *88*(1), 9–11.

Clark, H. W. (2001). Residential substance abuse treatment for pregnant and postpartum women and their children: Treatment and policy implications. *Child Welfare, 80,* 179–198.

Colantoni, A., Idilman, R., De Maria, N., La Paglia, N., Belmonte, J., Wezeman, F., et al. (2003). Hepatic apoptosis and proliferation in male and female rats fed alcohol: Role of cytokines. *Alcoholism Clinical Experimental Research, 27,* 1184–1189.

Copeland, J. (1997). A qualitative study of barriers to formal treatment among women who self-managed change in addictive behaviours. *Journal of Substance Abuse Treatment, 14,* 183–190.

Curry, S. J., Ludman, E. J. Grothaus, L. C., Donovan, D., & Kim, E. (2003). A randomized trial of a brief primary care-based intervention for reducing at-risk drinking practices. *Health Psychology, 22,* 156–165.

Dietary Guidelines for Americans (2005). Accessed January 5, 2009, http://www.health.gov/dietaryguidelines/dga2005/recommendations.htm.

Estes, C. L. (1995). Mental health services for the elderly: Key policy elements. In M. Gatz (Ed.), *Emerging issues in mental health and aging.* Washington, DC: American Psychological Association.

Fernandez-Sola, J., Estruch, R., Nicolas, J. M., Pare, J. C., Sacanella, E., Antunez, E., et al. (1997). Comparison of alcoholic cardiomyopathy in women versus men. *American Journal of Cardiology, 80,* 481–485.

Figdor, E., & Kaeser, L. (2005). Concerns mount over punitive approaches to substance abuse among pregnant women. *The Guttmacher Report on Public Policy, 1*(5), 3–5.

Fillmore, K. M., Golding, J. M., Leino, F. V., Motoyoshi, M., Shoemaker, C., Terry, H., et al. (1997). Patterns and trends in women's and men's drinking. In R. W. Wilsnack & S. C. Wilsnack (Eds.), *Gender and alcohol individual and social perspectives* (pp. 21–48). New Brunswick, NJ: Center of Alcohol Studies, Rutgers University.

Fleming, M. F., Barry, K. L., Manwell, L. B., Johnson, K., & London, R. (1997). Brief physician advice for problem alcohol drinkers: A randomized controlled trial in community-based primary care practices. *Journal of the American Medical Association, 277,* 1039–1045, editorial pp. 1079–1080.

Fleming, M. F., Manwell, L. B., Barry, K. L., Adams, W., & Stauffacher, E. A. (1999). Brief physician advice for alcohol problems in older adults: A randomized community-based trial. *Journal of Family Practice, 48,* 378–384.

Fleming, M. F., Mundt, M. P., French, M. T., Manwell, L. B., Stauffacher, E. A., & Barry, K. L. (2002). Brief physician advice for problem drinkers: Long-term efficacy and benefit-cost ratio. *Alcoholism: Clinical and Experimental Research, 26,* 36–43.

Flynn, H. A., Marcus, S. M., Barry, K. L., & Blow, F. C. (2003). Rates and correlates of alcohol use among pregnant women in obstetrics clinics. *Alcoholism: Clinical and Experimental Research, 27,* 81–87.

Gentilello, L. M., Rivara, F. P., Donovan, D. M., Villaveces, A., Daranciang, E., Dunn, C. W., et al. (2000). Alcohol problems in women admitted to a level I trauma center: A gender-based comparison. *The Journal of Trauma, 48,* 108–114.

Gilman, S. E., & Abraham, H. D. (2001) A longitudinal study of the order of onset of alcohol dependence and major depression. *Drug and Alcohol Dependence, 63,* 277–286.

Gladstone, J., Levy, M., Nulman, I., & Koren, G. (1997). Characteristics of women who engage in binge alcohol consumption. *Canadian Medical Association Journal, 156,* 789–794.

Grant, T. M., Ernst, C. C., & Streissguth, A. P. (1996). An intervention with high-risk mothers who abuse alcohol and drugs: The Seattle Advocacy Model. *American Journal of Public Health, 86,* 1816–1817.

Grazier, K. L. (2001). *Gender differences in the health status and services use: Consequences of mental health disorders: A longitudinal study.* Paper presented at Psychiatric Services for Women: Symposium conducted at the meeting of the First World Congress on Women's Mental Health, Berlin, Germany (D. Kohen & A. Wieck, chairs).

Green, C. A. (2006). Gender and use of substance abuse treatment services. *Alcoholism, Research and Health, 29,* 55–62.

Green, C. A., Polen, M. R., Dickinson, D. M., Lynch, F. L., & Bennett, M. D. (2002). Gender differences in predictors of initiation, retention, and completion in an HMO-based substance abuse treatment program. *Journal of Substance Abuse Treatment, 23,* 285–295.

Greenfield, S. F., Manwani, S. G., & Nargiso, J. E. (2003). Epidemiology of substance use disorders in women. *Obstetrics & Gynecology Clinics of North America, 30,* 413–446.

Grella, C. E., & Joshi, V. (1999). Gender differences in drug treatment careers among clients in the national drug abuse treatment outcome study. *American Journal of Drug and Alcohol Abuse, 25,* 385–406.

Grella, C. E., Joshi, V., & Hser, Y. I. (2000). Program variation in treatment outcomes among women in residential drug treatment. *Evaluation Review, 24,* 364–383.

Haller, D. L., Miles, D. R., & Dawson, K. S. (2002). Psychopathology influences treatment retention among drug-dependent women. *Journal of Substance Abuse Treatment, 23,* 431–436.

Hanna, E. Z., & Grant, B. F. (1997). Gender differences in DSM-IV alcohol use disorders and major depression as distributed in the general population: Clinical implications. *Comprehensive Psychiatry, 38,* 202–212.

Hser, Y. I., Evans, E., Huang, D., & Anglin, D. M. (2004). Relationship between drug treatment services, retention, and outcomes. *Psychiatric Services, 55,* 767–774.

Hser, Y. I., Huang, D., Teruya, C., & Anglin, D. M. (2003). Gender comparisons of drug abuse treatment outcomes and predictors. *Drug and Alcohol Dependence, 72,* 255–264.

Hubbard, R. L., Craddock, S. G, & Anderson, J. (2003). Overview of 5-year followup outcomes in the drug abuse treatment outcome studies (DATOS). *Journal of Substance Abuse Treatment, 25,* 125–134.

Ingersoll, K., Floyd, L., Sobell, M., & Velasquez, M. M. (2003). Project CHOICES Intervention Research Group. Reducing the risk of alcohol-exposed pregnancies: A study of a motivational intervention in community settings. *Pediatrics, 11*(5 Pt 2), 1131–1135.

Jacobson, J., & Jacobson, S. (1999) Drinking moderately and pregnancy. *Alcohol Research and Health, 23,* 25–33.

Jane-Llopis, E., & Matytsina, I. (2006). Mental health and alcohol, drugs and tobacco: A review of the comorbidity between mental disorders and the use of alcohol, tobacco and illicit drugs. *Drug and Alcohol Review, 25,* 515–536.

Kahan, M., Wilson, L., & Becker, L. (1995). Effectiveness of physician-based interventions with problem drinkers: A review. *Canadian Medical Association Journal, 152,* 851–859.

Kaltenbach, K., & Finnegan, L. (1998). Prevention and treatment issues for pregnant cocaine-dependent women and their infants. *Annals of the New York Academy of Sciences, 846,* 329–334.

Kandel, D. B., Warner, L. A., & Kessler, R. C. (1998). The epidemiology of substance use and dependence among women. In C. L. Wetherington & A. B. Roman (Eds.), *Drug addiction research and the health of women* (NIH Publication No. 98-4290, pp. 105–130). Rockville, MD: National Institute on Drug Abuse. (Available as a PDF within the full document (http://www.nida.nih.gov/WHGD/DARHW-Download2.html) at http://www.nida.nih.gov/PDF/DARHW/105-130_Kandel.pdf)

Kessler, R. C., Crum, R. M., Warner, L. A., Nelson, C. B., Schulenberg, J., & Anthony, J. C. (1997). Lifetime co-occurrence of DSM-III-R alcohol abuse and dependence with other psychiatric disorders in the National Comorbidity Survey. *Archives of General Psychiatry, 54,* 313–321.

Kilpatrick, D. G., Resnick, H. S., Saunders, B. E., & Best, C. L. (1998). Victimization, posttraumatic stress disorder, and substance use and abuse among women. In C. L. Wetherington & A. B. Roman (Eds.), *Drug addiction research and the health of women* (NIH Publication No. 98-4290, pp. 285–307). Rockville, MD: National Institute on Drug Abuse. (Available as a PDF within the full document (http://www.nida.nih.gov/WHGD/DARHW-Download2.html) at http://www.nida.nih.gov/PDF/DARHW/285-308_Kilpatrick.pdf)

Kissin, W. B., Svikis, D. S., Moylan, P., Haug, N. A., & Stitzer, M. L. (2004). Identifying pregnant women at risk for early attrition from substance abuse treatment. *Journal of Substance Abuse Treatment, 27,* 31–38.

Maisto, S. A., Conigliaro, J., McNeil, M., Kraemer, K., Conigliaro, R. L., & Kelley, M. E. (2001). Effects of two types of brief intervention and readiness to change on alcohol use in hazardous drinkers. *Journal of Studies on Alcohol, 62,* 605–614.

Mandayam, S., Jamal, M. M., & Morgan, T. R. (2004). Epidemiology of alcoholic liver disease. *Seminars in Liver Disease, 24,* 217–232.

Mann, R. E., Smart, R. G., & Govoni, R. (2003). The epidemiology of alcoholic liver disease. *Alcoholism Research and Health, 27,* 209–219.

Marsh, J. C., D'Aunno, T. A., & Smith, B. D. (2000). Increasing access and providing social services to improve drug abuse treatment for women with children. *Addiction, 95,* 1237–1247.

Martin, S. L., Beaumont, J. L., & Kupper, L. L. (2003). Substance use before and during pregnancy: Links to intimate partner violence. *American Journal of Drug and Alcohol Abuse, 29,* 599–617.

Martino, S. C., Collins, R. L., & Ellickson, P. L. (2005). Cross-lagged relationships between substance use and intimate partner violence among a sample of young adult women. *Journal of Studies on Alcohol and Drugs, 66,* 139–148.

McKenna, C., & Ross, C. (1994). Diagnostic conundrums in substance abusers with psychiatric symptoms: Variables suggestive of dual diagnosis. *American Journal of Drug and Alcohol Abuse, 20,* 397–412.

McMurtrie, C., Rosenberg, K. D., Kerker, B. D., Kan J., & Graham, E. H. (1999). A unique drug treatment program for pregnant and postpartum substance-using women in New York City: Results of a pilot project, 1990–1995. *American Journal of Drug and Alcohol Abuse, 25,* 701–713.

McPherson, M., Casswell, S., & Pledger, M. (2004). Gender convergence in alcohol consumption and related problems: Issues and outcomes from comparisons of New Zealand survey data. *Addiction, 99,* 738–748.

Merikangas, K. R., & Stevens, D. E. (1998). Substance abuse among women: Familial factors and comorbidity. In C. L. Wetherington & A. B. Roman (Eds.), *Drug addiction research and the health of women* (NIH Publication No. 98-4290, pp. 245–269). Rockville, MD: National Institute on Drug Abuse. (Available as a PDF within the full document (http://www.nida.nih.gov/WHGD/DARHW-Download2.html) at http://www.drugabuse.gov/PDF/DARHW/245-270_Merikangas.pdf)

Miranda, R., Meyerson, L. A., Long, P. J., Marx, B. P., & Simpson, S. M. (2002). Sexual assault and alcohol use: Exploring the self-medication hypothesis. *Violence and Victims, 17,* 205–217.

Mumenthaler, M. S., Taylor, J. L., O'Hara, R., & Yesavage, J. A. (1999). Gender differences in moderate drinking effects. *Alcohol Research and Health, 23,* 55–64.

Najavits, L. M., Weiss, R. D., & Shaw, S. R. (1997). The link between substance abuse and post-traumatic stress disorder in women. A research review. *American Journal on Addictions, 6,* 273–283.

National Institute on Alcohol Abuse and Alcoholism. (1999). *Alcohol Alert No. 46: Are women more vulnerable to alcohol's effects?* Retrieved December 5, 2003, from http://pubs.niaaa.nih.gov/publications/aa46.htm

National Institute on Alcohol Abuse and Alcoholism (2004a). *Self-reported amounts and patterns of alcohol consumption: Data from NSDUH 1994–2002.* Retrieved May 15, 2009, from http://www.niaaa.nih.gov/Resources/DatabaseResources/QuickFacts/AlcoholConsumption/dkpat3.htm and http://www.niaaa.nih.gov/Resources/DatabaseResources/QuickFacts/AlcoholConsumption/dkpat4.htm

National Institute on Alcohol Abuse and Alcoholism. (2004b). *Alcohol Alert No. 62: Alcohol: An important women's health issue.* Retrieved April 27, 2007, from http://pubs.niaaa.nih.gov/publications/aa62/aa62.htm

National Institute on Alcohol Abuse and Alcoholism. (2007). *What is a safe level of drinking?* Retrieved April 30, 2009, from http://www.niaaa.nih.gov/publications/alcoholalerts

Nilssen, O. (1991). The Toronto Study: Identification of and a controlled intervention on a population of early-stage risk drinkers. *Preventive Medicine, 20,* 518–528.

Ockene, J. K., Adams, A., Hurley, T. G., Wheeler, E. V., & Hebert, J. R. (1999). Brief physician- and nurse practitioner-delivered counseling for high-risk drinkers: Does it work? *Archives of Internal Medicine, 159,* 2198–2205.

Petry, N. M., & Bickel, W. K. (2000). Gender differences in hostility of opioid-dependent outpatients: Role in early treatment termination. *Drug and Alcohol Dependence, 58,* 27–33.

Piano, M. R. (2002). Alcoholic cardiomyopathy: Incidence, clinical characteristics, and pathophysiology. *Chest, 121,* 1638–1650.

Poikolainen, K. (1999). Effectiveness of brief interventions to reduce alcohol intake in primary health care populations: A meta-analysis. *Preventive Medicine, 28,* 503–509.

Ramlow, B. E., White, A. L., Watson, D. D., & Leukefeld, C. G. (1997). Needs of women with substance use problems: An expanded vision for treatment. *Substance Use and Misuse, 32,* 1395–1404.

Randal, C. (2001). Alcohol and pregnancy: Highlights from three decades of research. *Journal of Studies on Alcohol, 62,* 554–561.
Randall, C. L., Roberts, J. S., Del Boca, F. K., Carroll, K. M., Connors, G. J., Mattson, M. E., et al. (1999). Telescoping of landmark events associated with drinking: A gender comparison. *Journal of Studies on Alcohol, 60,* 252–260.
Redgrave, G. W., Swartz, K. L., & Romanoski, A. J. (2003). Alcohol misuse by women. *International Review of Psychiatry, 15,* 256–268.
Richmond, R., Heather, N., Wodak, A., Kehoe, L., & Webster, I. (1995). Controlled evaluation of a general medical practice-based brief intervention for excessive drinking. *Addiction, 90,* 119–132.
Riehman, K. S., Hser, Y.-I., & Zeller, M. (2000). Gender differences in how intimate partners influence drug treatment motivation. *Journal of Drug Issues, 30,* 823–838.
Riehman, K. S., Iguchi, M. Y., Zeller, M., & Morral, A. R. (2003). The influence of partner drug use and relationship power on treatment engagement. *Drug and Alcohol Dependence, 70,* 1–10.
Satre, D. D., Mertens, J. R., & Weisner, C. (2004). Gender differences in treatment outcomes for alcohol dependence among older adults. *Journal of Studies on Alcohol, 65,* 638–642.
Saxe, G., & Wolfe, J. (1999). Gender and posttraumatic stress disorder. In P. A. Saigh & J. D. Bremner (Eds.), *Posttraumatic stress disorder: A comprehensive text* (pp. 160–182). Boston, MA: Allyn and Bacon.
Sayre, S. L., Schmitz, J. M., Stotts, A. L., Averill, P. M., Rhoades, H. M., & Grabowski, J. J. (2002). Determining predictors of attrition in an outpatient substance abuse program. *American Journal of Drug and Alcohol Abuse, 28,* 55–72.
Scott, E., & Anderson, P. (1990). Randomized controlled trial of general practitioner intervention in women with excessive alcohol consumption. *Drug and Alcohol Review, 10,* 313–321.
Senft, R. A., Polen, M. R., Freeborn, D. K., & Hollis, J. F. (1997). Brief intervention in a primary care setting for hazardous drinkers. *American Journal of Preventive Medicine, 13,* 464–470.
Stein, M. D., & Cyr, M. G. (1997). Women and substance abuse. *Medical Clinics of North America, 81,* 979–998.
Substance Abuse and Mental Health Services Administration, Office of Applied Studies. (2004a). *Results from the 2003 National Survey on Drug Use and Health: National Findings* (DHHS Publication No. SMA 04-3964, NSDUH Series H-25). Rockville, MD: Substance Abuse and Mental Health Services Administration.
Substance Abuse and Mental Health Services Administration, Office of Applied Studies. (2004b). Treatment Episode Data Set (TEDS): 1992–2002. National Admissions to Substance Abuse Treatment Services (DASIS Series: S-23, DHHS Publication No. (SMA) 04-3965). Rockville, MD.
Substance Abuse and Mental Health Services Administration, Office of Applied Studies. (2004c). The DASIS Report: Pregnant women in substance abuse treatment, 2002. (Available at http://www.oas.samhsa.gov/facts.cfm and http://www.oas.samhsa.gov/2k4/pregTX/pregTX.cfm)
Sun, A. P. (2007). Relapse among substance-abusing women: Components and processes. *Substance Use and Misuse, 42,* 1–21.
Testa, M., Livingston, J. A., & Leonard, K. E. (2003). Women's substance use and experiences of intimate partner violence: A longitudinal investigation among a community sample. *Addictive Behaviors, 28,* 1649–1664.
Teusch, R. (2001). Substance abuse as a symptom of childhood sexual abuse. *Psychiatric Services, 52,* 1530–1532.
TOPPS-II Interstate Cooperative Study Group. (2003). Drug treatment completion and post-discharge employment in the TOPPS-II Interstate Cooperative Study. *Journal of Substance Abuse Treatment, 25,* 9–18.
Tracy, S. W., Kelly, J. F., & Moos, R. H. (2005). The influence of partner status, relationship quality and relationship stability on outcomes following intensive substance-use disorder treatment. *Journal of Studies on Alcohol, 66,* 497–505.
van Olphen, J., & Freudenberg, N. (2004). Harlem service providers' perceptions of the impact of municipal policies on their clients with substance use problems. *Journal of Urban Health, 81,* 222–231.

Wallace, P., Cutler, S., & Haines, A. (1988). Randomised controlled trial of general practitioner intervention in patients with excessive alcohol consumption. *British Medical Journal, 297,* 663–668.

Wallace, A. E., & Weeks, W. B. (2004). Substance abuse intensive outpatient treatment: Does program graduation matter? *Journal of Substance Abuse Treatment, 27,* 27–30.

Wasilow-Mueller, S., & Erickson, C. K. (2001). Drug abuse and dependency: Understanding gender differences in etiology and management. *Journal of the American Pharmaceutical Association, 41,* 78–90.

Wechsberg, W. M., Craddock, S. G., & Hubbard, R. L. (1998). How are women who enter substance abuse treatment different than men? A gender comparison from the drug abuse treatment outcome study (DATOS). *Drugs & Society, 13,* 97–115.

Whitlock, E. P., Polen, M. R., Green, C. A., Orleans, T., & Klein, J. (2004). U.S. preventive services task force. Behavioral counseling interventions in primary care to reduce risky/harmful alcohol use by adults: A summary of the evidence for the U.S. Preventive Services Task Force. *Annals of Internal Medicine, 140,* 557–568.

WHO Brief Intervention Study Group. (1996). A cross-national trial of brief interventions with heavy drinkers. *American Journal of Public Health, 86,* 948–955.

Wilk, A. I., Jensen, N. M., & Havighursy, T. C. (1997). Meta-analysis of randomized control trials addressing brief interventions in heavy alcohol drinkers. *Journal of General Internal Medicine, 12,* 274–283.

Young, A. M., Boyd, C., & Hubbell, A. (2002). Self-perceived effects of sexual trauma among women who smoke crack. *Journal of Psychosocial Nursing and Mental Health Services, 40,* 46–53.

Chapter 10
HIV/AIDS and Mental Disorders

Linda Rose Frank, Michael D. Knox and Annie M. Wagganer

Introduction

Despite advances in treatment that have resulted in decreased mortality and hospitalizations and improved quality of life, human immunodeficiency virus (HIV) infection leading to acquired immunodeficiency syndrome (AIDS) remains a life-long, life-threatening, infectious disease that requires ongoing medical intervention and monitoring as well as intervention to reduce risk of reinfection and transmission to others. Women with HIV face many challenges in obtaining medical care, accessing services, and dealing with life circumstances that often interfere with quality self-care. Women with HIV and mental illness face additional social, economic, and healthcare challenges that are different than those that occur for the general population, as well as an increased risk of infection and decreased ability to obtain proper treatment.

This chapter will outline general risks for women before addressing how mental health disorders can undermine a woman's ability to prevent contracting or infecting others, as well as complicate her access to HIV/AIDS treatment and care. The chapter will conclude with a discussion of a variety of prevention and intervention strategies. After finishing this chapter, readers should have (1) a general knowledge of the HIV/AIDS epidemic and risks specific to women for acquiring and transmitting the virus; (2) an understanding of how mental disorders further complicate the prevention and treatment of women with HIV; and (3) a list of proven ways to prevent new infections.

L. R. Frank (✉)
Department of Infectious Diseases and Microbiology, Graduate School of Public Health, University of Pittsburgh, 130 DeSoto Street, Pittsburgh, PA 15261, USA

B. L. Levin, M. A. Becker (eds.), *A Public Health Perspective of Women's Mental Health*,
DOI 10.1007/978-1-4419-1526-9_10, © Springer Science+Business Media LLC 2010

Women and HIV

For most of the world, the HIV/AIDS pandemic has had a fairly equal impact on women and men (United Nations Programme on HIV/AIDS (UNAIDS) 2004). That is, the rate of infection for males and females is about the same, as the major mode of transmission internationally is heterosexual transmission. In the USA, however, the epidemic began with infection among homosexual men.

Therefore, early HIV interventions focused on infected gay men since this community was initially most severely impacted. Considerable effort was focused on developing antiretroviral drugs and treatment for opportunistic infections. Members of the gay community who were infected became involved in participating in clinical trials, and made it possible for researchers and clinicians to successfully develop medications to treat HIV and opportunistic infections, as well as develop improved understanding of the complexities of HIV pathogenesis and immunology.

However, due to an increase in transmission from injection drug use, contaminated needles and syringes, as well as heterosexual sex between injection drug users and their female sexual partners, the percentage of women infected in the USA continues to grow as this epidemic moves toward reaching the kind of equilibrium that it has in other countries (Centers for Disease Control and Prevention (CDC) 2006a). Also, many men who have sex with men also have sex with women, particularly in communities where homosexuality is stigmatized. As the disease has matured (and is now well into its third decade), prevention, treatment, and care issues for women are requiring much more attention in the USA and throughout the world.

Gender Inequalities

Unequal socioeconomic status and an uneven distribution of power in intimate relationships between men and women are a common reality. In general, poverty is more widespread among women than among men. In addition, the lack of personal property and inheritance rights for women as well as domestic violence continue to be global issues. These inequalities only increase the threat of acquiring HIV. On becoming HIV-positive, access to care may be further complicated by the lack of property, domestic violence, discrimination in employment and salaries, child care, extended family responsibilities, and lack of power in intimate relationships.

In many countries, even though a woman's partner may become HIV-infected due to infidelity, if a woman divorces, she is often left without any money or a home (Rwomire 2001). General poverty and the lack of opportunities and education may result in women engaging in sex work to survive. Domestic violence also poses a serious issue for women with HIV; the related trauma can contribute to engagement in high-risk behaviors that put women at risk for HIV infection, reinfection, and transmission, as well as impair their ability to continue seeking treatment or refuse sexual relations with men. Although these issues have been a concern since the beginning of the pandemic, the progress that has been made to address these inequalities has not been at the same pace as the rapidly spreading disease. The lack of progress impedes access to healthcare information, services, and support, as well as contributes to low levels of participation by women in community organizations or social change institutions (Romero et al. 2006).

Access to Treatment and Care

More than 25 years after the first case of HIV occurred in the USA, the response to the epidemic has included both success and failure in mounting a coordinated effort for prevention, treatment, and care. The complexity of HIV/AIDS requires intensive and sophisticated intervention, treatment, and coordination of services (Remple et al. 2004). Therefore, clinical intervention is available only in countries and areas that have the funding to develop and support such services. In addition, the economics of governments, healthcare, and HIV treatment has resulted in an uneven availability of both prevention and treatment. In reality, most individuals around the world do not have access to comprehensive HIV care, antiretroviral treatment, and prevention technology.

These issues are complicated by the stigma associated with being HIV-infected, discrimination, homophobia, racism, sexism, violence against persons with HIV, and disparities in access to HIV treatment and care. Even when persons with HIV have access to treatment, they are faced with many challenges. These include adherence to complicated regimens, side effects, need for clinical monitoring, access to continuous coordinated and comprehensive clinical care, and comorbidities of mental illness, including substance abuse, and other diseases such as tuberculosis, hepatitis, and various sexually transmitted diseases (STDs).

While there are many issues related to the prevention, treatment, and care for persons with HIV that are similar for men and women, such as the importance to adhere to antiretroviral therapy, the support services needed by women to assure adherence to medications and their treatment plan may be different due to their often multiple roles in the workforce, as well as their having to care for children and family. Moreover, many studies have found that women are less likely than men to receive highly active antiretroviral therapy (HAART). In a report from the HIV Cost and Services Utilization Study, which included a national sample of persons with HIV receiving on-going clinical care, significant variation was found in medication and utilization of treatment for HIV infection. HIV-positive women (vis-à-vis HIV positive men) were more likely to use emergency rooms and be hospitalized, and less likely to receive antiretroviral treatment (Shapiro et al. 1999). Studies have also documented poorer access to HAART among racial/ethnic minorities (Turner and Fleishman 2006), leaving minority women further disadvantaged in accessing HIV care.

Women may also need access to specialized gynecological, obstetrical, and mental health services, including substance abuse treatment. Accessing these specialized services frequently requires several appointments at different locations and with different clinicians. Therefore, the demands on women to coordinate their own care are often overwhelming and may be compounded by the lack of fiscal resources, competing responsibilities for children and families, difficulty in accessing psychosocial supports, transportation, child care, and clinical services. Because there is no cure for HIV and the treatment of this disease is highly complicated by strict medical regimens and various social contexts, preventing transmission is essential to ending this epidemic.

Risk of Transmission to and by Women

Research shows that women are significantly more likely than men to contract HIV infection during vaginal intercourse (European Study Group on Heterosexual Transmission of HIV 1992; Padian et al. 1991). Unprotected, high-risk heterosexual contact was the source of 80% of newly diagnosed infections among US women in 2005 (CDC 2006a). Nevertheless, women of child-bearing age report fearing pregnancy more than STDs, including HIV (Carrieri et al. 2006). When the birth control pill is used for contraception, other methods of disease prevention, such as condom use, become much less of a prevention focus for women (Carrieri et al. 2006). Moreover, many social and personal obstacles prevent women from protecting themselves from HIV by using a male or female condom.

Male Condom

The context of a woman's relationship and the characteristics of her sexual partner are important when determining whether or not to use or suggest using a condom. Studies show that women are less likely to use condoms within a primary and stable relationship than with a secondary partner, as well as less likely to use a condom in an established relationship than in a new one. Finally, women are more likely to discuss or use a condom when less invested in their relationship rather than more invested (Perrino et al. 2005). Women are also more likely to use a condom when they attempt to negotiate its use with their sexual partner (Perrino et al. 2005). However, there are many reasons why women may not make this suggestion.

While women are more likely than men to initiate using a male condom (Perrino et al. 2005), its use still necessitates cooperation from the male partner. Therefore, some women may not insist on using a condom because it results in their partner's suspicion about HIV serostatus, other STDs, infidelity, or complaints that its use reduces sexual pleasure, or because they fear their partner will threaten to end the relationship or react violently (Perrino et al. 2005; Suarez-Al-Adam et al. 2000). In fact, even among HIV-positive women in relationships with uninfected men, the male's desire not to use a condom may be sufficient reason for inconsistent use (Carrieri et al. 2006).

Female Condom

Given the obstacles to negotiating the use of male condoms, the female condom offers another option for women. This alternative provides more control in the decision-making for women, as well as the opportunity to insert the condom hours before a plural encounter, thus offering protection in circumstances where drug or alcohol consumption could prevent the use of the male condom (UNAIDS 1997; UNAIDS and WHO Department of Reproductive Health and Research (RHR) 2002). While many studies report its acceptability, there has been a lack of wide-scale distribution due to its relatively high cost as a single use product, and women report a lack of awareness of the female condom as a prevention method. Furthermore a lack of information from their healthcare providers may reduce appropriate use (Corbett et al. 2003; UNAIDS and WHO RHR 2002).

Although effective in protecting oneself from acquiring HIV or preventing transmission to a sexual partner, relationship factors can also inhibit use of the female condom. For example, when a woman's real or perceived role is to please her partner regardless of her own risks, or when a woman perceives herself as having little or no risk of acquiring HIV, the female condom is rarely used. In addition, women who are married or remain monogamous may be unaware of their partner's high-risk behavior, such as sex with men, infidelity, or drug use.

Mother-to-Infant

Perinatal transmission accounts for 91% of all AIDS cases among children in the USA and carries a variety of economic, health, and mental health burdens for the family (CDC 2007; Quinn and Overbaugh 2005). However, with antiretroviral therapy during pregnancy, the chance of an infected mother transmitting HIV to her unborn child is reduced from 25% without antiretroviral treatment to being almost completely eliminated with combination antiretroviral treatment (CDC 2007).

HIV testing rates and awareness of the ability to prevent mother-to-infant transmission increase with federal HIV prevention spending (Linas et al. 2006). Therefore, we know that prevention is possible through behavioral interventions and policy changes that implement routine testing and increased access to prevention resources. Nevertheless, HIV continues to severely threaten the lives of women. Behavioral interventions and preventing HIV-positive women from transmitting the disease to others becomes much more complicated when mental disorders are added to the equation.

Women, HIV, and Mental Health

When mental illness occurs, a person's risk of acquiring or transmitting HIV increases. Those populations that are disproportionately affected by the co-occurrence of HIV and mental illness include women, racial and ethnic minorities, and socially and economically marginalized people (Parrya et al. 2007). In addition to the risk of women with mental illnesses contracting HIV, there is also the risk of women with no prior history of mental disorders developing affective, anxiety, and/or adjustment disorders, as well as dementia, following HIV infection (Parrya et al. 2007). As the rate of HIV infection continues to grow among women, so does the need for preventing and treating this disease within the field of mental health (Stoskopf et al. 2001).

HIV Risks for Women with Mental Disorders

Mental disorders may persist over time and cause extensive functional disability, cognitive disorganization, and social impairment which contribute to HIV risk (Parrya et al. 2007). Persons with mental disorders are also particularly vulnerable to contracting STDs and less likely to be diagnosed due to socioeconomic factors and limited access to medical care, further increasing their risk of HIV infection (Knox and Chenneville 2006). Persons with mental disorders may lack the ability to understand their risk and lack the capacity to engage in risk reduction. Their illness can directly or indirectly contribute to HIV risk-taking, such as homelessness, multiple sex partners, limited interpersonal skills, infrequent or inconsistent use of condoms, injection drug use, and sex with partners who use injection drugs (Parrya et al. 2007; Randolph et al. 2007; Collins et al. 2001). Substance use further heightens their risk of acquiring or transmitting HIV by impairing decision-making ability, lowering inhibitions, increasing impulsivity, reducing the perception of personal risk, decreasing the ability to negotiate safer sex practices, having sex with strangers, or having sex in exchange for money, goods, or shelter (Parrya et al. 2007; Randolph et al. 2007).

Women with severe mental disorders present significant challenges for the healthcare team. Mental illness contributes to the complexity of care, increased costs, and difficulty in adjusting to and coping with HIV infection. Persons dually diagnosed with HIV and mental disorders are often lost to follow-up because of delays in accessing care, lack of understanding by providers of their immediate needs, and insensitivity to the social and psychological factors that interfere with consistency in sustaining care. Accessing primary medical care, as well as timely and appropriate risk-reduction counseling, is often difficult for women dually diagnosed with HIV and mental illness (Andersen et al. 2005). Furthermore, research shows that their HIV outcomes are poor (Parrya et al. 2007). In a Detroit, Michigan study, nurses found that "mental health agencies sometimes require assessment by three different disciplines, necessitating three separate assessment dates that must be completed before clients are eligible for mental health services" or medication (Andersen et al. 2005). Consequently, obtaining treatment and prevention information is complicated and burdensome. Unless HIV-positive women who suffer from mental illness have adequate socioeconomic support and resources, they are left with few treatment and prevention options, are at greater risk for transmitting the virus to others, and result in poorer clinical outcomes.

HIV-Positive Women and Mental Disorders

Women who become HIV-positive are also at risk for developing various mental disorders due to the stress related, but not limited, to the following:

- dealing with issues of disclosure at their workplace and to their partner, family, and friends;
- struggling financially if too ill to continue working;
- facing discrimination from coworkers, family, or friends;
- taking pill-intensive medications that are often accompanied by side effects and toxicities;
- fearing discrimination against their children;
- worrying about caring for HIV-positive children;
- coping with feelings of guilt about passing the virus on to their children; and
- worrying about potentially not seeing their children grow (Remple et al. 2004; Cooperman and Simoni 2005).

Depression is a significant healthcare problem and in general, women have higher rates of depression than men. However, depression frequently goes undiagnosed in primary care settings due to a lack of knowledge by clinicians, time limitations, and inadequate assessment. This is of particular importance because women with HIV who are diagnosed with depression show higher mortality rates (Ickovics et al. 2001). Moreover, symptoms of depression can interfere with adherence to HIV medication and engagement in self-care, and contribute to poor self-esteem which can lead to risk-taking behaviors. For women with HIV, the need for mental health assessment, psychotherapeutic interventions, and the use of antidepressants to treat depression as necessary cannot be overemphasized.

Posttraumatic stress disorder (PTSD) is another important issue for consideration in the assessment and comprehensive treatment of women with HIV. Women in general, develop PTSD at twice the rate of men (Nakell 2007). PTSD is related to more rapid HIV disease progression and high-risk sexual behavior, putting women with HIV at risk of reinfection as well as at risk of transmitting the virus to others. This disorder is also particularly relevant to HIV/AIDS because of the traumatic impact of being infected (Kelly et al. 1998). Simply receiving a diagnosis of HIV infection is associated with the development of post-traumatic stress symptoms (Radcliffe 2007).

As a result, people living with HIV suffer from disproportionately high rates of PTSD compared to healthy individuals and individuals with other chronic diseases (Kelly et al. 1998; Gore-Felton et al. 2001; Kimmerling et al. 1999). This is significant when considering disease progression as PTSD is associated with lower CD4 to CD8 cell ratios (Kalichman et al. 2002). Furthermore, studies show that there is a strong relationship between PTSD, depression, HIV disease markers, and adherence to antiretroviral treatment, where women with comorbid PTSD and depression report the lowest adherence levels and lowest CD4 cell counts (Boarts et al. 2006).

PTSD also puts women at greater risk for engaging in unsafe sexual activity as well as other high-risk behaviors, such as injection drug use. In a study of women prisoners, there was a 15% rate of PTSD, which was associated with unprotected anal sex and sex work (Hutton et al. 2001). In another study, women with one lifetime occurrence of sexual assault reported greater emotional distress, more symptoms of personality disorders, and greater unprotected anal intercourse, which is considered a high-risk sexual behavior (Kalichman et al. 2002). Moreover, childhood sexual abuse and childhood physical abuse, often leading to PTSD, are confirmed to be common in women injection drug users (Plotzker et al. 2007). These types of high-risk behaviors increase the likelihood of becoming infected, re-infected, or infecting another individual.

Because PTSD is more common in women than in men, women may also be at an increased risk for new traumas and poor coping skills, leading to impaired participation in HIV treatment and increased need for mental health support. Healthcare providers must ensure the assessment for this disorder within the clinical process. Treatment planning that includes the initiation of specific intervention to address symptoms has the potential of increasing adherence to treatment, reducing HIV risk behavior, improving coping skills, improving adaptation to HIV disease, and decreasing depressive symptoms. In addition, PTSD intervention in clinical settings for women may serve a preventive function among those not yet infected.

Preventing Transmission to and by Women

The unique circumstances that often put women at an increased risk of acquiring or transmitting HIV must necessarily be considered when determining effective strategies for prevention. Such strategies include routine testing, healthcare provider education, patient education, as well as advocacy for appropriate funding, legislation, and the involvement of women in policy development and clinical trials. The following paragraphs present these prevention methods within the mental healthcare setting.

Testing

The current Centers for Disease Control and Prevention (CDC) guidelines on HIV testing recommend increased HIV screening of patients in healthcare settings, providing earlier detection of infection (CDC 2006b). Early detection is crucial for HIV-positive individuals in order to change behaviors that put others at risk and reduce future transmission and link individuals to clinical services. Since timely access to diagnostic test results improves health outcomes, rapid HIV testing is a key method of prevention (CDC 2006b). Results are available within minutes to hours which helps avoid the pitfall of patients not returning for their diagnosis. In the mental healthcare setting, both pre- and posttest counseling are particularly critical. Healthcare professionals must assess their patient's ability to comprehend the information presented before consent can be given for testing as well as their patient's capacity to cope with their test results (Knox and Chenneville 2006).

Because prevention of HIV transmission from mother to child can be greatly reduced through the use of antiretroviral medications during pregnancy, labor, and delivery, every pregnant woman should be encouraged to be tested and offered appropriate treatment if HIV-positive. Even in mental healthcare settings, routine voluntary screening of women who are pregnant or considering pregnancy is critically important to assist in identifying HIV-infected women before or shortly after pregnancy so that antiretroviral therapy may be initiated for the benefit of the woman and the mitigation of risk of HIV transmission to the child. Such screening also assists in preventing secondary infections by working with newly discovered HIV-positive women on risk reduction and behavior change with their sexual and drug sharing partners.

Best practice in this situation suggests that the health of the mother should be considered first by treating the woman's HIV infection by offering HAART during pregnancy. If the mother opts not to avail herself of treatment, she must be assured that other care and services will not be compromised. The mental health provider must be prepared to discuss the importance of treatment to the welfare of the fetus and infant.

Reinforcement of adherence to medication is vital. Discussion of plans for the use of HAART during labor and delivery must be included in their education and ongoing care. For women of unknown HIV status when labor begins, the CDC recommends the use of rapid HIV testing. Informed consent and comfort during labor and delivery are essential to providing support to the woman in this difficult and emotional life situation. Mental health professionals can explain reasons for HIV testing and offer reassurance that testing is voluntary and confidential.

Patient Education

As discussed earlier, persons with mental illness often engage in behaviors that put themselves and others at risk for HIV infection. Thus, patient counseling that increases HIV/AIDS risk reduction, covers proven prevention methods, and is behaviorally focused is of utmost importance. Given the inconsistent use of male condoms and the lack of awareness and distribution of female condoms, healthcare providers have the opportunity to provide explicit instructions on how to properly use condoms, as well as offer skills building on the negotiation and use of condoms for their female patients. Some patients who are living with mental disorders may become anxious or agitated in response to prevention education; however, normalizing these behaviors and offering empathy, respect, warmth, and genuineness will likely help patients relax (Knox and Chenneville 2006).

Furthermore, any HIV/AIDS education must consider the specific mental health needs of each patient. For example, a clinician treating a woman with schizophrenia who has a high level of HIV knowledge but whose adherence to psychotropic medication is low, must first address the medication issue so that symptoms of schizophrenia will not interfere with the woman's awareness of HIV risk and appropriate prevention methods (Knox and Chenneville 2006). In addition to working with individuals who have a mental disorder, support must also be available for their community caregivers to provide them with needed HIV/AIDS education, prevention strategies, and knowledge of resources for testing and medical treatment.

Provider Education

There is a continual need for mental health providers to advocate for services that meet the complex needs of their female patients with HIV/AIDS. However, healthcare providers may lack knowledge about the complexities of treating persons with HIV disease and the special considerations for women, particularly women with mental disorders.

Fear of stigma and lack of trust may result in denial of disease, avoidance of clinic visits, and nonadherence. Therefore, the use of support groups, peer advocates, and peer counselors who understand the woman's values and culture are helpful. Fear of partner violence could also hinder disclosure. Women may stay with a partner without disclosing their HIV status or fail to use a condom because of their economic dependency and fear of becoming homeless. Mental health professionals can help women by being aware of, and providing, the possibility of referral to a domestic violence counseling service, partner notification program, and legal assistance services.

Unfortunately, the lack of coordination between the medical and mental health delivery systems contributes to delays and inability to access appropriate and timely care for individuals with HIV disease and mental illness. Providers must be cognizant of these issues and provide support, case management, and transportation assistance in assuring that appropriate care is obtained. Education of the healthcare providers on these issues must occur to improve both the availability and quality of services for women. Cross-training of providers from the HIV clinical care system, mental health delivery systems, and women's services must take place in order to improve knowledge, efficiency, and coordination of services.

Advocacy for Women

Some countries have made efforts to pass important legislation on issues such as domestic violence, property and inheritance rights, equality in marriage, and HIV-related discrimination. However, approaches to enforcement and means of funding their implementation must also be in place. Otherwise, legislation can fail to meet the needs of individuals. Education of community leaders, police, judges, and social service providers about legal aspects of these issues is critical to protect the rights of women. Funding must be made available for the development and expansion of legal services for women with HIV, including those with mental disorders.

Since the enactment of the Ryan White Care Act in 1990, there has been targeted funding for HIV care for women, children, and adolescents. However, funding and logistical aspects of assuring mental healthcare for all women with HIV continue to remain a challenge. Inadequate federal funding and regular cuts to health and social service programs have often forced local HIV planning councils to withdraw monies for prevention and mental healthcare in order to maintain basic medical services for their patients. This must be rectified so that funds are made available for both the care and coordination of prevention and mental health services.

All medical and social interventions must be tailored to meet the specific needs of women of all ages as well as their children and families. Public health campaigns for women are needed to assist them in understanding their risk, the need for HIV testing, and the availability of HIV services for treatment, care, and ongoing support. Reproductive health services must be integrated into HIV care and mental healthcare for women. These services must include prevention education, sexual and reproductive health services, prevention of mother-to-child transmission, antenatal care, and HIV treatment.

Additionally, HIV/AIDS clinical treatment and prevention strategies must be reviewed and adapted to ensure that they work for all women, including those with mental disorders. Clinical trials for new antiretroviral agents must include women in order to assess the efficacy, side effects, and complications in women. Interactions between antiretroviral drugs and psychotropic medications must be better understood. Funding for prevention, such as microbicide development, must continue and be enhanced to be able to provide methods of prevention that are controlled by women.

Another critical component of advocacy is involving women in policy development for HIV/AIDS prevention, care, treatment, and research. Women are underrepresented in regional, national, and international policy and programming initiatives. Women must have equitable representation on committees that are involved in developing interventions, programs, and allocating funds for services and direct treatment. Membership of HIV/AIDS and mental health coordinating groups should be reviewed to ensure representation of women and individuals with gender expertise. Programs need to be developed to provide funding for leadership skills building for women of all socioeconomic groups, and investments must be made in training women to be effective advocates in their response to HIV/AIDS in the USA and worldwide.

Continued activism is needed to address poverty, disparities, and human rights issues. It is essential that approaches to developing care and treatment be cognizant of cultural diversity. Finally, developing mechanisms for training healthcare professionals must also be continually addressed when new healthcare providers are recruited worldwide to replace those lost due to aging, morbidity, and mortality. Ending this epidemic will take the coordination and cooperation of health and mental health professionals, community groups, political leaders, and individual women.

Implications for Women's Mental Health

Although there are significant barriers and challenges for the HIV-infected woman, particularly those with mental disorders, HIV infection can also be a motivator for positive change. For some HIV-positive women, learning of their serostatus becomes the turning point for sexual behavior change, engagement in substance abuse treatment, and serious consideration of improving organization and life goal-setting. But for HIV-positive women who also live with mental illness, the possibility of making such positive changes requires that additional education and resources are made available through our mental health and healthcare delivery systems.

HIV-positive women need continued and ongoing psychosocial and mental health assessment and intervention throughout the course of comprehensive clinical care. Mental health programs must include a focus on HIV prevention, including routine testing with pre- and posttest counseling, tailored patient education, and advocacy for women. Primary care clinicians must be trained to recognize mental illness and make referrals for treatment as necessary. Mental health providers must be educated about their role in risk assessment, early detection of HIV, and strategies for reducing infection rates among their patients, and become aware of local HIV treatment resources.

Moreover, funding for prevention must be increased and policy development must focus on methods that are under a woman's control and involve the input of women. Enacting and funding legislation that affirms and protects women's rights are essential to preventing the continued spread of HIV. Therefore, appropriate Ryan White funding for mental health and prevention programs must be restored. In addition, clinical trials should purposively recruit women, including those with mental illness. Steps must be taken to integrate reproductive healthcare, HIV treatment, education, and mental healthcare for women, as well as coordinate treatment between medical and mental health delivery systems. This necessarily includes the cross-training of caregivers in the fields of women's health, HIV, and mental health.

It is possible to prevent HIV. Mental health delivery systems are in a primary position to substantially decrease the number of new infections. More specifically, mental health professionals can provide education, resources, treatment, and advocacy that may ultimately save women's lives.

References

Andersen, M., Tinsley, J., Milfort, D., Wilcox, R., Smereck, G., Pfoutz, S., et al. (2005). HIV health care access issues for women living with HIV, mental illness, and substance abuse. *AIDS Patient Care and STDs, 19*(7), 449–459.

Boarts, J. M., Sledjeski, E. M., Bogart, L. M., & Delahanty, D. L. (2006). The differential impact of PTSD and depression on HIV dease markers and adherence to HAART in people living with HIV. *AIDS and Behavior, 10*(3), 253–261.

Carrieri, M. P., Rey, D., Serraino, D., Tremolieres, F., Moatti, J. P., Spire, B., & The Manif 2000 Study Group. (2006). Oral contraception and unprotected sex with occasional partners of women HIV-infected through injection drug use. *AIDS Care, 18*(7), 795–800.

Centers for Disease Control and Prevention. (2006a). *HIV/AIDS Surveillance Report, 2005, 17,* 1–46. Retrieved August 12, 2008, from http://www.cdc.gov/hiv/topics/surveillance/resources/reports/2005report/

Centers for Disease Control and Prevention. (2006b). Revised recommendations for HIV testing of adults, adolescents, and pregnant women in health-care settings. *Morbidity and Mortality*

Weekly Report, 55(RR14), 1–17. Retrieved August 12, 2008, from http://www.cdc.gov/mmwr/preview/mmwrhtml/rr5514a1.htm

Centers for Disease Control and Prevention. (2007). *One test, two lives: Prenatal HIV screening benefits mom and baby.* Retrieved August 12, 2008, from http://www.cdc.gov/hiv/topics/perinatal/1test2lives/default.htm

Collins, P. Y., Geller, P. A., Miller, S., Toro, P., & Susser, E. S. (2001). Ourselves, our bodies, our realities: An HIV prevention intervention for women with severe mental illness. *Journal of Urban Health: Bulletin of the New York Academy of Medicine, 78*(1), 162–175.

Cooperman, N. A., & Simoni, J. M. (2005). Suicidal ideation and attempted suicide among women living with HIV/AIDS. *Journal of Behavioral Medicine, 28*(2), 149–156.

Corbett, M., de Moura, C. H., Mosack, K., & Weeks, M. R. (2003). Adoption and rejection of female condom use among women at high risk for HIV. *Abstract Book of the 2003 National HIV Prevention Conference.* Atlanta, GA.

European Study Group on Heterosexual Transmission of HIV. (1992). Comparison of female to male and male to female transmission of HIV in 563 stable couples. *British Medical Journal, 304,* 809–813.

Gore-Felton, C., Butler, L. D., & Koopman, C. (2001). HIV disease, violence, and post-traumatic stress. *Focus, 16,* 5–6.

Hutton, H. E., Treisman, G. J., Hunt, W. R., Fishman, M., Kendig, N., Swetz, A., et al. (2001). HIV risk behaviours and their relationship to post-traumatic stress disorder among women prisoners. *Psychiatric Services, 52*(1), 508–513.

Ickovics, J. R., Hamburger, M. E., Vlahov, D., Schuman, P., Schoenbaum, E., Boland, R. J., & Moore, J. for the HIV Epidemiology Research Study Group. (2001). Mortality and CD4 cell count decline and depressive symptoms among HIV-Seropositive women: Longitudinal analysis from the HIV epidemiology research study. *Journal of the American Medical Association, 285,* 1466–1474.

Kalichman, S. C., Sikkema, K. J., DiFonzo, K., Luke, W., & Austin, J. (2002). Emotional adjustment in survivors of sexual assault living with HIV-AIDS. *Journal of Traumatic Stress, 15*(4), 289–296.

Kelly, B., Raphael, B., & Judd, F. K. (1998). Post traumatic stress disorder in response to HIV infection. *General Hospital Psychiatry, 20,* 345–352.

Kimmerling, R., Armistead, L., & Forehand, R. (1999). Victimization experiences and HIV infection in women: Associations with serostatus, psychological symptoms, and health status. *Journal of Traumatic Stress, 12* (1), 41–58.

Knox, M. D., & Chenneville, T. (2006). Prevention and education strategies. In F. Fernandez & P. Ruiz (Eds.), *Psychiatric aspects of HIV/AIDS* (pp. 395–403). Philadelphia, PA: Lippincott Williams and Wilkins.

Linas, B. P., Zheng, H., Losina, E., Walensky, R. P., & Freedberg, K. A. (2006). Assessing the impact of federal HIV prevention spending on HIV testing and awareness. *American Journal of Public Health, 96*(6), 1038–1043.

Nakell, L. (2007). Adult post-traumatic stress disorder: Screening and treating in primary care. *Primary Care Clinical Office Practice, 34,* 593–610.

Padian, N. S., Shiboski, S. C., & Jewell, N. P. (1991). Female to male transmission of HIV. *JAMA, 266,* 1664–1667.

Parrya, C. D., Blankc, M. B., & Pitheya, A. L. (2007). Responding to the threat of HIV among persons with mental illness and substance abuse. *Current Opinion in Psychiatry, 20,* 235–241.

Perrino, T., Fernández, M. I., Bowen, G. S., & Arheart, K. (2005). Main partner's resistance to condoms and HIV protection among disadvantaged, minority women. *Women & Health, 42*(3), 37–56.

Plotzker, R. E., Metzger, D. S., & Holmes, W. C. (2007). Childhood sexual and physical abuse histories, PTSD, depression, and HIV risk outcomes in women injection drug users: A potential mediating pathway. *The American Journal on Addictions, 16,* 431–438.

Quinn, T. C., & Overbaugh, J. (2005). HIV/AIDS in women: An expanding epidemic. *Science, 308,* 1582–1583. Retrieved August 12, 2008, from http://www.sciencemag.org/index.dtl

Radcliffe, J. (2007). Posttraumatic stress and trauma history in adolescents and young adults with HIV. *AIDS Patient Care and STDs, 21*(7), 501–508.

Randolph, M. E., Pinkerton, S. D., Somlai, A. M., Kelly, J. A., McAuliffe, T. L., Gibson, R. H., et al. (2007). Severely mentally ill women's HIV risk: The influence of social support, substance use, and contextual risk factors. *Community Mental Health Journal, 43*(1), 33–47.

Remple, V. P., Hilton, B. A., Ratner, P. A., & Burdge, D. A. (2004). Psychometric assessment of the multidimensional quality of life questionnaire for persons with HIV/AIDS (MQOL-HIV) in a sample of HIV-infected women. *Quality of Life Research, 13,* 947–957.

Romero, L., Wallerstein, N., & Lucero, J. (2006). Woman to woman: Coming together for positive change – using empowerment to prevent education to prevent HIV in women. *AIDS Education and Prevention, 18*(5), 390–405.

Rwomire, A. (2001). *African women and children: Crisis and response*. Westport, CT: Praeger Publishers.

Shapiro, M. F., Morton, S. C., McCaffrey, D. F., Senterfitt, J. W., Fleishman, J. A., Perlman, J. F., et al. (1999). Variations in the care of HIV-infected adults in the United States: Results of the HIV cost and services utilization study. *Journal of the American Medical Association, 281,* 2305–2315.

Stoskopf, C. H., Kim, Y. K., & Glover, S. H. (2001). Dual diagnosis: HIV and mental illness, a population-based study. *Community Mental Health Journal, 37*(6), 469–479.

Suarez-Al-Adam, M., Raffaelli, M., & O'Leary, A. (2000). Influence of abuse and partner hypermasculinity on the sexual behavior of latinas. *AIDS Education and Prevention,* 12, 263–274.

Turner, B. J., & Fleishman, J. A. (2006). Effect of dysthymia on receipt of HAART by minority HIV-infected women. *Journal of General Internal Medicine,* 21, 1235–1241.

UNAIDS. (1997). The female condom and AIDS: UNAIDS point of view. UNAIDS, Geneva.

UNAIDS and WHO Department of Reproductive Health and Research. (2002). The female condom: A guide for planning and programming. UNAIDS, Geneva.

United Nations Programme on HIV/AIDS (UNAIDS), UN Population Fund, UN Development Fund for Women. (2004). Women and HIV/AIDS: Confronting the crisis. UNAIDS, New York.

Part III
Services Delivery & Emerging Research

Chapter 11
Services in an Era of Managed Care

Elizabeth Levy Merrick and Sharon Reif

Introduction

The purpose of this chapter is to provide an overview of the organization, financing, and delivery of women's mental health services in the current managed care environment. This background on the essentials of managed care is critical to a full understanding of women's mental health services.

Background

In the early 1990s, managed care was still seen as a relatively new and controversial development in the US healthcare system, but it is now the norm. About 95% of privately insured individuals are in a managed care plan (Gabel et al. 2005), and most state Medicaid programs incorporate managed care approaches (Ridgely and Maglione 2006). Medicare has incorporated optional health maintenance organizations (HMOs) and preferred provider organizations (PPOs) into its largely unmanaged system, although most seniors do not enroll in these programs. Furthermore, additional change is occurring rapidly with its initiatives for pay-for-performance, disease management, and care coordination.

Mental health services have been fully included in this transition to managed care. Managed behavioral health care encompasses managed mental health and substance abuse services, which are often managed together under the rubric of "behavioral health." Managed behavioral health care is complex organizationally, given the phenomenon of "carve-outs" or behavioral health services provided by specialized managed behavioral health care organizations (MBHOs). The impact of this managed behavioral health care evolution on women is worthy of study for several reasons: women have a higher prevalence of some of the most common

E. L. Merrick (✉)
Institute for Behavioral Health, Heller School for Social Policy and Management,
Brandeis University, 415 South Street, MA 02454, Waltham, USA

B. L. Levin, M. A. Becker (eds.), *A Public Health Perspective of Women's Mental Health*,
DOI 10.1007/978-1-4419-1526-9_11, © Springer Science+Business Media LLC 2010

mental health problems (Hasin et al. 2005; Kessler et al. 1994, 2005a), are more likely to seek treatment for mental disorders (Wang et al. 2005b), are more often low-income so may experience cost-sharing requirements differently, and are disproportionately eligible for certain public-sector programs such as Medicaid that fund mental health services. It is noteworthy that little research has investigated the potentially differential impacts of managed mental health care on women, although there are many ways in which these could occur.

The rationale for managed care includes the goals of reining in healthcare costs, increasing access, and improving quality (by eliminating unnecessary or inappropriate care and increasing use of evidence-based practices). In mental health, these areas have been of particular concern. Only 41% of people with selected mental and substance use disorders receive any treatment, and only one-third of those receive minimally adequate care (Wang et al. 2005b). At the same time, concerns have been raised that cost reduction is too often the overriding objective in managed care. Managed mental health care has received a fair amount of scrutiny in relation to these goals and possible pitfalls, but less in terms of gender-specific effects.

It is crucial to recognize that managed care is not monolithic. Rather, it consists of a range of organizational forms and specific mechanisms. In this chapter, we first describe the key organizational features, financial mechanisms, and nonfinancial mechanisms that are common in contemporary managed care. We then examine key dimensions of service delivery systems, treatment settings, and approaches in the context of managed care. In this chapter we take a more detailed look at how mental health services operate in the managed care environment and note issues of special relevance to women. Next we highlight several important issues in mental health services within the managed care context, and conclude with implications for women's mental health.

Mental Health Services Under Managed Care: Key Features

In this section, important features of managed mental health services are described.

Organizational Arrangements

Carve-Out Versus Integrated Approaches

Carve-Outs

Purchasers such as employers can contract with health plans or other entities for comprehensive healthcare benefits, including mental health. In the past, this was the dominant way of purchasing mental health services. During the 1990s, a new way of organizing specialty mental health services became popular: "carving out" mental health benefits, i.e., contracting separately with a specialty MBHO. MBHOs have networks of specialty mental health professionals and facilities, and they provide a range of administrative and clinical services.

Behavioral health carve-outs can occur at two levels: either an employer or other healthcare purchaser can contract directly with an MBHO, or a general health plan can choose to contract with an MBHO to deliver mental health and substance abuse services (Hodgkin et al. 1997, 2000). Either way, covered individuals with mental health benefits would access specialty mental health services through an MBHO. By 2002, enrollment in programs offered by MBHOs was estimated at 164 million (Oss et al. 2002), and in 2003, MBHOs were used by three-quarters of private insurance products (Horgan et al. 2009).

Integrated Approaches

If there is no carve-out arrangement, then mental health specialists are available within the same organization as general medical providers within the health plan. In the current context, "integrated" simply means that the plan does not carve out specialty services, thus integrated plans vary in organizational structure. Managed care plans include HMOs, point-of-service plans, and preferred provider organizations (PPOs). HMOs are typically considered to be on the more-managed side and PPOs on the less-managed end of the spectrum. Research on health plan management of mental health services supports this view (Merrick et al. 2006). There are also traditional fee-for-service plans that are relatively unmanaged; this is now rare in the private sector, but typical in Medicare.

Comparison of Approaches

Strengths and weaknesses have been identified for carve-outs versus integrated approaches. Arguments in favor of carving out revolve around several points (Frank and Garfield 2007; Frank et al. 1996). First is the advantage of specialized expertise in managing and delivering mental health care. Second, having a separate budget for mental health allows a purchaser to specifically allocate resources for those services. In addition, having a single carve-out for an entire covered population can alleviate "adverse selection" problems in which health plans with better mental health benefits attract higher-need enrollees. Economies of scale may also increase efficiency, as MBHOs contract with multiple payers. The motivation for establishing a carve-out typically includes a cost-containment goal.

Concerns regarding carve-outs include the reinforcement of stigma, potential for increased fragmentation, and lack of coordination between general medical and mental health care. However, even an integrated arrangement can, in practice, be lacking in coordination. Furthermore, because financial risk for prescription drugs typically is not borne by the MBHO, it may have an incentive to rely more on psychotropic drugs and less on psychosocial treatments. However, a recent study found no evidence of such cost shifting (Zuvekas et al. 2007).

Reviews of the research on carve-outs have found that they typically reduce costs and maintain or increase access to services as compared to integrated approaches (Frank and Garfield 2007; Frank and Lave 2003; Grazier and Eselius 1999; Mauery et al. 2006; Sturm 1999). Carve-outs have usually been found to have no detrimental impact on quality of care, although some studies have raised concerns about quality problems especially for subpopulations such as persons with serious mental illness in Medicaid carve-outs (Frank and Garfield 2007; Grazier and Eselius 1999).

A literature review revealed that few carve-out evaluations have examined gender-specific effects (Volpe-Vartanian 2007). Reasons for potentially different effects by gender have been proposed, including higher prevalence in women of common mental disorders such as depression; a higher likelihood of accessing mental health services; and greater reliance on mental health services in primary care settings (Dailard 1999; Huskamp et al. 1998; Volpe-Vartanian 2007). Two studies have found no significant gender-specific effects on access, utilization, and overall costs (Huskamp et al. 1998; Volpe-Vartanian 2007), except for disproportionately reduced spending for outpatient services for women with depression in the second year after a carve-out was implemented (Huskamp et al. 1998).

Beyond the Behavioral Health Carve-Out: Other Specialized Managed Care Programs

Several other specialized organizational arrangements that are relevant to mental health services are increasingly common.

Disease Management has been defined as "a system of coordinated healthcare interventions and communications for populations with conditions in which patient's self-care efforts are significant" (Disease Management Association of America 2006). Specialized vendors offer disease management programs, usually telephonic, for specific chronic diseases such as diabetes or congestive heart failure, and more recently depression and other mental disorders. Because depression rates are higher among women, they are more likely to be eligible for depression disease management programs.

These programs, which are utilized in both public and private sectors, aim to identify the clinical population; encourage the use of evidence-based practice guidelines; utilize care managers (often nurses) to monitor, coach, and offer support to patients in terms of adherence to treatment; provide self-management education; measure treatment process and outcomes; and provide feedback to patients and/or providers. Disease management programs can also be provided by health plans themselves. In some healthcare settings, there are more intensive and integrated disease management approaches that are fully aligned with the Wagner Chronic Care Model, a comprehensive approach to improving care for patients with chronic illness, including more direct collaboration between care coordinators/managers and physicians (Wagner 1998).

Pharmacy benefit management is managed care targeted to the utilization of prescription drugs. Active management of pharmacy benefits is ubiquitous in managed care and is often conducted by pharmacy benefit managers (PBMs), which are vendors that specialize in the management of health plans' pharmacy benefits, including psychotropic medications (Garis et al. 2004; Olson 2002). Pharmacy benefit management includes deciding which drugs to include in the formulary (a list of medications covered by the plan).

The use of "tiers" to determine patient cost sharing is another aspect (Landsman et al. 2005; Nair and Valuck 2004). Drugs are designated to tiers (usually three) that each carry a different copayment level, typically corresponding to generic, "preferred" brand, and "non-preferred" brand medications. Even if a medication is on the formulary, the managed care plan may have "fail-first" policies that require specific medications to be tried before others may be covered, or it may require prior authorization for certain medications (Hodgkin et al. 2007a). Given women's prevalence of depression and anxiety disorders (increasingly treated with medication), pharmacy benefit management can have a major impact on women with mental health disorders.

Employee assistance programs (EAPs) are workplace-based programs designed to address mental health and other problems that can affect employees' well-being and job performance (Blum and Roman 1995). Most large companies have EAPs. While EAPs began as occupational alcohol programs, they have evolved into "broad-brush" programs that deal with a wide range of issues including mental health, substance use, work/life stress, and concrete needs around eldercare, childcare, legal and financial problems, as well as management consultation. EAPs typically provide 3–5 visits for assessment and/or short-term counseling, with no copayment. They refer rather than directly treat people in need of higher levels of care or ongoing, specialized treatment. Contemporary EAPs are typically operated off-site by outside vendors, often by the same MBHOs that deliver carve-out services. MBHOs may offer EAPs separately or in conjunction with carve-out services (Merrick et al. 2007).

Women may have less access to EAPs, as they are less likely to be in the workforce (Bureau of Labor Statistics 2007b). Women who do work are more likely to have jobs in the service sector, nonunion companies, and low-wage companies (Bureau of Labor Statistics 2007a), all of which have lower prevalence of EAPs (Bureau of Labor Statistics 2007b). However, women are more willing than men to seek help through EAPs (Delaney et al. 1998; Lightner and McConatha 1995), suggesting that EAPs may be a particularly useful resource for women.

Financial Managed Care Mechanisms

Managed care makes use of financial mechanisms that can influence services by targeting vendor, individual provider, or consumer behavior. In economic terms, these mechanisms act on the supply side (health plans, MBHOs, provider organizations, facilities, and individual providers) or on the demand side (consumers).

Financing and Payment Mechanisms

In the past, most healthcare services were paid on a fee-for-service basis, with payment made for each additional service, thus constituting an incentive to provide more services. When HMOs became popular, the use of capitation as a payment mechanism proliferated. With capitated payment, a purchaser (employer or government entity, such as a state Medicaid agency) pays a set amount per capita for each covered individual for a defined range of services. In pure capitation, if treatment costs exceed the capitation payment, the health care organization must absorb the loss. Thus, it follows that if treatment costs are below the capitation payment, the organization profits. Therefore, on a strictly financial basis, there is an incentive to deliver fewer, less expensive services. This can be accomplished not only by improving the health of the covered population through prevention and timely, quality treatment (the argument in favor of this approach), but also by avoiding enrolling sicker or higher-risk people and skimping on care.

"Risk-sharing" approaches attempt to moderate the incentives of pure capitation. Risk sharing in mental health contracts refers to the degree of the vendor's responsibility for cost overruns or cost savings (Frank et al. 1995). One variation involves setting "risk corridors" around the target payment level. If treatment costs fall short of the target payment level, the vendor may keep the profits, but only to a certain level (e.g., within 10% under target). Beyond that level of savings, the vendor has no incentive to reduce costs further, thus offering a degree of protection against excessive cost cutting by withholding needed care. A 2006 literature review found evidence that full capitation or poorly designed risk sharing can be problematic in managed mental health care within the public sector, creating the potential for access problems to higher levels of care among persons with severe mental illness (Mauery et al. 2006). It is important to note that individual mental health providers are typically paid on a fee-for-service basis, even if the MBHO or health plan is paid on a risk basis.

More recently, attention to linking quality or performance goals to payment mechanisms has increased. Rather than focusing simply on cost, value-based contracting and "pay-for-performance" approaches seek to maximize value, i.e., obtain the best quality care feasible for every dollar spent. This requires identifying performance standards or quality indicators, and linking payment to set levels of performance. Pay-for-performance approaches are becoming increasingly emphasized in the public and private sectors (O'Kane 2007), although they are still rather limited for mental health.

In the general healthcare sector, Medicare payment to hospitals is moving toward contingency upon meeting multiple performance goals. More than half of HMOs use pay-for-performance in their provider contracts (Rosenthal et al. 2006). In contracting with MBHOs, state Medicaid agencies, employers, and health plans often specify performance standards regarding both administrative and clinical responsibilities. The standards may range from requirements for the delivery of utilization reports to the achievement of specified satisfaction rates in patient surveys. Contracts can be structured so that vendors failing to meet performance standards forfeit a percentage of their payment, or so that vendors exceeding performance standards receive a bonus of some percentage or dollar amount.

Consumer Cost Sharing and Benefit Limits

Demand-side financial mechanisms, i.e., those which target consumers directly, are omnipresent in the private sector and in some publicly funded programs such as Medicare, and are not limited to managed care settings. These include cost-sharing and benefit limits. Not all services are always covered. For those that are, consumer cost sharing, such as copayments (a flat fee paid at each visit or service) or coinsurance (a percent of the charges for each visit or service), is almost universal and is imposed in an attempt to deter unnecessary care. Benefit limits pertain to the quantity of services covered, in terms of dollar limits or limits on outpatient visits or inpatient days, either annually or lifetime.

Historically, coverage for mental health services has been much more limited than for other medical care, primarily due to insurers' concerns about excessive and unnecessary service use when insurance coverage is provided ("moral hazard") and generous coverage attracting persons with costly conditions ("adverse selection") (Frank and McGuire 1998). Restrictive benefit packages present enrollees with at least three key problems: (1) limited ranges of covered services can mean that optimal treatment is not obtainable, (2) burdensome cost-sharing provisions may create financial barriers to accessing needed care, and (3) low coverage limits for behavioral health make those consumers subject to catastrophic expenses, which negates a main purpose of insurance coverage (Frank et al. 1992). This situation has given rise to the mental health parity movement, which we will discuss below.

These financial mechanisms may constitute barriers to receiving mental health services. Many studies have found that higher cost sharing is related to decreased use of services (Frank and McGuire 1986; Horgan 1986; Keeler et al. 1989; Simon et al. 1996). Women also have, on average, lower income and are more likely to live in poverty (DeNavas-Walt et al. 2007), which might amplify the effect of cost-sharing requirements on willingness to utilize mental health services, although little empirical work has examined this question.

Nonfinancial Managed Care Mechanisms

Managed care also makes use of nonfinancial techniques to influence the type and quantity of services delivered.

Provider Selection/Networks

MBHOs and other managed care organizations establish or lease provider networks, which limits the providers from whom enrollees can receive services in order for payment to be covered fully or at all under the benefit plan. In some plans, in-network care is the only care normally covered, while in others plans pay a greater proportion of in-network costs versus for out-of-network care. From the managed care organization viewpoint, the goal is often stated as selecting and retaining high-quality and efficient providers. An additional focus may be to steer patients to providers seen as more cost-effective, such as masters-level clinicians rather than psychologists or psychiatrists. The criteria by which managed care organizations select and continue to include facilities and individual practitioners in their networks may include credentialing level, education, specialized expertise in certain disorders or populations, and geographic location (Flaherty et al. 1996; Garnick et al. 2008; Sobelman 2001). Provider practice patterns are often monitored and may play a role in network retention decisions. Critics have raised the concern that deselection or the threat of deselection may be used inappropriately against providers who deliver needed care that exceeds what the organization wants, or who challenge authorization limits.

Women may benefit from the credentialing process which allows plans to identify providers by gender, which some women may prefer, and by expertise in particular conditions, such as posttraumatic stress disorder. This may remove some level of uncertainty as an individual seeks out a treatment provider. By virtue of provider networks, plans can steer clients to preapproved providers. The use of provider networks enables plans to better negotiate payment rates and to focus on provision of quality care.

The managed behavioral health care industry has been consolidating. Several large MBHOs may account for a substantial proportion of some providers' caseloads. On the other hand, plans have an opportunity to work with network providers to encourage services that are desirable because they are evidence based. Gender differences in treatment response or gender-specific precipitants (e.g., postpartum depression) could be addressed through guidelines that address women's specific issues. However, plans may be slow to implement such approaches (Oss et al. 1998).

In any case, consumers' choice of providers is often limited by the MBHO or managed care organization. The extent of limitations on provider choice depends on the network size, sufficiency of geographic and subspecialty representation, and other factors. Yet, networks are often large, and providers typically belong to multiple networks. Furthermore, in some health plans an out-of-network option allows enrollees to receive services from providers outside of the network at a higher cost-sharing rate.

Utilization Management

Utilization management refers to a constellation of approaches including gatekeeping and prior authorization, review of continuing care, and case management.

Gatekeeping is the requirement to obtain a referral or authorization before accessing specialty mental health services. When managed care first became popular, HMOs typically assigned primary care providers a gatekeeping role with regard to specialty care, presuming that they should play a key role in coordinating care. Yet questions arose regarding whether this might constitute a barrier to mental health services and whether frequently rote referrals actually saved money or reduced inappropriate specialty care. Over time, primary care gatekeeping has diminished (Horgan et al. 2009), and even in plans with some primary care gatekeeping, sometimes mental health is exempt.

The rise of MBHOs has brought with it the frequent requirement that persons seeking to enter mental health treatment must call a centralized phone center to obtain authorization, or have the specialty provider do so (Horgan et al. 2009). If prior authorization is not obtained, the service will be covered at a lower level or will not be covered at all.

The authorization process for regular outpatient care may or may not involve detailed clinical assessment over the phone. It has been hypothesized that requiring enrollees to call a phone center for care may be particularly difficult for some women, given the stigma attached to certain disorders such as posttraumatic stress disorder (often stemming from sexual or physical abuse) and eating disorders (Volpe-Vartanian 2007). Such a gender-specific effect for disorders other than depression has not been empirically examined, but women are consistently over-represented among treatment users, including in systems that use call centers. For higher levels of care, prior authorization procedures apply medical necessity and placement criteria to determine what kind of care is indicated. Following initial entry into care, continuing review is also common. This involves review of clinical status and progress to determine whether further care is indicated, and if so, at what level of care.

Case management is a collaborative process of assessment, planning, facilitation and advocacy for options and services to meet an individual's health needs and to promote quality cost-effective outcomes (Case Management Society of America 2007). It is often used in two ways (Mechanic et al. 1995). In the public sector, it typically focuses on people with serious and persistent mental illness and can be intensive, including approaches such as assertive community treatment. In the private sector, for example, as conducted by health plans, it focuses on high-cost or high-utilizing enrollees and typically uses telephonic rather than face-to-face communication. Case management is particularly relevant for persons with complex treatment needs and those whose clinical picture is complicated by psychosocial issues. Women with mental disorders who have responsibility for young children, for example, may find it difficult to access services, may be concerned about the impact of their disorder on their children and on custody issues, and may need adjunct treatment such as family therapy.

The above mechanisms and approaches, while not an exhaustive list, include those most commonly used in contemporary managed mental health care. It is important to note that the field is dynamic, and therefore evolution will certainly continue.

Mental Health Services Delivery System in the Context of Managed Care

The US mental health services "system" is really more of a patchwork of delivery systems and funding streams, within which there are multiple treatment settings and approaches. Recent calls have been made for the transformation of the mental health service delivery system, to enhance its focus on recovery and resilience for individuals with mental disorders (President's New Freedom Commission on Mental Health 2003). This section describes important dimensions of the mental health services landscape that managed care has helped to shape and in which it now operates, and from which transformation must proceed. Issues of particular relevance to women are noted throughout this section.

Public Versus Private

To some degree, the mental health service delivery system can be characterized by whether the payer for services is private or public, and each of these systems has been shaped at least in part by managed care. In 2003, 72% of private health plans' managed care products contracted with an MBHO (Horgan et al. 2009), indicating that the carve-out approach to behavioral health care has become the norm in the private sector. As of 2003, 35 states implemented some version of Medicaid managed care for mental health and substance abuse services (Robinson et al. 2005), and one-third of states had adopted behavioral health carve-outs for their Medicaid programs (Frank and Garfield 2007). Thus, both the public and private systems are largely characterized by managed care features with the exception of Medicare. It is important to note that both public and private payers may purchase services from private providers (either for-profit or not-for-profit).

Public payers include Medicaid, Medicare, and other federal, state, and local funding sources. Public payers fund 58% of mental health treatment, compared to 40% of general medical care, with the largest portions stemming from Medicaid (45% of public mental health expenditures) and state/local funding (36% of public mental health expenditures; Mark et al. 2007). The public sector initially lagged behind the private sector in adopting managed care, but it is now prevalent, with general Medicaid managed care programs in place in nearly all states, covering 65% of all Medicaid enrollees (Centers for Medicare and Medicaid Services 2007). Medicaid allows some eligibility categories and services covered to vary by state, often with substantial restrictions that resemble those used in private insurance (Robinson et al. 2005). Primarily due to eligibility under Temporary Assistance to Needy Families (TANF), women are the majority (69%) of adult Medicaid beneficiaries (Kaiser Family Foundation 2007).

Other public sources also substantially contribute to funding for mental health services. State mental health agencies typically provide a service continuum, including those designed for long-term support and recovery, to adults with serious and persistent mental illness and children with serious emotional disturbance. Unlike public or private insurance mechanisms where reimbursement is tied directly to the enrollee, public subsidies typically provide a fixed dollar amount to providers (Horgan and Merrick 2001) which functions as a global budget limit under which services must be allocated (Rogowski 1992). State systems often provide a safety net and serve people with or without insurance coverage. Some managed care financing mechanisms, such as performance-based contracting and contracting with MBHOs, are often used in these programs.

Medicare, the federal entitlement program that provides health insurance coverage to elders and eligible persons with disabilities, accounts for 7% of mental health spending (Mark et al. 2007). Although it is largely fee-for-service, it has incorporated some managed care techniques. Nevertheless, there are many restrictions and substantial cost sharing, including some that are more burdensome for mental health than for general medical care (e.g., 50% coinsurance rates for psychotherapy which federal legislation in 2008 finally mandated be reduced to 20% over several years). Medicare does not cover some mental health services, such as psychosocial rehabilitation. Only recently (in 2006) was prescription drug coverage added, a key element of treatment for many with mental health disorders. There may still be restrictions on which psychotropic medications are covered, and use of prior authorization or "fail-first" policies (Donohue and Frank 2007).

Nearly all individuals with private insurance are insured via employers or as the dependent of someone with employer-based insurance, although some people purchase insurance separately. Similar to men, more women are covered by private payers (68%) than public payers (13%), but women are more likely to be covered as a dependent than are men, thus having less control over their insurance choices (Kaiser Family Foundation 2007). Over 90% of persons with private employer-sponsored health insurance have some coverage for mental health services (Bureau of Labor Statistics 2007a). Despite the fact that more than two-thirds of the population has private insurance, it only pays for 24% of mental health expenditures (Mark et al. 2007).

Individuals receiving mental health services frequently pay out of pocket for at least some of that care, for a total of 14% of mental health expenditures (Mark et al. 2007). This may include expenditures for the uninsured as well as out-of-pocket costs for some insured persons as well. Insured individuals may pay out of pocket through copayments or coinsurance, or because they choose not to use their insurance due to stigma and confidentiality concerns, have elected to see a provider out of the network, need a service that is not a covered benefit, or have exceeded their benefit limits.

Both private and public treatment systems are also affected by other aspects of managed care. Disease management and case management programs are used by both systems to ensure that care is effective and efficient and to reduce the likelihood of mental health needs escalating to higher levels of care. Nearly all private managed care benefit plans require prior authorization for inpatient mental health care, and more than half do so for outpatient mental health care (Horgan et al. 2009).

Pay-for-performance programs have been instituted or are in development by all types of payers to ensure that providers are offering quality healthcare and that the payers are receiving the best value for their purchases. While current pay-for-performance initiatives are not necessarily specific to mental health care, these approaches can be adopted in this arena. For example, a large health plan has instituted pay-for-performance for specialty behavioral health providers, including psychiatrists and nonphysician mental health providers (Pelonero and Johnson 2007).

Mental Health Benefits

Many factors influence the nature of mental health benefits, but managed care arrangements play a major role. The breadth of benefits may vary greatly in terms of whether mental health is covered at all, the types of services covered, annual or lifetime dollar or visit/day limits, and cost-sharing features. The vast majority of large employers report annual limits on inpatient days or outpatient mental health visits (Teich and Buck 2007). Regardless of the insurer, certain ancillary services, such as case management or occupational therapy, may be excluded from coverage altogether. While the promise of managed care was to rely less on demand-side financial restrictions found in benefit packages, these have not disappeared.

Studies have examined variation in mental health benefits by type of managed care organization and whether coverage is carved out or integrated. In 2003, private managed care plans almost always covered inpatient, intensive outpatient, and regular outpatient mental health care; fewer, but still the vast majority, covered residential services (Horgan et al. 2009). Plans with carve-outs were more likely to offer residential treatment than other plans. Insurance plans with a mental health carve-out are more likely to have any benefit limit or annual outpatient dollar limits, but they are less likely to have an annual limit on outpatient visits (Salkever et al. 1999).

Cost-sharing arrangements also vary by type of plan and carve-out status, with carve-outs more likely to impose copayments rather than coinsurance (Salkever et al. 1999). The estimated out-of-pocket cost for enrollees with 20 behavioral health visits in a year did not differ between health plans that carved out to MBHOs and those that did not (Hodgkin et al. 2008). However, for heavy users of mental health services (50 visits per year), enrollees in health plans with carve-outs would pay significantly less out-of-pocket compared to integrated plans.

Public insurers may exclude certain services as a cost-saving method and often limit the medications available. Among 36 states with a Medicaid managed care plan in 2000, most provided emergency mental health care, outpatient care, and inpatient care. Only half provided residential care, and three-quarters offered day treatment or partial hospitalization; these options varied by the specific plan within the state (Ridgely and Maglione 2006).

Mental health benefits within a plan, whether public or private, do not vary based on gender. However, to the extent that women are disproportionately represented in certain plans (e.g., Medicaid), the benefits available to women may differ from those available to men. In addition, women have differential prevalence of certain disorders, such as depression. As different diagnoses require different treatment plans, women may be affected differently by managed care benefit features. On average, women have lower incomes, which could affect their response to cost-sharing requirements.

Parity

In 2005, about 90% of people with private insurance had different coverage for mental health services than for general medical care (Bureau of Labor Statistics 2007a). One-third of large employers report greater cost sharing amongst their enrollees for inpatient mental health care than for general medical care, and more than half report the same for outpatient mental health care (Teich and Buck 2007). Other differential benefits for mental health versus general medical care are prevalent (Barry et al. 2003). In order to address discriminatory mental health coverage, federal and state legislation aimed at establishing parity for mental health treatment has proliferated. The federal Mental Health Parity Act implemented in 1997 prohibited private health plans from using dollar limits that were lower for mental health than general medical care. However, it did not require equal visit or day limits or cost sharing, and it did not apply to substance abuse.

In October of 2008, *The Paul Wellstone and Pete Domenici Mental Health Parity and Addiction Equity Act of 2008* was passed by the U.S. Congress. Under this Federal legislation, group health plans with 50 or more employees which provide both physical and mental health/substance use benefits must provide the same mental health/substance abuse coverage as they do for general medical coverage in terms of limits, cost-sharing and other features. The Wellstone-Domenici Mental Health Parity Act amended and substantially increased the regulation of mental health benefits under the Federal Mental Health Parity Act of 1996, which only required parity coverage for lifetime and annual dollar limits and did not apply to benefits for substance use. This law will become effective on January 1, 2010. Regulations have yet to be issued at the time of this writing, thus some important aspects of the legislation remains to be clarified. Most states have also enacted parity laws prior to this federal legislation.

Parity laws are a large step toward equalizing the playing field for people seeking mental health services under their insurance and also serve to reduce the impact of stigma. However, to date, the inequities have not disappeared, due to many gaps in what the earlier federal and state parity legislation mandated and for which segments of the population. Many employers are exempt from state parity requirements (Buchmueller et al. 2007). One study found that 45% of private sector workers with employer sponsored insurance were potentially covered by a strong parity law, but this was reduced to 20% once exemptions for firm size and self-insured employers are considered (Buchmueller et al. 2007). In addition, some state parity laws are less comprehensive than others, focusing on "biologically-based" disorders, such as schizophrenia and bipolar disorder, and omitting other diagnoses such as anxiety disorders.

Managed mental health care has played an important role in the parity movement because it is expected that with managed care in place, removing discriminatory limits, as parity aims to do, would not greatly increase costs (Barry et al. 2006; Sturm et al. 1999). The numerous managed-care mechanisms other than benefit limits (utilization management, provider networks) also mean that nominal benefits do not by themselves ensure access.

As with mental health benefits in general, parity is applied equally to all individuals who are within plans or states that are bound by the legislation. To the extent that earlier parity laws focused on severe mental illness and biologically based disorders, they may have had a differential effect by gender. For example, with higher rates of major depression than men, many women may have been more likely to date to benefit from state parity laws; however, other disorders that are also more frequent for women, such as dysthymia, eating disorders, or anxiety disorders have not always been covered. The new federal parity law requires that for all mental health and substance abuse disorders covered by a plan, the coverage offered must be equal to that for other medical care. However, plans may choose to exclude particular diagnoses from coverage.

Treatment Settings, Approaches and Providers

Mental health services consist of varied modalities, settings, and types of providers. While mental health care may be provided outside of the general medical or specialty mental health sectors, such as in a school or in criminal justice settings, the following discussion will focus on healthcare settings, where managed care has helped to shape changes in mental health service delivery.

Treatment in Primary Care and Specialty Mental Health Settings

Both specialty mental health and general medical settings are important in delivering mental health services. Specialty mental health providers, such as psychiatrists, psychologists, and clinical social workers, provide care for 22% of people with mental disorders, or about half of those who receive any treatment (Wang et al. 2005b). Service delivery in primary care is increasingly common. The increasing reliance on psychotropic medications for mental health treatment has helped to foster this trend. Currently, just over half of individuals receiving mental health services are seen in the general medical sector (Wang et al. 2005b), a more than twofold increase since the early 1990s (Kessler et al. 2005b). Nearly half of privately insured behavioral health service users reported using only anti-depressants without other mental health care (Larson et al. 2006) and nearly half of adolescents who are prescribed antidepressants do not receive psychotherapy (Mark 2008). Prescription and medication management may be done by primary care or other practitioners who do not specialize in mental health, yet there are documented deficiencies in the treatment of depression, for instance, in primary care (Wang et al. 2005b). Many individuals with depression or anxiety prefer to be treated by their primary care physician and might not otherwise seek out treatment for mental health problems.

Mental health treatment in primary care or other nonspecialty settings is affected by managed care in two main ways. To the extent that treatment with medications and without formal psychotherapy is less expensive than psychosocial approaches, such treatment may be encouraged by managed care plans and may increase primary care utilization. Managed care organizations can also encourage or discourage quick referrals to specialty mental health care through guidelines for primary care providers. A carve-out may encourage specialty treatment by having a readily identifiable resource for both eligible persons and primary care providers. However, nonspecialty providers may not be able to bill for mental health services beyond medication management.

Treatment setting is relevant to the provision of mental health services for women because of their different help-seeking behaviors. Women are more likely than men to have a usual source of healthcare (Agency for Healthcare Research and Quality 2004a) and are more likely to make office-based visits in a given year (Agency for Healthcare Research and Quality 2004b), thus have greater opportunity to identify and treat a mental health problem. Women with mental health needs are more likely than men to seek help in primary care (Glied 1997). This may be because women prefer to be treated in primary care, or primary care providers may be more willing to provide mental health treatment to women directly rather than referring to a specialist. Women are also likely to see OB/GYN specialists for primary care treatment, with nearly one-fourth of OB/GYN visits estimated to address mental health problems (Scholle et al. 2004). Of individuals receiving mental health care only in the general medical sector, 71% were women versus 58% of those receiving specialty mental health care (Uebelacker et al. 2006).

Psychosocial and Pharmacological Treatment for Mental Health Problems

Although the specific treatment approach used varies with the type and severity of disorder, the most prevalent treatments for mental disorders involve psychotherapy or other psychosocial approaches, and/or the use of pharmacotherapy. Some evidence suggests that, among depressed primary care patients, women are more likely than men to prefer counseling to medication (Dwight-Johnson et al. 2000). Managed care has generally controlled psychotherapy visits more strictly than medication management, which can be provided by general physicians, not only by psychiatrists. Furthermore, in carve-outs, MBHOs are typically not responsible for the costs of psychotropic medications, which are covered by the main health plan. Longer-term psychotherapy usually involves utilization review or prior authorization of visits beyond a certain limit, based on a medical necessity determination.

In general, persons covered under managed care have coverage for mental health services in most levels of care (Bureau of Labor Statistics 2007a; Ridgely and Maglione 2006). However, managed care may impact quantity, length, or provider of the services a person receives, and whether and how medications are covered. As noted above, the use of pharmacy benefits management approaches means that medication coverage may vary in several ways under managed care plans: formulary restrictions, use of higher cost-sharing tiers, prior authorization, and fail-first policies that require certain medications to be tried prior to others. Private managed care plans are more likely to use cost-sharing techniques than administrative techniques to steer patients to preferred medications; only 25% of plans had no restrictions on newer brand-name antidepressants, and 17% had no restrictions on newer brand-name antipsychotics (Hodgkin et al. 2007a).

Levels of Care

With the advent of managed care in the 1990s, a major focus was to implement controls on inpatient care, as it is the most costly service. Prior authorization for treatment and concurrent review to ensure that the level of care remains necessary for ongoing treatment were designed to ensure that patients were not treated more intensively or longer than needed. These mechanisms ultimately became standard in many otherwise unmanaged, fee-for-service plans as well. Other managed care mechanisms, such as provider networks, also have contributed to shorter inpatient length of stay and expansion of intermediate levels of care, such as day treatment. Studies have found that the implementation of mental health carve-outs, for example, results in decreased inpatient utilization and increased use of intermediate care (Frank and Garfield 2007). These effects have occurred in both private and public sectors.

Inpatient treatment is now typically short-term and used primarily for individuals with acute problems (or exacerbations of chronic problems) that cannot be addressed in less restrictive settings and/or present a danger to themselves or others. These declines in inpatient care and an expanding continuum of care have also been enabled by better medications and the recognition of the importance of community integration. Thus, most mental health treatment today occurs in outpatient settings, including office-based private practice, group practice, hospital outpatient department or community mental health center. Consumer-run or peer-run services are increasingly used as an adjunct to services provided by traditional mental health providers.

The level of care in which an individual is treated is determined by diagnosis, severity, and specific treatment needs. Therefore, gender differences in these areas may mean that managed care approaches affect women differently. To the extent, for instance, that women are more likely to make suicide attempts or have severe eating disorders, they may be more likely to be hospitalized than men (Savoie et al. 2004). Treatment options for postpartum depression, affecting 10–22% of new mothers, must consider the needs of the newborn as well, so medication may not be prescribed to breast feeding mothers (Seyfried and Marcus 2003). Alternatively, men may delay care-seeking longer than women, thus may have more severe symptomatology once presenting for care and may need a higher level of care (Wang et al. 2005a).

Some treatment settings provide a targeted focus on specific populations or expanded service offerings. For instance, women-only therapies or treatment settings are often available, which are particularly useful for women who were traumatized by sexual or intimate partner violence, or for women who are uncomfortable disclosing their feelings in a mixed-gender group. Some treatment programs provide childcare on-site, removing a potential barrier to treatment. Programs may offer other targeted treatment services, such as treatment for co-occurring disorders, or ancillary services such as employment counseling or medical care. Managed care plans may determine the specific treatment settings or programs that are available to an individual, thus these options may or may not be available as a paid benefit.

Treatment Providers

In addition to treatment type, one must also consider the types of providers that treat individuals with a mental disorder. Managed care has fostered greater use of psychiatrists for medication management rather than for psychotherapy, and it has increased the use of masters-level clinicians for psychotherapy. Thus, expensive psychiatrists are mostly used where their specialized training is required. Primary care physicians and other authorized practitioners may also prescribe and offer medication management, but rarely provide more than brief counseling. Mental health consumers are increasingly acknowledged for their important role in all aspects of the treatment system, as service providers, case managers, administrators, and providing peer support (Institute of Medicine 2006; Oss et al. 1998; U.S. Surgeon General 1999).

Nonmedical care for mental health needs can include Employee Assistance Programs (EAPs), other human service settings, schools, or criminal justice settings, or more informal settings (through clergy or self-help groups). Many of these resources occur outside the realm of insurance and managed care benefit coverage.

Treatment for Co-occurring Substance Abuse

The co-occurrence of mental and substance use disorders is common. Unless both issues are addressed, it is likely that recovery from either problem will be hindered. However, the mental health and substance abuse treatment systems often work as "silos," with different providers, treatment settings, and funding. Regardless of the treatment system, there is a dearth of providers with specific expertise in treating the individuals with co-occurring disorders. It is unclear exactly how much managed care has integrated the treatment for individuals with co-occurring disorders, although case management and provision of integrated treatment are common in health plans (Horgan et al. 2003). Furthermore, both mental health and substance abuse services are covered within most carve-outs, ensuring coverage of both illnesses within the same MBHO. For more information on co-occurring disorders, the reader is encouraged to examine Chaps. 5, 9, and 10 in this volume.

The divide between the mental health and substance abuse delivery systems may be particularly salient for women because of their help-seeking behaviors and symptoms. Women with substance use problems may present with symptoms that are similar to depression or anxiety, and they may be more likely than men to seek help in the mental health system rather than the substance abuse system (Weisner and Schmidt 1992). Therefore, expertise in co-occurring disorders, within the mental health system, may be especially beneficial for women to ensure that they are not misdiagnosed or treated inappropriately.

Selected Issues in Managed Behavioral Health Care

Access

The effect of managed care approaches on access to mental health services is a key issue. We focus here on several of the nonfinancial managed care mechanisms.

A substantial body of research has examined the effects of mental health carve-outs in both private and public sector settings, indicating increased overall access to mental health services (Frank and Garfield 2007; Frank and Lave 2003; Grazier and Eselius 1999; Mauery et al. 2006; Sturm 1999). In these studies, access is usually measured as the percentage of enrollees who receive any mental health care. Fewer studies have examined access in terms of unmet need, but this type of study can be informative. One national survey found that fewer privately insured individuals in managed care plans reported unmet need (defined as receiving no care) for behavioral health services, compared to those in unmanaged plans (Sturm and Sherbourne 2000). However, higher percentages of managed care enrollees reported receiving less care than needed or delayed care.

Carve-outs have also been associated with a shift in care settings, significant decreases in inpatient utilization (including both admission rates and length of stay) and increased use of intermediate care settings. Results are mixed regarding changes in outpatient utilization. Overall, it appears that carve-outs most often preserve access to any of the services while reducing intensity of care. Gender-specific effects of carve-outs have rarely been studied, and existing studies have found little or no differential effect (Huskamp et al. 1998; Volpe-Vartanian 2007). However, it is possible that differences do exist but have not yet been uncovered.

Approaches such as prior authorization or case management have been found to reduce inpatient utilization (Frank and Brookmeyer 1995; Hodgkin 1992; Wickizer and Lessler 1998; Wickizer et al. 1996). Some have raised concerns that the reduction can lead to worse outcomes, such as rapid readmission. Fewer studies have analyzed the effects of utilization management for outpatient mental health care, and results regarding access are mixed. For example, some research has found that the number of outpatient visits initially authorized is related to total utilization or correlated with termination at times when reauthorization is required (Howard 1998; Liu et al. 2000), while others have found no relationship (Compton et al. 2000). A study of one national MBHO found that only 0.6% of outpatient treatment requests were denied and another 1.5% were approved at a lower number of visits than requested (Koike et al. 2000). Utilization management may nonetheless have a "sentinel effect" in which providers know that utilization is monitored and may be concerned that requesting additional treatment could jeopardize their retention in the network.

Because women may be more likely to seek help earlier or for less severe conditions, utilization management may disproportionately reduce utilization for women, but this has rarely been examined (Huskamp et al. 1998). An evaluation of carve-outs found no evidence of this occurring (Huskamp et al. 1998). As discussed earlier, many aspects of gatekeeping and treatment entry can vary, and not all have been studied in terms of their independent effects on access. For example, studies of a change in the gatekeeping model at a large HMO found that switching from in-person evaluation to routine authorization through a call center resulted in a modest increase in the proportion of enrollees accessing care (Hodgkin et al. 2007b), with no detrimental impacts on quality indicators (Merrick et al. 2008). Further studies of specific mechanisms related to access are needed, including differential effects by gender.

Coordination/Integration of Services

Echoing the call by the President's New Freedom Commission on Mental Health (2003), the Institute of Medicine has recently emphasized the need to coordinate care in the treatment of mental and substance use disorders, requiring communication and collaboration across multiple providers and systems of care (Institute of Medicine 2006). At least three types of issues drive the need for coordination or integration of services, two of which have been noted previously. First are the challenges of helping persons with dual mental health and substance use problems when the two treatment systems have historically been separated in terms of funding streams, types of provider, and treatment approaches. The development of integrated treatment approaches and use of case management to help coordinate care at the individual level are promising, as is the increasing understanding on the part of providers and policymakers that the "silo" approach is problematic.

Second, persons with mental disorders who have particularly complex needs or severe problems can be helped both by case management and disease management programs. Case management can assist individuals who need help accessing care, psychosocial treatment, medications, and other supports, and provide assistance in recovery skills. Disease management, which is often focused on a specific disorder, takes a more systemic approach to improving care and adherence to treatment. At the same time, disease management approaches provide education, self-management training, coaching and support to assist individuals in accessing the various services needed.

Third is the lack of coordination or integration between the general medical and specialty mental health sectors. Risk of mental health problems, such as depression, is elevated in persons with chronic medical illnesses, such as diabetes and congestive heart failure (Anderson et al. 2001; MacMahon and Lip 2002). Barriers to coordination of care across sectors include less than optimal identification of mental disorders in primary care, separate service systems, stigma, lack of time and reimbursement for coordination activities, and confidentiality concerns.

Early forms of general managed care, such as staff-model HMOs, aimed at better coordination of all specialty services through the primary care physician. However, the backlash against highly managed care resulted in the loosening of gatekeeping systems and larger provider networks (Robinson 2001).

Despite concerns that carve-outs may exacerbate the fragmentation of mental health and other medical care, little empirical evidence addresses this point. Managed care, as typically organized, may not significantly improve coordination and integration of mental health services with other medical services. However, some approaches include coordination as an integral feature. The Wagner Chronic Care

Model, which has been implemented in numerous practices and certain managed care organizations, is an example of truly integrated and coordinated care (Wagner 1998). The six elements of the chronic care model include (1) delivery system design (e.g., multidisciplinary team, case management), (2) decision support (e.g., training and reminders to support guideline adherence), (3) clinical information systems (e.g., to enable performance feedback to providers), (4) patient self-management support, (5) healthcare organization (e.g., leadership support, quality improvement processes), and (6) community resources.

Managed care organizations can also take other steps to foster coordination and communication across general medical and specialty mental health sectors. Most private managed care plans provide practice guidelines for primary care screening and treatment of specific mental disorders (Horgan et al. 2009). Some plans include performance standards on coordination with primary care in their contracts with MBHOs (Horgan et al. 2009; Institute of Medicine 2006). Other ways to facilitate coordination include colocation of services and use of shared electronic health records (Institute of Medicine 2006; President's New Freedom Commission on Mental Health 2003). While the challenges are now recognized, much remains to do to address the divide. Integration of mental health care into primary care should build on the strengths of each delivery system (Thielke et al. 2007).

Quality Management

Managed care has both provoked concerns about quality of care and provided structured organizations that may facilitate the measurement and improvement of quality. Measuring performance of mental health providers and systems can foster quality improvement within organizations, enable comparability across organizations, and promote accountability for delivering high-quality care. Quality of health and mental health care can be measured according to Donabedian's now-classic paradigm of *structure* (including resources and infrastructure), *process* of delivering care, and *outcomes* attributable to the services received (Donabedian 1988). Currently the focus is on capturing the process or outcomes of care.

In the private sector, accrediting organizations, such as the National Committee for Quality Assurance (NCQA), have helped to drive the adoption of various quality activities by managed care organizations. NCQA offers a performance measurement system, Healthcare Effectiveness Data and Information Set (HEDIS), which is required for accreditation purposes and includes several behavioral health measures (National Committee for Quality Assurance 2007).

In the public sector, an important recent development is the National Outcomes Measures (NOMs) initiative of the Substance Abuse and Mental Health Services Administration (SAMHSA), aimed at helping to improve quality through standardized performance measurement for all states. The NOMs contain 10 domains cutting across mental health, substance abuse treatment, and substance abuse prevention. NOMs implementation is not contingent upon the type or degree of managed care approaches that states may be using, but is taking place within the context of widespread adoption of managed care approaches.

Focus on capturing the mental health consumer point of view through surveys is increasing. SAMHSA's Mental Health Statistics Improvement Project (MHSIP) offers a consumer-oriented mental health report card based on its consumer survey (Mental Health Statistics Improvement Program 2000). The report card features performance measures of access, quality/appropriateness, outcomes, and prevention, and it has been used extensively in public mental health settings. Another example is the Modular Survey initiative, also sponsored by SAMHSA, in conjunction with the Forum on Performance Measures in Behavioral Health and the Washington Circle. This initiative aims to develop and promote a common set of performance measures supported by a consumer survey that can be used widely across settings and populations, including public and private sectors (Bartlett et al. 2006).

Implications for Women's Mental Health

The era of managed care has brought major changes to the organization, financing, and delivery of mental health services. Managed care approaches, including mental health carve-outs and specific managed care mechanisms, have strongly shaped mental health services at every level and throughout various service systems. Managed mental health care has, at least indirectly, also contributed to developments such as the mental health parity movement. Thus, some benefits, but also new challenges, have resulted from the evolution of managed care. Because managed care is not a monolithic entity, it is difficult to characterize its effects upon mental health services categorically. Carve-outs are among the better-studied forms of managed care for mental health, and in general, they have been associated with improved initial access to care (use of any of the services), cost reductions, and reduced reliance on inpatient services, with some mixed findings regarding quality of care, though most studies do not find a detrimental impact.

Women seeking or in mental health treatment have been affected by these changes, as have all members of the population. Certainly, purely on the basis of numbers, women have been particularly affected as they are more likely than men to utilize mental health services. They are also likely to be affected differentially when managed care approaches particularly impact treatment of disorders more prevalent among women. Furthermore, women's greater likelihood of being low-income means that any financial management mechanism (such as cost sharing, which is used by, but not at all unique to, managed care) may have a stronger effect.

It is important to recognize that the era of managed mental health care also brings with it opportunities, such as increasing access, measuring and improving quality, and improving coordination of care. These are areas in which women stand to gain significantly, for the reasons noted earlier as well as their greater tendency to seek mental health treatment in primary care settings.

Further research is needed regarding gender-specific effects of various managed mental health care approaches, including studies that focus on the consumer experience of care as well as service utilization. This falls within the broader domain of women's mental health needs and services, which present many significant public health issues warranting additional women-focused research (Blehar 2003). To date, it is accurate to acknowledge that women have undoubtedly shared fully in the benefits and problems found to be associated with managed care, have been particularly affected as the higher-utilizing gender, and may, given the same clinical picture, experience managed care effects more, or somewhat differently, than men, but this largely remains to be determined.

Acknowledgments The authors thank Deborah W. Garnick, Sc.D., Dominic Hodgkin, Ph.D., and Constance M. Horgan, Sc.D., for review and helpful discussion of the manuscript, and Bernard McCann, MS, CEAP for research assistance.

References

Agency for Healthcare Research and Quality. (2004a). Table 1: Usual Source of Health Care and Selected Population Characteristics, United States, 2004. Medical Expenditure Panel Survey Component Data. Retrieved December 11, 2007, from www.meps.ahrq.gov/mepsweb

Agency for Healthcare Research and Quality. (2004b). Table 8: Office-based Medical Provider Services – Median and Mean Expenses per Person with Expense and Distribution of Expenses by Source of Payment, United States, 2004. Medical Expenditure Panel Survey Component Data. Retrieved December 11, 2007, from www.meps.ahrq.gov/mepsweb

Anderson, R. J., Freedland, K. E., Clouse, R. E., & Lustman, P. J. (2001). The prevalence of comorbid depression in adults with diabetes: A meta-analysis. *Diabetes Care, 24*(6), 1069–1078.

Barry, C. L., Frank, R. G., & McGuire, T. G. (2006). The costs of mental health parity: Still an impediment? *Health Affairs, 25*(3), 623–634.

Barry, C. L., Gabel, J. R., Frank, R. G., Hawkins, S., Whitmore, H. H., & Pickreign, J. D. (2003). Design of mental health benefits: Still unequal after all these years. *Health Affairs, 22*(5), 127–137.

Bartlett, J., Chalk, M., Manderscheid, R. W., & Wattenberg, S. (2006). Finding common performance measures through consensus and empirical analysis: The Forum on performance measures in behavioral healthcare. In R. W. Manderscheid (Ed.), *Mental health, United States 2004.* Rockville, MD: Center for Mental Health Services, Substance Abuse and Mental Health Services Administration.

Blehar, M. C. (2003). Public health context of women's mental health research. *Psychiatric Clinics of North America, 26*(3), 781–799.

Blum, T. C., & Roman, P. M. (1995). *Cost effectiveness and preventive implications of employee assistance programs* (No. DHHS RP-0907). Rockville, MD: Substance Abuse and Mental Health Services Administration, Center for Substance Abuse Prevention.

Buchmueller, T. C., Cooper, P. F., Jacobson, M., & Zuvekas, S. H. (2007). Parity for whom? Exemptions and the extent of state mental health parity legislation. *Health Affairs, 26*(4), w483–w487.

Bureau of Labor Statistics. (2007a). *National compensation survey: Employee benefits in private industry in the United States, 2005.* Washington, DC: U.S. Department of Labor, Bureau of Labor Statistics.

Bureau of Labor Statistics. (2007b). *Women in the labor force: A databook* (2007 edition). Retrieved December 11, 2007, from www.bls.gov/cps/wlf-databook2007.htm

Case Management Society of America. (2007). Definition of case management. Retrieved July 29, 2007, from http://www.cmsa.org/ABOUTUS/DefinitionofCaseManagement/tabid/104/Default.aspx

Centers for Medicare and Medicaid Services. (2007). Medicaid Managed Care Enrollment as of December 31, 2006. Retrieved November 18, 2007, from http://www.cms.hhs.gov/MedicaidDataSourcesGenInfo/Downloads/mmcpr06.pdf

Compton, S. N., Cuffel, B. J., Burns, B. J., & Goldman, W. (2000). Datapoints: Effects of changing from five to ten preauthorized outpatient sessions. *Psychiatric Services, 51*(10), 1223.

Dailard, C. (1999). Gender-specific approaches to mental health policy. *Journal of Gender Specific Medicine, 2*(3), 32–34, 39–40.

Delaney, W., Grube, J. W., & Ames, G. M. (1998). Predicting likelihood of seeking help through the employee assistance program among salaried and union hourly employees. *Addiction, 93*(3), 399–410.

DeNavas-Walt, C., Proctor, B., & Smith, J. (2007). *Income, poverty and health insurance coverage in the U.S., 2006.* Washington, DC: U.S. Government Printing Office.

Disease Management Association of America. (2006). DMAA Definition of Disease Management. Retrieved March 20, 2008 from www.dmaa.org/dm_definition.asp.

Donabedian, A. (1988). The quality of care. How can it be assessed? *JAMA, 260*(12), 1743–1748.

Donohue, J. M., & Frank, R. G. (2007). Estimating Medicare Part D's impact on medication access among dually eligible beneficiaries with mental disorders. *Psychiatric Services, 58*(20), 1285–1291.

Dwight-Johnson, M., Sherbourne, C. D., Liao, D., & Wells, K. B. (2000). Treatment preferences among depressed primary care patients. *Journal of General Internal Medicine, 15*(8), 527–534.

Flaherty, R. A., Rashbaum, R. F., Triano, J. J., Hansen, D. T., Mootz, R. D., Coile, R. C., et al. (1996). Healthcare credentialing and qualifications commission: An alternative to "any willing provider"? *American Journal of Managed Care, 2*(5), 559–566.

Frank, R. G., & Brookmeyer, R. (1995). Managed mental health care and patterns of inpatient utilization for treatment of affective disorders. *Social Psychiatry and Psychiatric Epidemiology, 30*(5), 220–223.

Frank, R. G., & Garfield, R. L. (2007). Managed behavioral health care carve-outs: Past performance and future prospects. *Annual Review of Public Health, 28,* 303–320.

Frank, R. G., Goldman, H. H., & McGuire, T. G. (1992). A model mental health benefit in private health insurance. *Health Affairs, 11*(3), 98–117.

Frank, R. G., Huskamp, H. A., McGuire, T. G., & Newhouse, J. P. (1996). Some economics of mental health "carve-outs". *Archives of General Psychiatry, 53*(10), 933–937.

Frank, R. G., & Lave, J. (2003). Economics. In S. Feldman (Ed.), *Managed behavioral health services: Perspectives and practice* (pp. 146–165). Springfield, IL: Charles C. Thomas, Ltd.

Frank, R. G., & McGuire, T. G. (1986). A review of studies of the impact of insurance on the demand and utilization of specialty mental health services. *Health Services Research, 21*(2 Pt 2), 241–265.

Frank, R. G., & McGuire, T. G. (1998). Parity for mental health and substance abuse care under managed care. *Journal of Mental Health Policy and Economics, 1*(4), 153–159.

Frank, R. G., McGuire, T. G., & Newhouse, J. P. (1995). Risk contracts in managed mental health care. *Health Affairs, 14*(3), 50–64.

Gabel, J., Claxton, G., Gil, I., Pickreign, J., Whitmore, H., Finder, B., et al. (2005). Health benefits in 2005: Premium increases slow down, coverage continues to erode. *Health Affairs, 24*(5), 1273–1280.

Garis, R. I., Clark, B. E., Siracuse, M. V., & Makoid, M. C. (2004). Examining the benefit of pharmacy benefit management companies. *American Journal of Health-System Pharmacy, 61,* 81–85.

Garnick, D., Horgan, C., Reif, S., Merrick, E., & Hodgkin, D. (2008). Management of behavioral health provider networks in private health plans. *Journal of Ambulatory Care Management, 31*(4), 330–341.

Glied, S. (1997). The treatment of women with mental health disorders under HMO and fee-for-service insurance. *Women & Health, 26*(2), 1–16.

Grazier, K. L., & Eselius, L. L. (1999). Mental health carve-outs: Effects and implications. *Medical Care Research & Review, 56*(Suppl. 2), 37–59.

Hasin, D. S., Goodwin, R. D., Stinson, F. S., & Grant, B. F. (2005). Epidemiology of major depressive disorder: Results from the National Epidemiologic Survey on Alcoholism and Related Conditions. *Archives of General Psychiatry, 62*(10), 1097–1106.

Hodgkin, D. (1992). The impact of private utilization management on psychiatric care: A review of the literature. *Journal of Mental Health Administration, 19*(2), 143–157.

Hodgkin, D., Horgan, C. M., & Garnick, D. W. (1997). Make or buy: HMOs' contracting arrangements for mental health care. *Administration and Policy in Mental Health, 24*(4), 359–376.

Hodgkin, D., Horgan, C. M., Garnick, D. W., & Merrick, E. L. (2008). *Benefit limits for behavioral healthcare in private health plans.* Waltham, MA: Brandeis University.

Hodgkin, D., Horgan, C. M., Garnick, D. W., Merrick, E. L., & Goldin, D. (2000). Why carve out? Determinants of behavioral health contracting choice among large U.S. employers. *Journal of Behavioral Health Services and Research, 27*(2), 178–193.

Hodgkin, D., Horgan, C. M., Garnick, D. W., Merrick, E. L., & Volpe-Vartanian, J. (2007a). Management of access to branded psychotropic medications in private health plans. *Clinical Therapeutics, 29*(2), 371–380.

Hodgkin, D., Merrick, E. L., Horgan, C. M., Garnick, D. W., & McLaughlin, T. J. (2007b). Does type of gatekeeping model affect access to outpatient specialty mental health services? *Health Services Research, 42*(1 Pt 1), 104–123.

Horgan, C. M. (1986). The demand for ambulatory mental health services from specialty providers. *Health Services Research, 21*(2 Pt 2), 291–319.

Horgan, C. M., Garnick, D. W., Merrick, E. L., & Hodgkin, D. (2009). Changes in how health plans provide behavioral health services. *Journal of Behavioral Health Services and Research, 36*(1), 11–24.

Horgan, C. M., & Merrick, E. L. (2001). Financing of substance abuse treatment services. In M. Galanter (Ed.), *Recent developments in alcoholism, Vol. XV: Services research in the era of managed care.* New York, NY: Plenum Publishing.

Horgan, C. M., Merrick, E. L., Garnick, D. W., Hodgkin, D., Cenczyk, R. E., Lusenhop, R. W., et al. (2003). *The provision of mental health services in managed care organizations* (DHHS Publication No. (SMA) 03-3797). Rockville, MD: Center for Mental Health Services, Substance Abuse and Mental Health Services Administration.

Howard, R. (1998). The sentinel effect in an outpatient managed care setting. *Professional Psychology Research and Practice, 29*(3), 262–268.

Huskamp, H. A., Azzone, V., & Frank, R. G. (1998). Carve-outs, women, and the treatment of depression. *Womens Health Issues, 8*(5), 267–282.

Institute of Medicine. (2006). *Improving the quality of health care for mental and substance-use conditions.* Washington, DC: National Academies Press.

Kaiser Family Foundation. (2007). Women's Health Policy Facts: Women's Health Insurance Coverage. Retrieved November 18, 2007, from http://www.kff.org/womenshealth/upload/6000_05.pdf

Keeler, E. B., Manning, W. G., & Wells, K. (1989). The demand for episodes of mental health services. *Journal of Health Economics, 7,* 369–392.

Kessler, R. C., Berglund, P., Demler, O., Jin, R., Merikangas, K. R., & Walters, E. E. (2005a). Lifetime prevalence and age-of-onset distributions of DSM-IV disorders in the National Comorbidity Survey Replication. *Archives of General Psychiatry, 62*(6), 593–602.

Kessler, R. C., Demler, O., Frank, R. G., Olfson, M., Pincus, H. A., Walters, E. E., et al. (2005b). Prevalence and treatment of mental disorders, 1990 to 2003. *New England Journal of Medicine, 352*(24), 2515–2523.

Kessler, R. C., McGonagle, K. A., Zhao, S., Nelson, C. B., Hughes, M., Eshleman, S., et al. (1994). Lifetime and 12-month prevalence of DSM-III-R psychiatric disorders in the United States. Results from the National Comorbidity Survey. *Archives of General Psychiatry, 51*(1), 8–19.

Koike, A., Klap, R., & Unutzer, J. (2000). Utilization management in a large managed behavioral health organization. *Psychiatric Services, 51*(5), 621–626.

Landsman, P. B., Yu, W., Liu, X., Teutsch, S. M., & Berger, M. L. (2005). Impact of 3-tier pharmacy benefit design and increased consumer cost-sharing on drug utilization. *American Journal of Managed Care, 11*(10), 621–628.

Larson, M. J., Miller, K., & Fleming, K. J. (2006). Antidepressant medication use in private insurance health plans, 2002. *Psychiatric Services, 57*(2), 175.

Lightner, E., & McConatha, J. T. (1995). Factors affecting supervisory referrals to employee assistance programs: The impact of race and gender. *Journal of Social Behavior and Policy, 10,* 179–188.

Liu, X., Sturm, R., & Cuffel, B. J. (2000). The impact of prior authorization on outpatient utilization in managed behavioral health plans. *Medical Care Research & Review, 57*(2), 182–195.

MacMahon, K. M., & Lip, G. Y. (2002). Psychological factors in heart failure: A review of the literature. *Archives of Internal Medicine, 162*(5), 509–516.

Mark, T. L. (2008). Half of adolescents who are prescribed antidepressants don't receive psychotherapy. *Thomson Healthcare Research Brief March 2008.* Retrieved April 9, 2008, from http://research.thomsonhealthcare.come/articles/view/?id=1629

Mark, T. L., Levit, K. R., Coffey, R. M., McKusick, D. R., Harwood, H. J., King, E. C., et al. (2007). *National expenditures for mental health services and substance abuse treatment, 1993–2003* (No. SMA 07-4227). Rockville, MD: Substance Abuse and Mental Health Services Administration.

Mauery, D. R., Vaquerano, L., Sethi, R., Jee, J., & Chimento, L. (2006). *Managed mental health care: Findings from the literature, 1990–2005* (No. SMA-06-4178). Rockville, MD: Substance Abuse and Mental Health Services Administration, Center for Mental Health Services.

Mechanic, D., Schlesinger, M., & McAlpine, D. D. (1995). Management of mental health and substance abuse services: State of the art and early results. *Milbank Quarterly, 73*(1), 19–55.

Mental Health America. (2007). What Have States Done to Ensure Insurance Parity. Retrieved April 9, 2008, from http://www.nmha.org/go/parity/states

Mental Health Statistics Improvement Program. (2000). MHSIP Consumer Survey version 1.1. Retrieved December 5, 2007, from http://www.MHSIP.org/

Merrick, E. L., Hodgkin, D., Horgan, C. M., Garnick, D. W., & McLaughlin, T. J. (2008). Changing mental health gatekeeping: Effects on performance indicators. *Journal of Behavioral Health Services and Research, 35*(1), 3–19.

Merrick, E. L., Horgan, C. M., Garnick, D. W., & Hodgkin, D. (2006). Managed care organizations' use of treatment management strategies for outpatient mental health care. *Administration and Policy in Mental Health, 33*(1), 104–114.

Merrick, E. L., Volpe-Vartanian, J., Horgan, C. M., & McCann, B. (2007). Alcohol & drug abuse: Revisiting employee assistance programs and substance use problems in the workplace: Key issues and a research agenda. *Psychiatric Services, 58*(10), 1262–1264.

Nair, K. V., & Valuck, R. J. (2004). Impact of three-tier pharmacy benefit structures on consumer attitudes, pharmacy, medical utilization and costs: A critical review. *Disease Management and Health Outcomes, 12*(2), 81–92.

National Committee for Quality Assurance. (2007). Retrieved December 11, 2007, from http://web.ncqa.org/tabid/59/Default.aspx

O'Kane, M. E. (2007). Performance-based measures: The early results are in. *Journal of Managed Care Pharmacy, 13*(2 Suppl.), S3–S6.

Olson, B. M. (2002). Approaches to pharmacy benefit management and the impact of consumer cost-sharing. *Clinical Therapeutics, 25,* 250–272.

Oss, M. E., Jardine, E., & Pesare, M. J. (2002). *OPEN MINDS Yearbook of managed behavioral health and employee assistance program market share in the United States, 2002–2003.* Gettysburg, PA: OPEN MINDS.

Oss, M. E., Yennie, H., & Birch, S. (1998). Managed care approaches and models for the treatment and management of depression: Specific issues for women. *Womens Health Issues, 8*(5), 283–292, discussion 293–303.

Pelonero, A. L., & Johnson, R. L. (2007). Economic grand rounds: A pay-for-performance program for behavioral health care practitioners. *Psychiatric Services, 58*(4), 442–444.

President's New Freedom Commission on Mental Health. (2003). Achieving the Promise: Transforming Mental Health Care in America. Retrieved December 7, 2007 from www.mentalhealthcommission.gov.

Ridgely, M. S., & Maglione, M. A. (2006). Managing Medicaid behavioral health care: Findings of a national survey in the year 2000. *Psychiatric Services, 57*(7), 1000–1006.

Robinson, J. C. (2001). The end of managed care. *The Journal of the American Medical Association, 285*(20), 2622–2628.

Robinson, G., Kaye, N., Bergman, D., Moreaux, M., & Baxter, C. (2005). State Profiles of Mental Health and Substance Abuse Services in Medicaid. Retrieved April 9, 2008, from http://mentalhealth.samhsa.gov/Publications/allpubs/State_Med/StateProfiles.pdf

Rogowski, J. A. (1992). Insurance coverage for drug abuse. *Health Affairs, 11*(3), 137–148.

Rosenthal, M. B., Landon, B. E., Normand, S. L., Frank, R. G., & Epstein, A. M. (2006). Pay for performance in commercial HMOs. *New England Journal of Medicine, 355*(18), 1895–1902.

Salkever, D. S., Shinogle, J., & Goldman, H. (1999). Mental health benefit limits and cost sharing under managed care: A national survey of employers. *Psychiatric Services, 50*(12), 1631–1633.

Savoie, I., Morettin, D., Green, C. J., & Kazanjian, A. (2004). Systematic review of the role of gender as a health determinant of hospitalization for depression. *International Journal of Technology Assessment in Health Care, 20*(2), 115–127.

Scholle, S. H., Chang, J., Harman, J., & McNeil, M. (2004). Characteristics of patients seen and services provided in primary care visits in obstetrics/gynecology: Data from NAMCS and NHAMCS. *American Journal of Obstetrics & Gynecology, 190*(4), 1119–1127.

Seyfried, L. S., & Marcus, S. M. (2003). Postpartum mood disorders. *International Review of Psychiatry, 15*(3), 231–242.

Simon, G. E., Grothaus, L., Durham, M. L., VonKorff, M., & Pabiniak, C. (1996). Impact of visit copayments on outpatient mental health utilization by members of a health maintenance organization. *American Journal of Psychiatry, 153*(3), 331–338.

Sobelman, J. S. (2001). Managed care credentialing of physicians. *Physician's News Digest.* Retrieved May 19, 2006, from http://www.physiciansnews.com/business/601sobelman.html

Sturm, R. (1999). Tracking changes in behavioral health services: How have carve-outs changed care? *Journal of Behavioral Health Services and Research, 26*(4), 360–371.

Sturm, R., & Sherbourne, C. D. (2000). Managed care and unmet need for mental health and substance abuse care in 1998. *Psychiatric Services, 51*(2), 177.

Sturm, R., Zhang, W., & Schoenbaum, M. (1999). How expensive are unlimited substance abuse benefits under managed care? *Journal of Behavioral Health Services and Research, 26*(2), 203–210.

Teich, J. L., & Buck, J. A. (2007). Mental health benefits in Employer-sponsored Health Plans, 1997–2003. *Journal of Behavioral Health Services and Research, 34*(3), 343–348.

Thielke, S., Vannoy, S., & Unutzer, J. (2007). Integrating mental health and primary care. *Primary Care, 34*(3), 571–592, vii.

Uebelacker, L. A., Wang, P. S., Berglund, P., & Kessler, R. C. (2006). Clinical differences among patients treated for mental health problems in general medical and specialty mental health settings in the National Comorbidity Survey Replication. *General Hospital Psychiatry, 28*(5), 387–395.

U.S. Surgeon General. (1999). Mental Health: A Report of the Surgeon General. Retrieved December 11, 2007 from www.surgeongeneral.gov/library/mentalhealth/home.html.

Volpe-Vartanian, J. (2007). Are there gender differences in the effects of a managed behavioral health carve-out? Evidence from Puerto Rico. Dissertation, Brandeis University.

Wagner, E. H. (1998). Chronic disease management: What will it take to improve care for chronic illness? *Effective Clinical Practice, 1*(1), 2–4.

Wang, P. S., Berglund, P., Olfson, M., Pincus, H. A., Wells, K. B., & Kessler, R. C. (2005a). Failure and delay in initial treatment contact after first onset of mental disorders in the National Comorbidity Survey Replication. *Archives of General Psychiatry, 62*(6), 603–613.

Wang, P. S., Lane, M., Olfson, M., Pincus, H. A., Wells, K. B., & Kessler, R. C. (2005b). Twelve-month use of mental health services in the United States: Results from the National Comorbidity Survey Replication. *Archives of General Psychiatry, 62*(6), 629–640.

Weisner, C., & Schmidt, L. (1992). Gender disparities in treatment for alcohol problems. *The Journal of the American Medical Association, 268*(14), 1872–1876.

Wickizer, T. M., & Lessler, D. (1998). Do treatment restrictions imposed by utilization management increase the likelihood of readmission for psychiatric patients? *Medical Care, 36*(6), 844–850.

Wickizer, T. M., Lessler, D., & Travis, K. M. (1996). Controlling inpatient psychiatric utilization through managed care. *American Journal of Psychiatry, 153*(3), 339–345.

Zuvekas, S. H., Rupp, A., & Norquist, G. (2007). Cost shifting under managed behavioral health care. *Psychiatric Services, 58*(1), 100–108.

Chapter 12
Evidence-Based Medicine

Gina Perez, Lisa Dixon and Deanna L. Kelly

Introduction

Ensuring the quality of medical care has not always been a priority or even a consideration for providers and purchasers of health care. However, awareness of tremendous regional variations in care provided as well as increasing awareness of poor access and suboptimal healthcare practice have brought about efforts to improve the quality of care.

The identification and implementation of best practices to standardize procedures and approaches in the treatment of health care, including mental health care, has been an important strategy to improve the quality of care. The field of medicine is ever-expanding in its development of new procedures and techniques for the care of patients. With the growing body of research studies, the challenge arises of deciphering which studies are most applicable to clinical care and most valid for particular patients. This quest for finding the most effective treatments impacts all fields of medicine, including psychiatry. Similar to other fields of medicine, psychiatry has developed general guidelines for the treatment of various disorders through information gleaned from controlled research studies.

In this chapter, the authors review some of the basic concepts associated with evidence-based medicine (EBM). In addition, the authors discuss the treatment of depression, a major cause of morbidity and mortality in women residing in the USA, to illustrate the use of EBM for the development of evidence-based clinical practice or "best practice" treatment guidelines. The authors also discuss factors to consider when making a clinical treatment decision about depression in women.

G. Perez (✉)
School of Medicine, University of Maryland, 655 West Baltimore Street,
Baltimore, MD 21201, USA

B. L. Levin, M. A. Becker (eds.), *A Public Health Perspective of Women's Mental Health*,
DOI 10.1007/978-1-4419-1526-9_12, © Springer Science+Business Media LLC 2010

What is Evidence-Based Medicine?

The concept of EBM has existed for several decades, though its absorption into the practice of medicine has dramatically increased over the past two decades. EBM is most commonly defined as "the conscientious, explicit, and judicious use of current best evidence in making decisions about the care of individual patients" (Sackett et al. 1996). EBM provides the foundation of evidence-based practice (EBP). It is useful to think about EBP as the clinician's way of applying EBM in the care of their patients. EBP is the integration of individual clinical expertise with EBM (Sackett et al. 1996).

Incorporating the right balance of clinical experience with current research and patient preferences allows for the best medical care. However, given the plethora of research studies on medical care, including psychiatric illnesses, practitioners do not have the time to read, let alone synthesize and analyze, this wealth of information. Evidence-based research offers a logical solution to the management of this information overload.

Evidence-based research constitutes the building blocks of EBM. Limitations in evidence-based research also constrain the range and scope of EBM. Challenges in the evaluation of this body of research are discussed later in this chapter, but rarely are there sufficient research initiatives to answer all of the important clinical questions that require answers. Evidence-based research is not meant to serve as a written set of inflexible rules or a user's guide to medicine, since clinical experience, understanding of the research available, patient preferences, and additional factors must be incorporated into the clinical decision-making process (Sackett et al. 1996). It is important to have a systematic way to synthesize all of the research and evidence being produced to help guide patient care and understand psychiatric illnesses.

Randomized Controlled Trials and Meta-analyses

Randomized trials or meta-analyses often provide the best clinical information (Sackett et al. 1996). A randomized controlled trial is designed in such a way that participants are assigned to one so-called arm of a study that provides a specific treatment by random assignment and compared to a group of similar individuals who do not receive the assigned intervention.

Meta-analyses use specific statistical methods designed to combine information from different studies (Hatala et al. 2005) to address a specific clinical question. There are times when randomized controlled trials are not feasible, most commonly when certain treatment options could pose an unknown serious risk to the patient or lack of a specific treatment could lead to negative consequences for the patient (Sackett et al. 1996). There are additional practical barriers to conducting randomized controlled trials, including lack of funding, lack of resources needed to manage the study, and lack of time to oversee such a time-intensive project.

The advantage of a randomized control design is that patients are randomly assigned to receive a certain intervention. This limits bias from the investigator in deciding what treatment a patient will get. For example, if the investigator is researching the effectiveness of a drug on depression and only selects patients with mild depression to receive the treatment versus patients with more severe depression to receive the placebo, the investigator might falsely conclude that the treatment is more effective than the placebo. Additionally, in a double-blind randomized control study, the patient and the investigator do not know what treatment is being given, decreasing the chance for bias on the part of either. However, the benefits of a randomized control trial do not negate the potential usefulness of case reports and studies with less stringent designs. Studies that do not utilize randomized experimental designs may not be able to offer as definitive of an answer for the clinician trying to figure out what to do for a particular patient's problem, but they still hold value in shedding light on a particular medical topic.

Many of the larger randomized controlled studies are conducted by pharmaceutical companies seeking FDA approval for their particular medication. Drug company sponsored studies can be biased, however, in other ways. These sponsored studies often have limited follow-up periods and may be restricted to patients without any comorbidity. Reducing the follow-up period saves on the cost of the study, but is not always as helpful to the clinician who will be treating the patient for a more extended period of time. Selecting patients with no comorbid illnesses allows for more precise interpretation of the study, but often in the clinical practice of medicine, patients present with many illnesses simultaneously (For more information on co-occurring disorders, see Chap. 5). There remains a need for longitudinal outcome research and study designs that include more representative samples of participants. The medical community must try to understand how to evaluate the validity of a study and detect any potential biases.

Randomized controlled trials are needed when constructing a meta-analysis. Many strict inclusion criteria are needed for the studies included in a meta-analysis so that the information can be combined, if possible, to help answer a particular clinical question with more certainty. The study design is the most critical factor: the patients chosen to participate in a study, the interventions that are employed, the outcomes that are measured, and the methods of measurement. The authors of the meta-analyses try to understand the results of each study to see if information can, in fact, be combined (Hatala et al. 2005).

There are numerous methods for conducting studies on treatment effectiveness. EBM aims to decipher and weigh the scientific validity of various studies with a goal of providing the best available research evidence to guide the development of evidence-based clinical practice guidelines for the optimal treatment of patients.

Navigating Through Evidence-Based Medicine

How can patients and treatment teams navigate through the growing body of literature to best understand whether EBM exists for a particular medical issue? Patients are advised to utilize their medical team initially to help guide them through the research literature. Blindly searching topics on the Internet often results in the review of mixed quality sites. In the quest for answers, misinformation can be confusing and at times even harmful to a patient eager to learn more about a particular illness.

Both patients and treatment teams can also refer to one of the most well-known EBM sites, the Cochrane Library (www.thecochranelibrary.com). This site focuses on digesting data related to a specific clinical question and reviewing all of the available research pertaining to the topic. The Cochrane Library is made up of numerous teams dedicated to appraising the medical literature on a particular topic and then, if possible, organizing it into meta-analyses or reviews.

Other information sites for patients and medical professionals include the American College of Physicians Journal (www.acpjc.org), the Cochrane Database of Systematic Reviews, Cochrane Central Registrar of Randomized Controlled Trials (CENTRAL), Britain's Centre for Review and Dissemination, and the Cochrane Effective Practice and Organization of Care (EPOC). Many journals now exist for the purpose of synthesizing medical information, including EBM and evidence-based nursing. Although other sites exist for EBM, in this chapter, the recent meta-analyses conducted through the Cochrane Library will be highlighted in addition to other pertinent research studies and case reports.

Applying Evidence-Based Practice for the Management of Depression

Incorporating EBM into clinical decision making is much more complicated than simply knowing the most recent meta-analysis or expert consensus on "best clinical practice" guidelines. In this next section, we will explore the EBM available for the treatment and understanding of depression, an illness which impacts a person's emotional well-being as well as cognitive and physical functioning.

Depression is a leading cause for long-term disability, afflicting men and women across the world. The lifetime prevalence of major depression is variable depending on the study, but it is consistently higher for women versus men. According to the Epidemiologic Catchment Area Study, in the USA the lifetime prevalence of a major depressive disorder for men and women over 18 years of age is 5.8%. Some studies show that women have a lifetime prevalence of major depression approaching 26%. In men, the lifetime prevalence tends to be lower, but may still be as high as 12%. The peak age of onset for women is in their 30s and 40s, though some women will experience depressive symptoms in childhood or later in life.

Major depression consists of a period lasting at least 2 weeks with persistently low mood or inability to experience pleasure. In addition, during a depressive episode, it may be difficult to concentrate, eat regularly, sleep, or complete usual daily activities. During a depressive period, people can also be burdened by feelings of worthlessness or excessive guilt about their life or past decisions. Thoughts of death or suicide may also be prominent. A person can even experience psychotic symptoms during depression, which refers to a break from reality in some way: perceiving things that are not there, harboring beliefs that are false, and suffering from behavior or thoughts that are grossly disorganized.

What information should be taken into account when deciding on treatment for an individual with depression? When choosing a strategy for treating depression in women, the most important factor is actually establishing a collaborative approach that respects the patient's goals and wishes in combination with the suggestions of the rest of the mental health treatment team and the clinical judgment of the responsible medical provider. Many people only have one provider who is most often a primary care physician. The patient is a critical partner in the treatment decision-making process and, along with involved family members, should be considered part of the treatment team. Figure 12.1 identifies major areas to address, including EBM, when deciding on a specific treatment or level of support for an individual with depression.

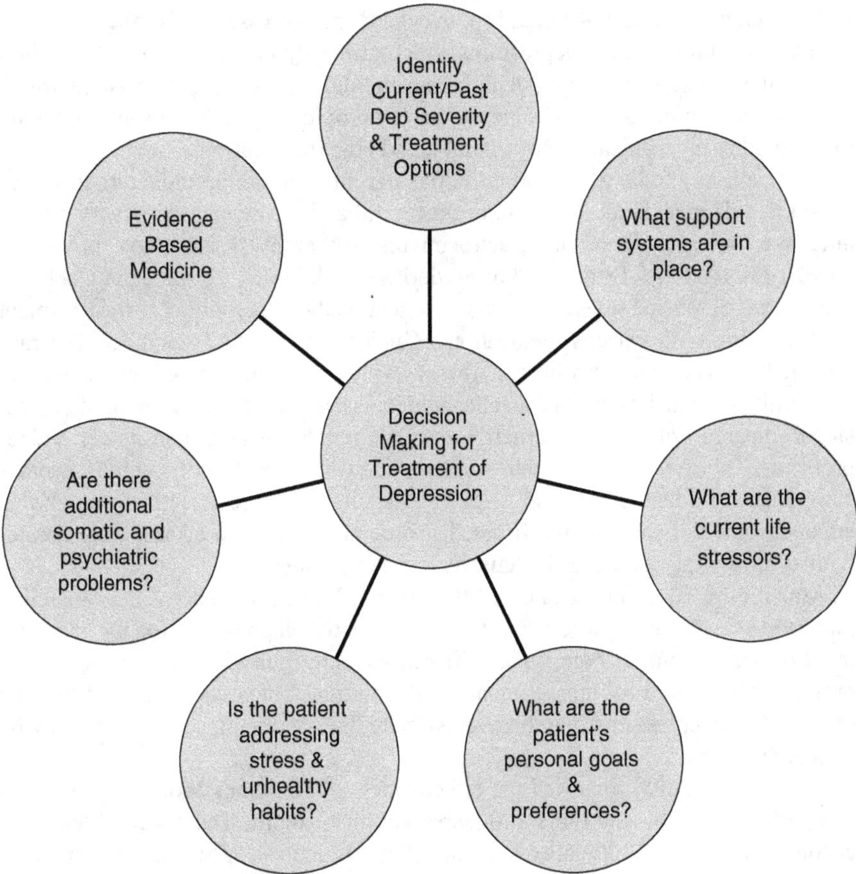

Fig. 12.1 Decision-making factors for the management of depression

Medication Options for Depression

If the treatment team feels medications may be helpful, there are many options. The most basic and commonly used of the antidepressants are serotonin reuptake inhibitors: fluoxetine (Prozac), sertraline (Zoloft), citalopram (Celexa), escitalopram (Lexapro), paroxetine (Paxil), and fluvoxamine (Luvox). About half of the people will show a reduction of symptoms with an initial trial of a serotonin reuptake inhibitor. However, studies evaluating the complete remission of symptoms demonstrate lower rates (Trivedi et al. 2006; Entsuah et al. 2001). The effect of any of these antidepressants takes 4–6 weeks. Sometimes the benefits are noticed first by loved ones rather than the person experiencing the symptoms. People often say that their problems have not gone away with medication, but they feel less burdened by them and less overwhelmed. This may allow them to take a fresh look at strategies to approach their major life issues. Some women may require more than one trial of medication or a combination of treatment modalities to find relief from symptoms.

There are other medication options aside from serotonin reuptake inhibitors which include, but are not limited to, tricylclic antidepressants (TCAs), monoamine oxidase inhibitors, antidepressants which primarily increase the levels of norepinephrine and serotonin (e.g., venlafaxine and duloxetine), antidepressants which increase dopamine and norepinephrine (Bupropion), antidepressants working through other mechanisms (Mirtazapine), and other medications.

Medications can be an important initial step in overcoming moderate to severe depression. If medication trials are unsuccessful and the depression is very severe, alternate strategies, including electroconvulsive therapy (ECT), have proven to be very effective (McDonald 2006; Frederikse et al. 2006). To date, the Cochrane Library has published several reviews and meta-analyses pertaining to the treatment of depression with various medications. Guaiana et al. (2007) included 194 randomized controlled studies in their review which examined the effectiveness and tolerability of amitriptyline, a tricyclic antidepressant, in the management of depression compared with other alternative tricylcic antidepressants and newer antidepressants. The results showed that amitriptyline was at least as efficacious as other comparison antidepressants and perhaps even slightly more effective, though this edge was not statistically significant. Unfortunately, the side effects were greater with amitriptyline compared with newer antidepressants.

Moncrieff et al. (2004) examined the effect of antidepressants versus an active placebo (i.e., mimics side effects, but has no active ingredient) for the management of depression. Of note, small differences were found in favor of the antidepressant with regard to improvements in depression. The authors suggest that the effects of antidepressants may be overestimated, while the placebo effects may be underestimated.

Linde et al. (2008) reviewed the effectiveness of St. John's Wort for depression compared to placebo and other antidepressant medications. There were 29 studies, encompassing over 5,000 patients, included in this analysis. The authors concluded that extracts from St. John's Wort were better than placebo in patients with major depression, similar in efficacy compared to standard antidepressants, and had fewer side effects than standard antidepressants. The authors emphasized that some of the studies from German-speaking areas may have overestimated the benefit of St. Johns Wort. In addition, the authors warn that all formulations of St. Johns Wort are not the same, and thus the results of the studies only apply to the specific extract examined.

A meta-analysis by Furukawa et al. (2001) evaluated the positive effects and potential harm when using benzodiazepines concomitantly with an antidepressant versus just prescribing an antidepressant alone. For those individuals receiving combined treatment, the drop-out rates were less and there also seemed to be an increased medication response during the first 4 weeks compared to those receiving an antidepressant alone. However, these benefits must be weighed with the increased risk of benzodiazepine dependence, the increased propensity for accidents, and the decline in drug effect over time associated with benzodiazepine use. The authors conclude that there are pros and cons to using this combination approach.

Therapy for the Treatment of Depression

Depression treatment is not focused simply on medications alone. Oftentimes a doctor will recommend that a person seek psychotherapy alone or in addition to medication. Cognitive-behavioral therapy (CBT) is a time-limited therapy proven to be effective in reducing symptoms of depression (in addition to other illnesses). In a study conducted by Goldapple et al. (2004), treatment response to CBT was associated with functional brain changes in certain regions commonly associated with emotion. Though this was a small study, it highlights the promising effects of CBT. Other types of therapy modalities also exist, and the treatment team can individually tailor what approach makes the most sense for each individual.

Alternative Strategies for the Management of Depression

Cochrane reviews have also examined alternate approaches to depression management, such as exercise and acupuncture. For example, Mead et al. (2008) examined randomized trials reviewing the effect of exercise on depression. Patients with postpartum depression (PPD) were excluded. Twenty-five trials were included in the meta-analysis, which showed that exercise did seem to help with symptoms of depression. However, the extent to which exercise improves mood is not well-defined, and the types of helpful exercise are not yet clearly delineated. The authors conclude that exercise needs to be continued over a longer period of time to show benefit on mood symptoms.

Smith and Hay (2004) systematically reviewed the randomized controlled studies on acupuncture for depression and revealed that there currently is insufficient evidence to demonstrate that acupuncture may help in the management of depression. Nevertheless, additional studies are needed in this area.

Future Evidence-Based Studies for the Management of Depression

Many additional protocols are underway through the Cochrane Library to further glean evidence-based clinical information on the treatment of individuals with depression. For example, there are protocols for studies looking into the effectiveness of various modes of individual therapy, light therapy, various newer antidepressants (citalopram, sertraline, fluoxetine, paroxetine, bupropion, mirtazapine, and venlafaxine), omega-3 fatty acids, and the impact of collaborative care in the treatment of depression and anxiety in the primary care setting. These are in addition to the clinical trials being conducted by other institutions and centers and individual practitioners.

Treatment Response Based on Gender or Age

Few studies have examined the symptom and treatment response differences between men and women. Kornstein et al. (2000) demonstrated a difference between men and women suffering from chronic depression with regard to antidepressant treatment response and side effects. In this study, premenopausal women with depression showed a better response and tolerability to sertraline (a selective serotonin reuptake inhibitor (SSRI)) versus imipramine (a TCA). Men, on the other hand, showed a better response and tolerability to imipramine instead of sertraline. Postmenopausal women had responses more similar to the men in the study.

Entsuah et al. (2001) conducted a meta-analysis to examine whether gender or age affected response rates and remission of depression with SSRI or venlafaxine treatment. No differences were found between men and women with regard to the response to these antidepressants.

Option of No Treatment for Depression

When people weigh the various treatment options, the option of no treatment can be overlooked. If a depression is severe, this is not a safe route. In a study by Cohen et al. (2006), 26% of women who remained on their antidepressant medications during pregnancy experienced a relapse of depression during pregnancy versus 68% of women who stopped their antidepressants. Untreated depression can lead to death. On the other hand, if depression is mild, not recurrent, or if the diagnosis remains unclear, the decision may be to try therapy without medication.

Patients also need to understand the potential outcomes of an untreated episode of depression. The course of illness can also be worsened with no treatment. Making these treatment decisions is sometimes overwhelming and complicated, particularly if a woman is pregnant or breastfeeding. It is best to incorporate the support of loved ones and the advice of a trusted treatment team.

Evidence-Based Treatment of Premenstrual Dysphoric Disorder

When addressing depressive symptoms associated with premenstrual dysphoric disorder (PMDD), antidepressants often provide relief. Yonkers et al. (1997) completed a double-blind placebo-controlled study comparing sertraline to placebo for the treatment of premenstrual dysphoria and found that sertraline was significantly better than placebo in improving depressive symptoms. In a meta-analysis by Shah et al. (2008), SSRIs were shown to be effective in the treatment of PMDD and possibly more effective when given consistently throughout the month, rather than splitting the dose to correspond with the menstrual phase.

Evidence-Based Treatment of Depression During Pregnancy

Treating depression during pregnancy can be a complicated decision. Pregnant women considering antidepressant medications should weigh the severity of their depression, potential serious consequences of untreated depression, exposure of the infant to medications, potential adverse birth outcomes, neonatal withdrawal syndrome, child development, personal level of comfort with potential risk, normal rates for negative pregnancy outcomes, and risks for untreated depression (Suppaseemanont 2006; Wisner et al. 2000). Wisner et al. (2000) propose a helpful, structured approach to this decision-making process. A major downside to interpreting the literature on antidepressant use in pregnancy is that many studies lack adequate sample size or design from which to draw clear conclusions. The literature is filled with case reports and uncontrolled studies, limiting the patient and the doctor in the decision-making process. Often practitioners will recommend nonpharmacologic strategies for mild depression and strongly encourage medications for moderate to severe depression.

Antidepressant Use in Pregnancy

Several studies have examined the extent to which antidepressants cross into the fetus, either through the blood stream or possibly through the gastrointestinal tract and lungs of the fetus. Research comparing the amount of antidepressant crossing the placenta shows that nortriptyline may lead to less fetal exposure than amytriptyline (Heikkinen et al. 2001). Both of these medications are tricyclic medications and currently are not often used as first-line agents for the management of depression.

All SSRIs seem to cross the placenta leading to fetal exposure; however, at much lower levels than in the maternal blood stream. Fluoxetine may leave higher levels of drug in the umbilical cord at delivery compared to sertraline and paroxetine, raising the possibility of higher infant exposure particularly around the time of delivery, though the clinical relevance of this is not clear (Hendrick et al. 2003; Hallberg and Sjöblom 2005).

Hallberg and Sjöblom (2005) offer a summary of antidepressant use in pregnancy based on the reports available before 2005. In this summary, all studies noted found no increase in major malformations for infants exposed to SSRIs during pregnancy. However, Paxil exposure compared to other antidepressants during the first trimester has since been associated with "a trend toward an increased risk for cardiovascular malformations and increased risk of overall major congenital malformations," including cardiovascular defects (Bar-Oz et al. 2007; *Use of Paxil CR or Paxil during pregnancy* 2005).

There are conflicting studies about whether SSRIs lead to decreased maternal weight gain and secondary decreased prenatal growth. It is not clear if these findings are more reflective of the complications of untreated depression, which can cause poor appetite and poor weight gain during pregnancy. Other studies noted some instances of lower birth weight or lower gestational age, though most did not confer this difference (Hallberg and Sjöblom 2005). In addition, there is not a clear link between SSRI exposure and children having behavioral or developmental deficits. Some studies reported more neonatal complications, particularly for infants exposed in the third trimester, but not all studies supported this finding (Hallberg and Sjöblom 2005). Hallberg and Sjöblom (2005) point out that the possibility of premature labor or minor malformations associated with SSRI exposure in utero cannot be completely ruled out, though the data on which this is based are lacking in several areas. There may also be a link between exposure to SSRIs later in pregnancy and a neonatal withdrawal syndrome (Hallberg and Sjöblom 2005).

The data regarding the treatment of depression during pregnancy are quickly changing and can often be complicated to interpret. Any woman who is considering pregnancy or is currently pregnant should sit down with her healthcare provider to review the most up-to-date literature to help with this sensitive decision-making process.

Treatment of Postpartum Depression

More studies are emerging to help clinicians, researchers, and women better understand what treatment options can be effective for mothers suffering from Postpartum Depression (PPD). A study by Appleby et al. (1997) showed that treating PPD with fluoxetine was more effective than a placebo. Furthermore, treatment with six cognitive behavioral counseling sessions was more effective than just one session.

Another study, looking at 24 US women suffering from PPD, evaluated sertraline as a treatment option and found that the vast majority of women experienced symptom improvement or resolution of the depression (Stowe et al. 1995). However, this study was limited in size and methodology. A small-scale study by Dennis and Stewart (2004) showed a positive treatment response with fluvoxamine.

Some researchers suggest that women with PPD tend to have more anxious features and may require higher doses of antidepressants and take longer to respond to medications (Hendrick et al. 2000). Estrogen replacement may also serve as a useful treatment option or augmentation strategy.

The effects of breastfeeding a child and the effects of estrogen in combination with antidepressants are not yet known (Dennis and Stewart 2004). A study of 16 pregnant women with depression examined the potential effect of daily exposure to light therapy and found that it yielded a positive response on depression scales. There were several limitations to the study including lack of a control group, small sample size, and possible confounding effects of the study design (Oren et al. 2002).

Electroconvulsive therapy also remains a last resort option for mothers experiencing severe depression associated with suicidal impulses, homicidal impulses, psychosis, or severe treatment-resistant symptoms. One advantage is the lack of exposure of the breastfeeding child to antidepressants. No randomized controlled trials have been conducted on ECT for PPD (Dennis and Stewart 2004) (For more information on depression and postpartum disorders, see Chap. 6). As with many studies pertaining to pregnancy or the postpartum period, the ability to extract useful clinical information is often limited by the study design.

The Cochrane Library offers a few reviews to date regarding the management of PPD. The reader is referred to www.thecochranelibrary.com for the most up-to-date reviews. Howard et al. (2005) reviewed the effectiveness of antidepressant medications versus alternate interventions or placebo in women at risk for PPD. Only two studies met the inclusion criteria for this analysis, involving a total of 73 patients. Nortriptyline failed to offer more benefit compared to a placebo, and sertraline did reduce the risk of PPD compared to a placebo, leaving the authors to conclude that not enough evidence exists to clearly comment on the effectiveness of antidepressants in the prevention of PPD. Larger trials are needed to clarify differences among drug classes or alternative strategies and to assess potential harm to the fetus and infant.

Dennis et al. (2008) conducted a systematic review of the literature to assess the use of estrogens and progesterones in the prevention and treatment of PPD. Only two trials with 229 women participants met the inclusion criteria. Synthetic progesterone, given within 48 hours of delivery, was associated with an increase in PPD. Conversely, giving estrogen led to some improvement in depressive symptoms. The authors concluded that progesterone should be used with caution in the postpartum period and that estrogen may offer a moderate benefit in cases of severe depression, but there are not enough data to conclude if estrogen has the ability to prevent depression. More studies are needed before conclusions can be drawn regarding the role of estrogen or progesterone in the management or prevention of PPD.

A 2001 Cochrane Database review examined randomized trials of women up to 6 months postpartum to evaluate the effectiveness of various antidepressants, medication alternatives, or a placebo. Only one trial met the inclusion criteria, thus exemplifying the challenge in reaching a firm conclusion in the management of PPD treatment. The authors note that PPD is a research area that has been neglected and is in need of larger trials comparing various treatment options (Hoffbrand et al. 2001). For additional information on PPD, see Chap. 6 in this volume.

Antidepressant Use and Breastfeeding

Obviously, when treating an episode of PPD, many mothers may be breastfeeding, which brings to light an additional complicating factor: exposure of the nursing child to antidepressants. Deciding whether to take antidepressants during breastfeeding is another critical decision in the treatment of depression for new mothers. Hallberg and Sjöblom (2005) present an excellent review of case reports and studies pertaining to breastfeeding with SSRI medications. Most of the drugs, except paroxetine, have been detected in the plasma of the children exposed. The maximum infant weight-adjusted exposure varies among SSRIs, with fluoxetine and citalopram yielding the greatest exposure at 12% and 10.6% respectively. The clinical significance of this is not known. No adverse outcomes have been reported with paroxetine, though only a total of 77 children were studied in all case reports and studies cited in this review. With fluoxetine, there were some cases of colic, withdrawal symptoms, irritability, and convulsions. With fluvoxamine, there was one case of icterus, which cannot be definitively linked to the medication. With citalopram, there was one report of disturbed sleep, which seemed to resolve once the mother lowered the dose and eventually stopped breastfeeding. With sertraline, there was one reported case of benign sleep disturbance.

It is difficult for breastfeeding mothers and their treatment teams to sift through such limited data when making the decision of whether or not to treat depression with medications. Another essential piece in this decision-making process is the impact of the depression on the mother, since this is such a critical time for her to bond with her child and endure the challenges of raising a child.

Implications for Women's Mental Health

Though there are obvious potential benefits to be gained from EBM, turning EBM into clinical practice still poses many barriers: practitioner resistance to change; difficulty with implementation secondary to the need for acquisition of new skills; lack of equipment; and delayed dissemination of the latest EBM findings. Knowledge translation research is an area of research geared to understand the barriers between what evidence is available in the literature and what is actually being practiced in clinical settings (Zwarenstein and Reeves 2006). Less attention has been paid to how EBM is disseminated and then translated into practice for an interdisciplinary team as a whole. Often different disciplines function autonomously rather than sharing knowledge of EBPs as a more ideal approach to collaboration of care (Zwarenstein and Reeves 2006). Barriers to communication may be complicated by poor interdisciplinary interactions, poor establishment of boundaries within professions, and poor team leadership (Zwarenstein and Reeves 2006).

Future Directions

What are critical directions for future evidence-based studies in women's mental health? While there remains a need for more general research comparing various treatments of different psychiatric conditions, one area that is repeatedly neglected is the management of any psychiatric illness during pregnancy, in the postpartum period, and during breastfeeding. This gap in EBM leaves practitioners and patients to fend for themselves with regard to the interpretation of studies with a limited number of patients and inadequate study design.

Often women are faced with very difficult decisions regarding their mental health during one of the most vulnerable times of their lives with little EBM to guide them toward the healthiest and safest decision. In addition, limited information is available regarding the treatment response differences between men and women suffering from various mental health problems. Overall, much progress has been made toward the development of EBM pertaining to mental health issues, but more is still needed, particularly for women.

References

Appleby, L., Warner, R., Whitton, A., & Faragher, B. (1997). A controlled study of fluoxetine and cognitive-behavioural counselling in the treatment of postnatal depression. *British Medical Journal, 314,* 932–936.

Bar-Oz, B., Einarson, T., Einarson, A., Boskovic, R., O'Brien, L., Malm, H., et al. (2007). Paroxetine and congenital malformations: Meta-analysis and consideration of potential confounding factors. *Clinical Therapeutics, 29*(5), 918–926.

Cohen, L. S., Altshuler, L. L., Harlow, B. L., Nonacs, R., Newport, D. J., Viguera, A. C., et al. (2006). Relapse of major depression during pregnancy in women who maintain or discontinue antidepressant treatment. *The Journal of the American Medical Association, 295*(5), 499–507.

Dennis, C. L., Ross, L. E., & Herxheimer, A. (2008). Oestrogens and progestins for preventing and treating postpartum depression. *Cochrane Database of Systematic Reviews,* Issue 4. Art. No.: CD001690. doi:10.1002/14651858.CD001690.pub2.

Dennis, C. E., & Stewart, D. (2004). Treatment of postpartum depression, part 1: A critical review of biological interventions. *The Journal of Clinical Psychiatry, 65,* 1242–1251.

Entsuah, A. R., Huang, H., & Thase, M. (2001). Response and remission rates in different subpopulations with major depressive disorder administered venlafaxine, selective serotonin reuptake inhibitors or placebo. *The Journal of Clinical Psychiatry, 62,* 869–877.

Frederikse, M., Petrides, G., & Kellner, C. (2006). Continuation and maintenance electroconvulsive therapy for the treatment of depressive illness: A response to the National Institute for Clinical Excellence Report. *The Journal of ECT, 22,* 13–17.

Furukawa, T. A., Streiner, D. L., Young, L. T., & Kinoshita, Y. (2001). Antidepressants plus benzodiazepines for major depression. *Cochrane Database of Systematic Reviews,* Issue 3. Art. No.: CD001026. doi: 10.1002/14651858.CD001026.

Goldapple, K., Segal, Z., Garson, C., Lau, M., Bieling, P., Kennedy, S., et al. (2004). Modulation of cortical-limbic pathways in major depression. Treatment specific effects of cognitive behavioral therapy. *Archives of General Psychiatry, 61,* 34–41.

Guaiana, G., Barbui, C., & Hotopf, M. (2007). Amitriptyline for depression. *Cochrane Database of Systematic Reviews,* Issue 3. Art. No.: CD004186. doi: 10.1002/14651858.CD004186.pub2.

Hallberg, P., & Sjöblom, V. (2005). The use of selective serotonin reuptake inhibitors during pregnancy and breast-feeding: A review and clinical aspects. *Journal of Clinical Psychopharmacology, 25*(1), 59–73.

Hatala, R., Keitz, S., Wyer, P., & Guyatt, G. (2005). Tips for learners of evidence-based medicine: 4. Assessing heterogeneity of primary studies in systematic reviews and whether to combine their results. *Canadian Medical Association Journal, 172*(5), 661–665.

Heikkinen, T., Ekblad, U., & Laine, K. (2001). Transplacental transfer of amitriptyline and nortriptyline in isolated perfused human placenta. *Psychopharmacology, 153,* 450–454.

Hendrick, V., Altshuler, L., Strouse, T., & Grosser, S. (2000). Postpartum and nonpostpartum depression: Differences in presentation and response to pharmacologic treatment. *Depression and Anxiety, 11,* 66–72.

Hendrick, V., Stowe, Z. N., Altshuler, L. L., Hwang, S., Lee, E., & Haynes, D. (2003). Placental passage of antidepressant medications. *The American Journal of Psychiatry, 160,* 993–996.

Hoffbrand, S. E., Howard, L., & Crawley, H. (2001). Antidepressant treatment for post-natal depression. *Cochrane Database of Systematic Reviews,* Issue 2. Art. No.: CD002018. doi: 10.1002/14651858.CD002018.

Howard, L. M., Hoffbrand, S., Henshaw, C., Boath, L., & Bradley, E. (2005). Antidepressant prevention of postnatal depression. *Cochrane Database of Systematic Reviews,* Issue 2. Art. No.: CD004363. doi: 10.1002/14651858.CD004363.pub2.

Kornstein, S. G., Schatzberg, A. F., Thase, M. E., Yonkers, K. A., McCullough, J. P., Keitner, G. I., et al. (2000). Gender differences in treatment response to sertraline versus imipramine in chronic depression. *The American Journal of Psychiatry, 157,* 1445–1452.

Linde, K., Berner, M. M., & Kriston, L. (2008). St John's wort for major depression. *Cochrane Database of Systematic Reviews,* Issue 4. Art. No.: CD000448. doi:10.1002/14651858.CD000448.pub3.

McDonald, W. (2006). Is ECT cost-effective? A review of the National Institute of Health and Clinical Excellence's report on the economic analysis of ECT. *The Journal of ECT, 22,* 25–29.

Mead, G. E., Morley, W., Campbell, P., Greig, C. A., McMurdo, M., & Lawlor, D. A. (2008). Exercise for depression. *Cochrane Database of Systematic Reviews,* Issue 4. Art. No.: CD004366. doi: 10.1002/14651858.CD004366.pub3.

Moncrieff, J., Wessely, S., & Hardy, R. (2004). Active placebos versus antidepressants for depression. *Cochrane Database of Systematic Reviews,* Issue 1. Art. No.: CD003012. doi: 10.1002/14651858.CD003012.pub2.

Oren, D. A., Wisner, K. L., Spinelli, M., Epperson, C. N., Peindl, K. S., Terman, J. S. et al. (2002). An open trial of morning light therapy for treatment of antepartum depression. *The American Journal of Psychiatry, 159,* 666–669.

Sackett, D., Rosenberg, W., Gray, J., Haynes, R., & Richardson, W. (1996). Evidence based medicine: What it is and what it isn't. *British Medical Journal, 312,* 71–72.

Shah, N. R., Jones, J. B., Aperi, J., Shentov, R., Karne, A., & Borenstein, J. (2008). Selective serotonin reuptake inhibitors for premenstrual syndrome and premenstrual dysphoric disorder. A meta-analysis. *Obstetrics and Gynecology, 111,* 1175–1182.

Smith, C. A., & Hay, P. P. J. (2004). Acupuncture for depression. *Cochrane Database of Systematic Reviews,* Issue 3. Art. No.: CD004046. doi: 10.1002/14651858.CD004046.pub2.

Stowe, Z. N., Casarella, J., Landry, J., & Nemeroff, C. B. (1995). Sertraline in the treatment of women with postpartum major depression. *Depression, 3,* 49–55.

Suppaseemanont, W. (2006). Depression in drug safety and nursing management. *American Journal of Maternal Child Nursing, 31*(1), 10–15.

Trivedi, M. H., Rush, A. J., Wisniewski, S. R., Nierenberg, A., Warden, D., & Ritz, L. (2006). Evaluation of outcomes for depression using measurement-based care in Star*D: Implications for clinical practice. *The American Journal of Psychiatry, 163,* 28–40.

Use of Paxil CR or Paxil during pregnancy. (2005). Retrieved December 10, 2008, from http://www.gsk.com/media/paroxetine/mi_letter_paroxetine_pregnancy.pdf

Wisner, K. L., Zarin, D. A., Holmboe, E. S., Appelbaum, P. S., Gelenberg, A. J., Leonard, H. L., et al. (2000). Risk-benefit decision making for treatment of depression during pregnancy. *The American Journal of Psychiatry, 157,* 1933–1940.

Yonkers, K. A., Halbreich, U., Freeman, E., Brown, C., Endicott, J., & Frank, E. (1997). Symptomatic improvement of premenstrual dysphoric disorder with sertraline treatment: A randomized controlled trial. *The Journal of the American Medical Association, 278,* 983–988.

Zwarenstein, M., & Reeves, S. (2006). Knowledge translation and interprofessional collaboration: Where the rubber of evidence-based care hits the road of teamwork. *The Journal of Continuing Education in the Health Professions, 26,* 46–54.

Chapter 13
Mental Health Issues of Incarcerated Women

Bonita M. Veysey

Introduction

This chapter discusses the specific needs of women who are held in US jails. While many of the characteristics of these women are shared by women who are incarcerated in prison, the nature of the jail as a short-term facility that processes and must treat vast numbers of people with many acute medical, mental health, and addiction problems in a short period of time makes this setting a particularly difficult place to provide good treatment. This chapter begins with a discussion of the magnitude of the problem and the rates of mental illnesses of women in jail, followed by other common characteristics of women with mental illnesses in jail. Building upon the argument that experiences of severe interpersonal violence across the lifecourse are central to the emergence of many mental illnesses, health problems, and addictions, the chapter presents principles of trauma-informed care, followed by trauma-informed mental health treatment. The chapter concludes with a discussion of the implications of trauma-informed mental health services in jail settings.

Jails are short-term facilities that hold persons awaiting trial and persons serving short sentences, generally of less than 1 year (Sabol et al. 2007). Many of those booked into jail are released pending trial. Their time in jail is very brief, from several hours to a few days. The average stay in jail for a sentenced inmate is about 3 months (92 days; Camp and Camp 2000). As such, jails are best characterized as people-processing institutions. On any given day, 766,010 persons are held in US jails (Sabol et al. 2007). However, this number cannot capture the vast numbers of persons processed through jails. Over 12 million adults are admitted to jails during

B. M. Veysey (✉)
School of Criminal Justice, Rutgers University, 123 Washington Street,
Newark, NJ 07102, USA

B. L. Levin, M. A. Becker (eds.), *A Public Health Perspective of Women's Mental Health*,
DOI 10.1007/978-1-4419-1526-9_13, © Springer Science+Business Media LLC 2010

an average year (Camp and Camp 2000; Sabol et al. 2007).[1] Jails, nevertheless, are 24-hour secure facilities and incur a substantial Constitutional mandate to assure that people held pretrial and those who have been sentenced do not suffer beyond the punishment they receive.

While men still represent the largest proportion of those in jail, the number of women continues to increase. In 1996, the mid-year census of women in jail was 55,700 (Gilliard and Beck 1997). In 2006, it was 98,577 (Sabol et al. 2007). Further, women's incarceration rate in jail has outpaced that of men. In 1996, women represented 10.8% of the jail population (Gilliard and Beck 1997).Today women represent 12.9% (Sabol et al. 2007). This means that approximately 1.5 million women will be processed through jails this year alone, and this number is likely to continue to increase.

It is no longer possible to discuss mental health issues for incarcerated women without acknowledging the multiple problems they bring with them. Incarcerated women are not single-issue people. A majority of women entering jails have mental health problems. They also have addictions, chronic and acute health conditions, parenting and relationship concerns, poor educational and vocational preparation, and long and extensive histories of violence. It is neither ethical nor practical to provide mental health treatment to incarcerated women as if this were the sole problem.

This chapter will review the major issues that incarcerated women with mental health problems have and how they are associated. Jail management and treatment practices for women with mental health problems will then be discussed.

Incarcerated Women with Mental Health Problems

Prevalence of Mental Disorders

Although women represent a small proportion of jail inmates, studies consistently find that they are more likely to exhibit mental problems and be diagnosed with serious mental illnesses. Seventy-five percent of women in jail exhibit symptoms of mental disorder compared to 63% of men (James and Glaze 2006). Seventy percent of incarcerated women had acute symptoms, while 40% had a recent treatment episode (James and Glaze 2006). In a prevalence study of mental illnesses among female and male admissions to a large urban jail, Teplin et al. (1996) found that 15% of women compared to 6.1% of men met the criteria for an acute mental illness (18.5% vs. 8.9% lifetime prevalence). Women and men had comparable rates of

[1] Estimates were derived from 1999 summaries of admissions and census totals for US jails (Camp and Camp 2000). The average number of admissions to all jails was 23,364 and the average daily census was 1,480. Admissions exceeded census numbers by a factor of 15.8. Using this estimate on 2006 census numbers (Sabol et al. 2007; $n = 759{,}906$) results in an estimated admission population of 12,006,514 persons.

acute schizophrenia and bipolar disorder (1.8% females vs. 3.0% males met criteria for schizophrenia; 2.2% females vs. 1.2% males for bipolar disorder). However, 13.7% of women met the criteria for depression compared to only 3.4% of men. In addition, a notable 22.3% of women in jail met the criteria for posttraumatic stress disorder (PTSD), an additional 6.5% for dysthymia, and approximately 3.5% for anxiety and panic disorders.

Teplin et al. (1997) found that 10.7% of women needed mental health treatment. Of these women, only 23.5% received treatment in the 6 months following the research assessment compared to 37% of men. Further, depression is much less likely to be treated in comparison to other diagnoses, thus compounding the treatment differences between women and men.

Co-occurring Substance Use and Abuse

In the most recent 2003 Arrestee Drug Abuse Monitoring (ADAM) Program report, 68% of arrested women tested positive for one or more drugs similar to the 67% of men (Zhang 2004). The most common drugs for women were cocaine and marijuana, the same drugs of choice as men. However, a staggering 86.4% of women tested positive for alcohol at arrest compared to 9.5% of men. According to the ADAM data and based on a standardized screen of the past year's behavior, 23.8% of women are at risk of dependence to alcohol and 40.5% to other drugs, again similar to men (28.6% for alcohol and 40.5% for other drugs; Zhang 2004).

The gender treatment gaps are also narrowing among arrestees. Twenty-three percent of women and 20.9% of men reported having received outpatient substance abuse treatment during the previous year (Zhang 2004).

The Teplin et al. (1996) study also found that a large percentage (70.2%) of female admissions to jail had a diagnosable substance use disorder (32.3% alcohol abuse/dependence and 63.5% other drug abuse/dependence) compared to 61.3% of men (51.1% alcohol abuse/dependence and 32.4% other drug abuse/dependence). These rates are even higher for persons with a diagnosed mental illness. Among jail detainees with serious mental illnesses, 74.9% of women and 72.0% of men have a co-occurring substance use disorder (Teplin et al. 1996). For additional information on multiple morbidities, see Chap. 5 in this volume.

Acute and Chronic Health Conditions

In 2002, 52.6% of women in jails reported a current medical problem compared to only 34.8% of men (Maruschak 2006). The most common medical problems of women in jails were asthma (19.4%), arthritis (19.4%), and hypertension (14.1%). Among contagious diseases, including sexually transmitted diseases (STDs), 5% reported hepatitis, 4% tuberculosis (lifetime), 2.3% HIV, and 2% STDs. In a single jail study, 59.8% of women rated their health as poor (Finckensher et al. 2001). Approximately 5% of women were pregnant at the time of arrest (Bell et al. 2004; Maruschak 2006).

Childhood and Adult Experiences of Violence

Experiences of abuse are the norm among women in jails. Green et al. (2005) found that nearly all women (98%) in jail had experienced at least one traumatic event. Ninety percent reported at least one incident of interpersonal violence and 71% reported having been a victim of domestic violence. In a California jail, 80% of women reported abuse, with two-thirds having been abused within the past year (Pennell and Burke 2003). Finckenscher et al. (2001) reported that 67% of the women in the jail sample had a history of sexual abuse and 79% had a history of physical abuse.

An Organizing Paradigm: The Adult Consequences of Childhood Trauma

The multiple problems that incarcerated women have can be understood as symptoms and consequences of traumatic childhood experiences. Using a trauma paradigm as an organizing principle, mental illnesses and emotional problems, addiction, infectious and chronic disease, risk behaviors, and even intergenerational violence and criminality may be integrated.

A decade-long, community-based investigation of over 17,000 respondents, the Adverse Childhood Events (ACE) Study, is arguably the most important study investigating the relationship of negative childhood events to adult health. This study found that childhood traumatic events, particularly abuse and neglect, are associated with many adolescent and adult emotional, health, and behavioral problems. The health consequences include obesity, STDs, liver disease, ischemic heart disease, and chronic obstructive pulmonary disease. Adverse childhood events are related to poor mental health in general (Edwards et al. 2003), hallucinations (Whitfield et al. 2005), depression (Chapman et al. 2004), and suicide attempts (Dube et al. 2001). They are also related to alcohol use in general as well as age of first use (Dube et al. 2006), illicit drug use (Dube et al. 2003), adolescent pregnancy and fetal death (Hillis et al. 2004), and sexual risk behaviors (Hillis et al. 2001).

The ACE study findings suggest that early childhood trauma leads to impaired neuro-development, adoption of risk behaviors in adolescence, the development of chronic health problems in adulthood, and early death. As the number of adverse childhood events increase, the odds of displaying specific problems in a number of domains, including mental health, addiction, sexuality, risk behaviors, and health, also increase (Anda et al. 2006). Compared to persons without negative childhood events, the odds of any given problem typically increase by a factor of 2–10 times when four or more adverse childhood events are present (Anda et al. 2006). Sexual abuse in particular is related to increased suicide attempts (Dube et al. 2005). Adverse childhood events include many childhood events beyond physical and sexual abuse. They also reflect adverse events, such as parental loss, neglect, and serious illness. Increasingly, research demonstrates that various types of negative childhood events rarely occur in isolation. When one is present, typically others are as well. As the number of negative events increase, the number of health and behavioral problems as well as the severity of those problems associated with them increase, not in an additive fashion, but multiplicatively (Dong et al. 2004).

Commonly, the justification for gender specific services for incarcerated women focuses on the experiences of physical and sexual abuse. These have long been thought to be more damaging to children than neglect or emotional abuse. However, emerging research in human and animal studies is now showing that profound neglect, particularly in the earliest years of life, has severe and direct effects on brain development, and consequently, on the ability to form attachments as well as on intellectual functioning (Perry 2002). The nature of harm (i.e., neglect vs. physical threat) and the timing, duration, and intensity of the harm are related to the specific neurological dysfunction (Perry 2002). Similarly, emotional abuse has long been overlooked as an unfortunate but unimportant factor in abused persons' lives. Childhood negative events in general are related to increased risk of mental health problems. When comparing the relative damage of various types of abuse, recent research suggests that emotional abuse is a significant predictive factor of mental health problems (Teicher et al. 2006). In fact, it has comparable effects to witnessing domestic violence and nonfamilial sexual abuse and effects larger than familial physical abuse. When found in combination with witnessing family violence, emotional abuse exceeded the effects of familial sexual abuse on several of the mental health outcome measures.

This research collectively suggests that attention to specific conditions, whether it is mental illness or addiction, may be successful in symptom reduction but will not address the underlying cause, thus reducing the probability of long-term recovery. Integrated, trauma-informed care focuses on the woman as a whole person and tends to address the concerns that are of greatest importance to women.

Principles of Trauma-Informed Treatment

Correctional settings and treatment environments, by their very nature, may cause distress to women with trauma histories. This may occur through institutional triggers (i.e., sensory perceptions that remind the woman of abuse) or retraumatization (i.e., practices that recreate the experience of the original trauma). In jail treatment settings, attention should be given to assessments, therapist interactions, coercion (or lack of autonomy) in treatment decisions, and emergency interventions (e.g., forced medication, seclusion, and restraint). Within the security domain, attention should be given to routine interviews and assessments; the use of cuffs, shackles and restraints; searches, pat-downs and clothing removal; lack of autonomous action; privacy; lock downs and the use of administrative segregation; authoritarian control and threats of violence; and critical incidents and institutional responses.

Jail facilities differ in resources and correctional philosophies. Each jail must make decisions regarding what services and supports will be dedicated to a particular need. To the degree that jails focus attention on female offenders, the following principles may be used to guide the development and operation of assessment and treatment services.

- **Symptom-based assessments**
  There are many reasons that event-based assessments are less desirable than symptom-based assessment, including (1) refusal to disclose because of shame, lack of trust, fear of reprisal; (2) memory and recall (i.e., the event may be repressed); (3) denial or minimalization; and (4) retraumatization and emotional safety. Further, the degree of trauma reaction to any given event is individual. Some women may have few or no reactions and, therefore, treatment would not be indicated. Distress comes not from the event per se, but from the persistent stress symptoms. Symptoms, therefore, should be the target of intervention. For women with trauma reactions, assessors should anticipate disruptions in cognition, emotion, and behavior that not only cause distress to the individual, but may present security concerns. Also, because of the nature of abuse, indicators of neurological problems resulting from head trauma and STDs should be screened.
- **Noncoercive and empowering**
  Because the essential nature of trauma is powerlessness, coercion of any sort is damaging at worst and not helpful at best. Wherever possible, women should be involved in decisions in a substantive way (i.e., not simply asking her to sign off on a treatment plan). This may take the form of (1) informing the woman about all procedures and possible outcomes, (2) specifying what information will be used for and respecting her wishes not to disclose, (3) partnering with the individual in treatment planning and goal setting, and (4) maximizing a woman's control over crisis interventions through advance directives.
- **Safety**
  Emotional and physical safety is a first duty in treatment. Assessment of safety is critical. It is important to know whether the woman was in a violent situation or relationship prior to arrest and to attend to the possibility of continuing violent victimization within the facility.
- **Treatment continuity**
  Continuity of care is critical in this population. The assessment process should be considered initial "treatment." To the degree possible, assessment staff should also be treatment staff, so that the women (1) can create trusting, stable relationships, and (2) do not have to recount their stories repeatedly.
- **Trauma-informed**
  Given the high incidence of abuse among incarcerated women, all services and staff, including medical, psychological, substance abuse, social work, and

security, should be trauma-informed. All personnel must be able to identify symptoms of trauma, interact with women appropriately, and refer as needed. Since substance use, mental health issues, and medical problems are intimately related to trauma and each other, treatment services, in particular, should be trauma-informed. In addition, trauma specific services should be developed to address trauma reactions.

- **Integrated care**
  Because trauma reactions are intertwined with substance use and mental health problems, assessment and treatment for any one of these issues should address the interactions of all issues. Integrated mental health and substance abuse treatment for persons with histories of trauma is superior to both parallel and sequential treatment. To the degree possible, women should be provided opportunities to explore the relationships among these problems to identify new and more functional adaptive strategies to trauma.
- **Security involvement**
  Security staff spend many more hours of each day with the inmates than do assessment or treatment providers. Involvement of these staff in behavior and crisis management is critical. Like assessment and treatment staff, they must be trained in trauma issues. Standard operating procedures (SOPs) for physical management should be reviewed, and all staff should work together to identify and implement concrete behavioral management plans. At a minimum, security staff should refrain from the use of excessive force and shaming.
- **Gender and cultural responsiveness**
  Assessments and treatment must reflect the gender and various cultural affiliations of inmates. To a large degree, symptom-based assessments avoid some of the gender and cultural pitfalls of the meaning of events. Assessments and treatment can be improved to the degree that staff persons reflect the characteristics of those with whom they work. Individuals are embedded in networks in which the meanings of events are socially constructed. To the degree that assessors/treatment personnel share those networks, rapport, empathy, and understanding are increased.

Trauma-Informed Mental Health Treatment

Building upon these principles, jail-based mental health services must be trauma-informed. Jails are short-term facilities. Because of this fact, jail mental health services focus on stabilization, particularly through crisis management and short-term treatment. Given the growing awareness of traumatic experiences among women offenders, trauma-specific services are now strongly indicated. In jail settings, these services fall into medications, physiological interventions, and cognitive-behavioral group modalities. Both trauma-informed practices and trauma-specific treatment are discussed below.

Trauma-Informed Supervision and Clinical Practice

First and foremost is the need to understand and value the high rate of trauma, particularly childhood abuse and neglect, among female offenders. Second is a philosophical acceptance that our correctional and treatment settings have a significant capacity to retraumatize these same individuals in a myriad of ways. Effort needs to be put forth by leaders who implement trauma-informed principles to objectively evaluate how persons with trauma histories experience booking procedures, incarceration in general, treatment within a secure facility, and release into the community. This task includes a review of the environment, the overt and covert messages, policies and procedures, staff attitudes and language, noise levels, and perceptions of objective safety. Because of the high rates of PTSD and other disorders directly linked to trauma (e.g., substance abuse, depression, and other anxiety disorders) in populations of incarcerated women, screening for trauma symptoms is important. A component of a trauma assessment procedure would include some education about trauma, its effects, its prevalence, and the availability of treatment for signs and symptoms.

Depending on the facility environment, other changes will need to be made, starting with a vision or policy statement on trauma communicated to staff and resultant workforce development and training activities. In many, if not most, jails this may call for a very different view of women in custody and an overall culture change. Trauma-informed systems of care strive to prevent conflicts, immediately intervene when conflicts occur, and place a great deal of attention on staff negotiation skills. Staff must view the women being served as human beings first, often terribly traumatized, and be able to see institutional misbehavior as behaviors that are survival focused and learned over time in chaotic environments outside of the jail. In addition, all efforts must be made to avoid the use of coercive techniques, such as seclusion, restraint, and forced medication as well as basic autocratic behaviors by staff. Assuring environmental safety is a priority. Trauma-specific services and interventions will not be nearly as effective or as sustainable in a system of care that is not trauma-informed.

Screening, Assessment, and Evaluation

Screening, assessment, and evaluation are critical points in the services delivery system for the provision of appropriate services to female offenders. Information uncovered at these points affects classification (i.e., housing) decisions and whether women will receive mental health and other treatment services. Screening instruments used by booking officers should include a minimum set of questions related to symptoms of mental health problems, history of mental health treatment, current use of prescribed psychotropic medication, and risk of suicide. For these screens to encompass the characteristics of women diagnosed with mental illnesses, questions should also ask specifically about (1) symptoms of depression; (2) current intoxication (legal and illegal substances); (3) whether the woman was recently injured; and (4) whether she has minor children and, if so, whether they are currently being cared for and by whom.

In addition to more detailed information regarding the areas noted above, mental health assessments (and standard medical history protocols) and psychiatric evaluations should be the points where information about physical and sexual abuse is gathered. This requires that medical and mental health staff receive training in assessing women with histories of abuse. This information is critical for the correct diagnosis and the development of appropriate mental health, health care, and substance abuse treatment plans.

Medication and Psychiatric Follow-Up Services

Medication and medication monitoring of women are major issues for the delivery of mental health services in jails. Women are diagnosed with unipolar depression at a much higher rate than men. However, some jails do not allow the prescription of certain antidepressants because of their potential for abuse. Despite indications or previous treatment, some women cannot receive the medication of choice due to standing policies. On the other hand, these policies exist for good reason. Women (and men) with significant addictive disorders may request antidepressants as a substitute for their drug of choice. Each individual case must be reviewed carefully prior to the prescription of medication, and at regular intervals thereafter, to assure that the medications are appropriate to the specific need of each individual.

Overprescription of medication is as problematic as underprescription. Because women's housing is limited and because women are not as easily managed as men in general (Veysey et al. 1998), there is a tendency to overprescribe medications for the sole purpose of tranquilizing the detainee. From the jail's perspective, this is a reasonable policy because it enhances the jail's security. From a human rights perspective, it is an unjustified use of chemical restraints and violates constitutional rights. In addition, the medication may interfere with the detainee's ability to participate in her adjudication process.

Crisis Intervention and Suicide Precautions

Women diagnosed with mental illnesses in jail do not typically exhibit the same symptoms as men, nor should the crisis intervention responses be the same (Veysey et al. 1998). Clinicians must be trained to identify suicide risk in women and how to appropriately intervene in mental health crises without retraumatizing a woman who typically has been repeatedly traumatized.

The policies and procedures governing the use of physical and chemical restraints should be carefully reviewed for their application on all female detainees, including those diagnosed with mental illnesses and those without. Because histories of abuse are so prevalent among women in jail, these procedures should be developed for all women. Some mental health systems are beginning to review these issues in response to a growing awareness of the damage that these procedures have on individuals' physical and emotional well-being. This is critically important when managing women with significant histories of physical and sexual abuse.

If staff of jail mental health services expect to have a continuing relationship with a female detainee, it may be helpful to understand what actions or events cause distress and what interventions staff can use that will help to calm the detainee. It is also helpful to tell women diagnosed with mental illnesses, who might require restraint, what procedures are used in the facility early on in their confinement.

Other Mental Health and Substance Abuse Treatment

In jails where other kinds of mental health and substance abuse treatment are available, several considerations for women should be addressed. First, single-gender groups are critically important. Women who have been victims of abuse do not function well in mixed-gender treatment groups. Second, most treatment modalities operate within an expert/passive patient paradigm; some are built upon direct confrontation and shaming. These modalities do not work as well with women as they do with men, and this is especially true when women have significant trauma experiences. In addition, women who have experienced physical or sexual abuse as well as women diagnosed with mental illnesses appear to benefit from peer-support groups. Given the prohibitive costs of professional services and the benefit of peer support, jails may want to consider using community resources to supplement core mental health services.

Trauma-Specific Services

A broad array of interventions exists that are designed to affect symptoms related to traumatic events. Interventions can be loosely categorized as (1) pharmacological, (2) behavioral/physiological, (3) cognitive-behavioral, and (4) other psychological strategies. These interventions target different aspects of trauma symptoms (i.e., biological, physiological, or cognitive) and assume different pathways to recovery, particularly with regard to the use of traumatic memories in the intervention (e.g., habituation vs. cognitive restructuring).

Medications

Of all the possible interventions for trauma, medications are the most prevalent in correctional settings. Posttraumatic stress disorder (PTSD) is the diagnostic classification for the array of symptoms commonly associated with traumatic events (i.e., it is a medical disorder characterized by a set of psychobiological dysfunctions; Stein et al. 2003). As such, it is amenable to pharmacological intervention. The biological processes underlying trauma symptoms are, at a minimum, complex. As basic research in this area grows, resulting information provides new insights into potential targets for intervention. In the literature, however, several cautionary notes are offered for the use of medications for trauma-related symptoms. First, research suggests that clinical practice be done in a stepwise approach using broad spectrum medications first (Donnelly and Amaya-Jackson 2002). Further, medications have limited utility in reducing perceptions of distress. Even when medications suppress symptoms, these symptoms are not the problems that cause women the most distress. The impact of medications can be greatly enhanced by using them in conjunction with other supports, most notably cognitive-behavioral groups (Popper 1993).

Physiological Interventions

Behavioral and physiological interventions involve the targeting of specific physiological responses to trauma (e.g., rapid heartbeat, panic reactions) or the biological mechanisms thought to be associated with the encoding of trauma memories (e.g., rapid eye movement). All therapies in this class involve exposure to traumatic memories as an essential component of treatment. The therapies include, but are not limited to, prolonged exposure (PE), stress innoculation training (with prolonged exposure) (SITPE), flooding therapy, image habituation training (IHT), eye movement desensitization and reprocessing (EMDR), relaxation and biofeedback methods, and hypnosis. It is important to note that in most cases, a cognitive component is added to provide cognitive restructuring and skills training. The research demonstrates that these are effective in community populations and for those exposed to single traumatic events (Cahill et al. 1999; Davidson and Parker 2001; Shepard et al. 2000). Because exposure therapies often trigger distressing PTSD symptoms (Ehlers 2004), there is concern that exposure therapies have limited use with individuals with complex PTSD (i.e., victims of chronic abuse; Allen 2003; Colosetti and Thyer 2000).This is a particularly important concern since female offenders have high rates of interpersonal violence across the lifespan and often evidence symptoms consistent with chronic trauma. This class of interventions is not recommended for use in correctional settings in general, but particularly with women or those in short-term facilities.

Cognitive-Behavioral Group Interventions

Cognitive-behavioral therapies, as the title suggests, focus on the cognitive and behavioral consequences of trauma. There are several manualized trauma recovery models. One is a generic model designed for both women and men, and others are designed specifically for women. Seeking Safety (Najavits et al. 1998) is a general model, while the Trauma Recovery and Empowerment Model (TREM; Fallot and Harris 2002), the Addiction and Trauma Recovery Integration Model (ATRIUM; Miller and Guidry 2001), and *Beyond trauma: A healing journey for women* (Covington 2003) were developed on, and with, women. Further, one model that was initially designed to address problems common to persons diagnosed with borderline personality disorder (i.e., dialectic behavior therapy; Linehan 1993) has also been applied to trauma survivors. All of these models have been implemented in correctional settings.

These group therapies share several characteristics. First, they focus heavily on concrete strategies to cope with trauma symptoms. They also do not place an emphasis on, or even necessarily attend to, traumatic memories. Second, they are designed for groups of people who typically have long histories of abuse, often beginning in childhood. Therefore, they tend to be more responsive to complex PTSD. They also are designed for multiproblem individuals (i.e., persons with substance use or mental disorders) and address issues in a holistic and integrated fashion.

Considerations When Adapting Community-Based Trauma Treatment to Corrections

Adapting effective community-based models to correctional settings requires an understanding of the likely differences between correctional populations and the populations for which the models were originally designed. Even pharmacological interventions based on human biology must be used cautiously, taking into consideration the high rates of comorbid mental disorders, physical health status (e.g., high rates of HIV+/AIDS, Hepatitis C) and the consequent multiple drug interactions, and chronic substance use. While all of the issues raised below are also present in community populations, the prevalence suggests that models be responsive in a systematic way, instead of on an *ad hoc* basis.

First, a diagnosis of PTSD is based on a single-incident model (e.g., single rape in adulthood), and many treatments for trauma were designed specifically to respond to this type of event, most notably the behavioral/physiological (i.e., exposure) therapies. Given the high rates of abuse and violence over offenders' lifetimes, there must be an appreciation of the difference between single-event trauma and complex PTSD. Allen (2003) notes that "complex trauma requires a multifaceted treatment approach" that balances the processing of traumatic memories with strategies to contain intense (and dys-regulated) emotions (p. 213). Further, when the trauma occurs in childhood, not only does it produce chronic physiological symptoms, but it also interrupts important developmental stages (Herman 1992) and creates cognitive and emotional dysfunction. The most profound statement in this regard is that trauma "forms and deforms the personality" (Herman 1992). Trauma treatment for these individuals must therefore include extensive habilitation, noting that these persons may never have possessed some basic skills, particularly relational skills.

Second, correctional populations experience an overlay of persistent and chronic stressors that may exacerbate trauma symptoms. These stressors include racial and social discrimination, living in violent neighborhoods, and adapting to correctional environments. For example, Rittenhouse (2000) asserts that persistent discrimination and trauma responses interact; therefore, treatment should focus on the effects of discrimination and prejudice as well as the traumatic event(s).

Finally, as a general caveat, the treatments noted above have been shown to reduce trauma symptom severity and psychological distress. There is no evidence to suggest that these interventions improve other life domains, many of which are of more concern to survivors than the symptoms (e.g., relationship or employment problems; Robertson et al. 2004). Nor is there any guidance about what intervention works best for whom under what circumstances, or whether components should be offered sequentially or in a parallel fashion (Robertson et al. 2004).

Implications for Women's Mental Health

Jails are required to provide medical and psychiatric care to persons in distress. However, in correctional facilities, security is always paramount. This means that treatment and services are constrained in the degree of flexibility and autonomy granted to individual inmates. Further, correctional environments are hostile at best and violent and dangerous at worst. Any unnecessary treatment that might make an individual more vulnerable to victimization may be counterproductive. A primary question remains as to whether trauma issues *could* or *should* be addressed directly during confinement.

Further, trauma reactions are complicated and interrelated with many other problems. It is clear that when violence occurs repeatedly, the consequences are broad ranging and commonly include addictions, mental health and health problems, relationship disruption, and loss of self-efficacy. In fact, in most cases, trauma is central and these other problems may be better understood as the symptoms of this underlying trauma. This fact has two important implications for treatment in correctional settings. First, no single issue should be treated as a stand-alone problem. That is, treatment and support should be provided in an integrated manner. Second, all treatment and services should be trauma-informed.

There are four priority areas which need to be developed and disseminated across states and localities. These include information use, training, developing trauma-informed practices, and adapting effective trauma interventions for use within differing settings and with different populations.

Research and Evaluation Information

The most significant need is information. First, little is known about the rate and nature of trauma experiences among female offender groups. Second and more importantly, when it is available, this information is neither systematically nor routinely gathered. Without this basic information, it is difficult to justify the use of resources for the creation of trauma programs. Further, clinical information on trauma and its effects is not routinely gathered; therefore, persons exhibiting behaviors that are consistent with a trauma history may be misdiagnosed and poorly treated. Finally, as models of trauma treatment are implemented in correctional settings, evaluation of program performance is critical. Therefore, it is strongly recommended that jurisdictions and facilities develop an administrative and clinical information gathering capacity to address these deficits.

Training of Correctional and Behavioral Health Staff

Training of correctional and clinical staff is also a high priority. These professionals should be trained on the nature of trauma, its effects, and known effective or promising interventions. Emphasis should also be placed on clinical and supervisory practices that are both gender-specific and trauma-informed. In general, training for direct-care staff should not be limited to this information, but should also include practical techniques for physical custody, de-escalation, and interpersonal communication.

Review and Revision of Supervisory Practices

Criminal justice settings are, by their very nature, coercive and controlling. However, within the mandate of security and safety, procedures can be adapted to decrease the probability of trauma reactions and increase safety for staff and the women they supervise. This process should include the review of standard operating procedures (SOPs), as well as the informal norms and practices at the unit level. This review should investigate information sharing (i.e., what information is disclosed to an offender), use of force and crisis intervention protocols, coercion and decision-making opportunities, and victimization risks and safety.

Adaptation and Wide Dissemination of Trauma Interventions

At this time, effective trauma interventions are available for use with offender groups. These and other promising models should be widely disseminated and implemented in a variety of justice settings with different offender groups. Based on this knowledge, adaptations should be considered to improve the outcomes for specific subgroups of offenders.

References

Allen, J. G. (2003). Challenges in treating post-traumatic stress disorder and attachment trauma. *Current Women's Health Reports, 3,* 213–220.

Anda, R. F., Felitti, V. J., Bremner, J. D., Walker, J. D., Whitfield, C., Perry, B. D., et al. (2006). The enduring effects of abuse and related adverse experiences in childhood A convergence of evidence from neurobiology and epidemiology. *European Archives of Psychiatry and Clinical Neuroscience, 256,* 174–186.

Bell, J. F., Zimmerman, F. J., Cawthorn, M. L., Huebner, C. E., Ward, D. H., & Schroeder, C. A. (2004). Jail incarceration and birth outcomes. *Journal of Urban Health, 81,* 630–644.

Cahill, S. P., Carrigan, M. H., & Frueh, B. C. (1999). Does EMDR work? And if so, why?: A critical review of controlled outcome and dismantling research. *Journal of Anxiety Disorders, 13,* 5–33.

Camp, C. G., & Camp, G. M. (2000). *The 2000 corrections yearbook: Jails.* Middletown, CN: Criminal Justice Institute.

Chapman, D. P., Whitfield, C. L., Felitti, V. J., Dube, S. R., Edwards, V. J., & Anda, R. F. (2004). Adverse childhood experiences and the risk of depressive disorders in adulthood. *Journal of Affective Disorders, 82,* 217–225.

Colosetti, S. D., & Thyer, B. A. (2000). The relative effectiveness of EMDR versus relaxation training with battered women prisoners. *Behavioral Modification, 24,* 719–739.

Covington, S. (2003). *Beyond trauma: A healing journey for women.* Center City, MN: Hazelden Publishing.

Davidson, P. R., & Parker, K. C. (2001). Eye movement desensitization and reprocessing (EMDR): A meta-analysis. *Journal of Consulting and Clinical Psychology, 69,* 305–316.

Dong, M., Anda, R. F., Felitti, V. J., Dube, S. R., Williamson, D. F., Thompson, T. J., et al. (2004). The interrelatedness of multiple forms of childhood abuse, neglect, and household dysfunction. *Child Abuse and Neglect, 28,* 771–784.

Donnelly, C. L., & Amaya-Jackson, L. (2002). Post-traumatic stress disorder in children and adolescents: Epidemiology, diagnosis and treatment options. *Paediatric Drugs, 4,* 159–170.

Dube, S. R., Anda, R. F., Felitti, V. J., Chapman, D., Williamson, D. F., & Giles, W. H. (2001). Childhood abuse, household dysfunction and the risk of attempted suicide throughout the life span: Findings from Adverse Childhood Experiences Study. *Journal of the American Medical Association, 286,* 3089–3096.

Dube, S. R., Anda, R. F., Whitfield, C. L., Brown, D. W., Felitti, V. J., Dong, M., et al. (2005). Long-term consequences of childhood sexual abuse by gender of victim. *Journal of Preventive Medicine, 28,* 430–438.

Dube, S. R., Felitti, V. J., Dong, M., Chapman, D. P., Giles, W. H., & Anda, R. F. (2003). Childhood abuse, neglect and household dysfunction and the risk of illicit drug use: The adverse childhood experience study. *Pediatrics, 111,* 564–572.

Dube, S. R., Miller, J. W., Brown, D. W., Giles, W. H., Felitti, V. J., Dong, M., et al. (2006). Adverse childhood experiences and the association with ever using alcohol and initiating alcohol use during adolescence. *Journal of Adolescent Health, 38,* 444.e1–444.e10.

Edwards, V. J., Holden, G. W., Anda, R. F., & Felitti, V. J. (2003). Relationship between multiple forms of childhood maltreatment and adult mental health: Results from the adverse childhood experiences study. *American Journal of Psychiatry, 160,* 1453–1460.

Ehlers, A. (2004). CBT of PTSD in severe mental illness: A promising approach with possibilities for further development. *American Journal of Psychiatric Rehabilitation, 7,* 201–204.

Fallot, R. D., & Harris, M. (2002). The trauma recovery and empowerment model (TREM): Conceptual and practical issues in a group intervention for women. *Community Mental Health Journal, 38,* 475–485.

Finckenscher, A., Lapidus, J., Silk-Walker, P., & Becker, T. (2001) Women behind bars: Health needs of inmates in a county jail. *Public Health Reports, 116,* 191–196.

Gilliard, D. K., & Beck, A. J. (1997). Prison and jail inmates at midyear 1996. *Bureau of justice statistics bulletin* (NCJ-162843). Washington, DC: U.S. Department of Justice.

Green, B. L., Miranda, J., Daroowalla, A., & Siddique, J. (2005). Trauma exposure, mental health functioning, and program needs of women in jail. *Crime and Delinquency, 51,* 133–151.

Herman, J. (1992). *Trauma and recovery: The aftermath of violence—from domestic abuse to political terror*. New York, NY: Basic Books.

Hillis, S. D., Anda, R. F., Dube, S. R., Felitti, V. J., Marchbanks, P. A., & Marks, J. S. (2004). The association between adolescent pregnancy, long-term psychosocial outcomes, and fetal death. *Pediatrics, 113,* 320–327.

Hillis, S. D., Anda, R. F., Felitti, V. J., & Marchbanks, P. A. (2001). Adverse childhood experiences and sexual risk behaviors in women: A retrospective cohort study. *Family Planning Perspectives, 33,* 206–211.

James, D. J., & Glaze, L. E. (2006). Mental health problems of prison and jail inmates. *Bureau of justice statistics bulletin* (NCJ-213600). Washington, DC: U.S. Department of Justice.

Linehan, M. M. (1993). *Cognitive behavioral treatment of borderline personality disorder.* New York, NY: The Guilford Press.

Maruschak, L. M. (2006). Medical problems of jail inmates. *Bureau of justice statistics special report* (NCJ-210696). Washington, DC: U.S. Department of Justice.

Miller, D., & Guidry, L. (2001). *Addictions and trauma recovery: Healing the body, mind and spirit.* New York, NY: WW Norton.

Najavits, L. M., Weiss, R. D., Shaw, S. R., & Muenz, L. (1998). "Seeking Safety": Outcome of a new cognitive-behavioral psychotherapy for women with posttraumatic stress disorder and substance dependence. *Journal of Traumatic Stress, 11,* 437–456.

Pennell, S., & Burke, C. (2003). *The incidence and prevalence of domestic violence victimization among female arrestees in San Diego county.* San Diego, CA: San Diego Association of Governments (SANDAG).

Perry, B. D. (2002). Childhood experience and the expression of genetic potential: What childhood neglect tells us about nature and nurture. *Brain and Mind, 3,* 79–100.

Popper, C. W. (1993). Psychopharmacological treatment of anxiety disorders in adolescents and children. *Journal of Clinical Psychiatry, 54*(Suppl.), 52–63.

Rittenhouse, J. (2000). Using eye movement desensitization and reprocessing to treat complex PTSD in a biracial client. *Cultural Diversity and Ethnic Minority Psychology, 6,* 399–408.

Robertson, M., Humphreys, L., & Ray, R. (2004). Psychological treatments for posttraumatic stress disorder: Recommendations for the clinician based on a review of the literature. *Journal of Psychiatric Practice, 10,* 106–118.

Sabol, W. J., Minton, T. D., & Harrison, P. M. (2007). Prison and jail inmates at midyear 2006. *Bureau of justice statistics bulletin* (NCJ-217675). Washington, DC: U.S. Department of Justice.

Shepard, J., Stein, K., & Milne, R. (2000). Eye movement desensitization and reprocessing in the treatment of post-traumatic stress disorder: A review of an emerging therapy. *Psychological Medicine, 30,* 863–871.

Stein, D. J., Davidson, J., Seedat, S., & Beebe, K. (2003). Paroxetine in the treatment of post-traumatic stress disorder: Pooled analysis of placebo-controlled studies. *Expert Opinion on Pharmacotherapy, 4,* 1829–1838.

Teicher, M. H., Samson, J. A., Polcari, A., & McGreenery, C. E. (2006). Sticks, stones and hurtful words: Relative effects of various forms of childhood maltreatment. *American Journal of Psychiatry, 163,* 993–1000.

Teplin, L. A., Abram, K. M., & McClelland, G. M. (1996). Prevalence of psychiatric disorders among incarcerated women. *Archives of General Psychiatry, 53,* 505–512.

Teplin, L. A., Abram, K. M., & McClelland, G. M. (1997). Mentally disordered women in jail: Who receives services. *American Journal of Public Health, 87,* 604–609.

Veysey, B. M., De Cou, K., & Prescott, L. (1998). Effective management of female jail detainees with histories of physical and sexual abuse. *American Jails, 12,* 50–54.

Whitfield, C. L., Dube, S. R., Felitti, V. J., & Anda, R. F. (2005). Adverse childhood experiences and hallucinations. *Child Abuse and Neglect, 29,* 797–810.

Zhang, Z. (2004). *Drug and alcohol use and related matters among arrestees 2003.* Washington, DC: U.S. Department of Justice.

Chapter 14
Services in the Workplace

Alicia G. Dugan and Vicki J. Magley

Introduction

It has been said that in the course of our lives, we spend more time working than doing any other activity except sleeping. Therefore, it stands to reason that the ways in which we spend that enormous amount of our time (i.e., what we do for work, how we carry out our work tasks, when and how long we work, with whom we work, the environment in which we work, and how we feel about our work) are powerful factors influencing our experience of daily living.

This chapter aims to shed light on the ways in which well-being may be affected by aspects of one's work experience, and likewise how work may be influenced by one's level of well-being. Moreover, the chapter will focus on women, as the workplace confronts them with obstacles not faced by men, resulting in a unique set of challenges that place their well-being at risk. In the course of this chapter, the variety of organizational experiences that shape women's work lives will be examined, as well as the aspects of their personal lives that interact with their work situations, the consequences of their work lives on well-being, and the variety of workplace programs and services that help women enjoy a better quality of life.

Unfortunately, not all people have satisfactory work lives. Studies indicate that the percentage of people reporting work-related stress ranges from 26 to 40% (National Institute of Occupational Safety and Health 1999). Research has identified several specific sources of workplace stress, including aspects of the job itself (i.e., is the task too complex or too monotonous?), the work role (i.e., do I know what is expected of me; is my workload too heavy?), the physical environment (i.e., is the lighting poor or the temperature uncomfortable?), and interpersonal relationships (i.e., do I get along with my supervisor and coworkers?) (Barling et al. 2005; Kahn and Byosiere 1992; National Institute of Occupational Safety and Health 1999).

A. G. Dugan (✉)
Department of Psychology, University of Connecticut,
406 Babbidge Road, Storrs, CT 06269, USA

B. L. Levin, M. A. Becker (eds.), *A Public Health Perspective of Women's Mental Health*,
DOI 10.1007/978-1-4419-1526-9_14, © Springer Science+Business Media LLC 2010

Just as aspects of the job or work environment can contribute to employees' experiences of stress, individuals themselves also play a role in the stress process. That is, a person will experience a situation as stressful depending on the individual's perception of that situation. When one appraises that a circumstance is a threat beyond her or his ability to cope (Lazarus and Folkman 1984), or it places an excessive drain on her or his personal resources (Hobfoll 1989), distress may result, and if prolonged, it may become chronic.

In addition to appraising sources of stress differently, individuals have their own unique ways of responding to stress, whether psychological, physical, or behavioral. In responding to workplace stressors, people may experience psychological symptoms including anxiety, depression, burnout, dissatisfaction, emotional exhaustion, frustration, resentment, poor self-esteem, and boredom (Buunk et al. 1998; Kahn and Byosiere 1992; National Institute of Occupational Safety and Health 1999). Physiological responses are also common, such as cardiovascular symptoms (i.e., high blood pressure, increased heart rate, and cholesterol levels), biochemical effects (i.e., elevated stress hormones such as catecholamines, corticosteroids, and uric acid), and gastrointestinal symptoms (i.e., abdominal pain, diarrhea, and ulcers; Kahn and Byosiere 1992; Lovallo 2005; National Institute of Occupational Safety and Health 1999).

People may also respond behaviorally by engaging in counterproductive acts at work (i.e., stealing, sabotage, property damage, rumors), flight from the job (i.e., absenteeism, turnover, early retirement), damage to one's work role (i.e., poor performance, work accidents, workplace alcohol/drug use), damage to one's other life roles (i.e., abuse or neglect of spouse, family, friends, neighbors), and self-damage (use and/or abuse of alcohol, drugs, cigarettes, caffeine; Bruk-Lee and Spector 2006; Kahn and Byosiere 1992; Kouvonen et al. 2007). These symptoms clearly indicate the widespread implications that the work experience has, not only on the lives of employees, but on organizational functioning as well.

The fact that such a huge portion of our lives is dedicated to working, that the workplace is full of potential stressors, and that distress can have such substantial implications on emotional, physical, and social health makes the workplace a highly appropriate setting in which to address questions of personal well-being. For the purposes of this chapter, an integrative view of health will be adopted, with the term "well-being" used to refer to the state of being that results when a person's emotional, physical, and social systems are operating at optimal levels.

Women's Work and Well-Being

The following section will briefly cover the breadth of challenges faced by women in the workplace as a result of gender inequality. (For additional material on these topics, please see Anderson (2000); Cleveland et al. (2000); Nelson and Burke (2002)).

The First Shift: Women's Experiences at Work

To fully understand people's work experiences and the implications for their well-being, we must recognize that some sources of workplace distress affect only certain groups of people. Most of us are aware of the socio-cultural factors such as sexism, ethnocentrism, homophobia, classism, and ageism that pose constant challenges to our contemporary society. Likewise, these forms of discrimination pervade the work environment, as workers and managers do not leave their personal social biases at home when they begin their workday. Prejudice can cause one workplace to feel like different worlds for different employees, depending on their own experiences within that environment. We must take this into consideration when examining the body of work research, which has primarily been based on studies of middle class white males. Because their experiences are only representative of a subset of the entire working population, it is misguided to expect that such research can yield an accurate portrayal of all people's work experiences. For example, women's life experiences, and therefore their work experiences, are qualitatively different from those of men and require a dedicated body of research (Armstrong and Armstrong 1990; Davidson and Fielden 1999).

In exploring the ways in which women experience the work role differently from men, we must consider how the work environment is different for women, resulting primarily from the pervasive belief in "gender differences." To be clear, we are not talking about sex differences, which are biological, but gender differences, which are sociocultural. In western culture, gender differences are socially constructed notions that result in the perception that inborn differences exist in the psychology and behavior of women and men, despite research findings showing that women and men show more similarities among these variables than differences (Hyde 2005). That is, women are traditionally considered to have more "feminine" qualities, including being passive, emotional, and relationally oriented, whereas men are traditionally deemed to have more "masculine" qualities, including being aggressive, rational, and individually oriented. On an individual level, these beliefs, which children learn from the time they are very young, shape (and potentially limit) the lives of both women and men in terms of their self-concepts and enactment of life roles. On a social level, they pervade every aspect of the cultural environment, public institutions, and societal practices of our world, including work organizations (Nelson and Burke 2002).

The persistent belief in gender differences unfortunately gives rise to stereotyping and discrimination. Both women and men are confronted daily with socially prescribed expectations (about their abilities, preferences, behavior, appearance, strengths, and weaknesses), which may or may not have a basis in reality. In the workplace, this has led to such problems as occupational gender segregation, or the phenomenon that women and men, because they are "different," are predisposed to work in different types of jobs. For example, we do not often see male elementary school teachers or female plumbers. However, this may be due less to individual choice and more to the social forces that dictate which educational opportunities, career paths, and job prospects are designated as "appropriate" and openly available, depending on one's social classification as "woman" or "man" (Anderson 2000). Unfortunately this has relegated a large population of women to "pink collar" jobs, which involve a high degree of emotional labor or caregiving (i.e., daycare worker, health aid, and administrative assistant; Cleveland et al. 2000; Guy and Newman 2004). These traditionally "female" positions are oftentimes associated with adverse outcomes, such as burnout (Morris and Feldman 1997). Moreover, they require less training, are low-status, and have low levels of pay. A telling illustration of this is that while women comprise 74% of all employees in the healthcare industry, they have the least status and pay in the field; the most highly paid and prominent physicians and medical administrators are men (Anderson 2000).

Because of enduring notions that there is a certain "place" for women in organizations, they have been limited in career opportunities. Many women have found it difficult to enter male-dominated professions, and oftentimes they have been driven out of such environments by the daunting level of hostility and social isolation encountered once there. Sexual harassment is perhaps the most widely discussed form of gender discrimination and is defined by behavior that denigrates a person (usually a woman) based on her gender. In a sociocultural system with an inherent gender hierarchy, harassers (usually men) seek to preserve or enhance their own social and economic gender-based status. Therefore, sexual harassment is motivated by power rather than sexual desire (Berdahl 2007) and is characterized by behavior that is uninvited, unreciprocated, one-sided, and imposed (Rubenstein 1989, 1992). Two forms of sexual harassment have been identified: quid pro quo and hostile environment (Fitzgerald et al. 1988). Quid pro quo workplace harassment is explicit sexual coercion, where the harasser is an agent of the employer (often a supervisor) who asserts her or his authority (i.e., to hire, fire, discipline, or promote) in exchange for sexual favors from a subordinate. The employee may be asked either directly or indirectly to submit to a sexual advance as a condition of getting or keeping some tangible job benefit controlled by the harasser. Hostile environment harassment is the more common, and often more subtle, form of sexual harassment and may occur even if the harassing behavior is not directed or targeted at the complainant. A hostile working environment is one in which the harasser (e.g., a supervisor or coworker) does or says things that make the victim feel uncomfortable because of her or his gender. These unwelcome words or actions of a sexual nature thereby create an intimidating and offensive atmosphere.

Whether quid pro quo or hostile environment, sexual harassment is not without its consequences. Many studies have demonstrated the relationship between frequency of sexual harassment and morale-related job outcomes such as job satisfaction (Fitzgerald et al. 1997) and organizational commitment (Schneider et al. 1997). These relationships between sexual harassment and job-related outcomes persist even when general job stress and negative affectivity are statistically controlled (Glomb et al. 1999). Further, the long-term effects of sexual harassment on job satisfaction have been found with 2-year lagged data (Glomb et al. 1999; Munson et al. 2000). In addition to the consequences associated with lower morale, sexual harassment poses financial costs related to litigation and decreases in productivity.

Sexual harassment can also be damaging to a victim's well-being: psychological symptoms include anger and fear as well as more severe emotional problems such as depressive disorder, anxiety disorder, and posttraumatic stress disorder, while physical symptoms include headache, insomnia, gastrointestinal difficulty, and decreased appetite (Willness et al. 2007).

Gender differences can also result in restricted access to positions that garner both power and authority. For example, the old stereotype that women lack the strength and rationality required of a good leader has historically kept women from rising above the "glass ceiling" to the senior-most levels in organizations, from private industry to the military and to the world of politics. This invisible and often unacknowledged barrier has been kept in place within the work environment by biased recruiting, selection, and promotion practices, as well as the unavailability of formal and informal networking and mentoring opportunities that grant men the advantage of social and informational resources that help them get ahead (i.e., the "old boys network"; Cleveland et al. 2000; Nelson and Burke 2002). This explains why women comprise 46% of the workforce (Toossi 2005) in Fortune 500 companies but hold only 16% of corporate officer positions, 12% of board seats, and 6% of the top-paying positions (Catalyst 2006a, b). This parallels the situation of women leaders in government, where women make up 51% of the US population (Spraggins 2005) and exceed the number of men voting in recent elections (Center for American Woman and Politics 2005) but hold only 16% of seats in the US Congress and 24% of statewide elective executive offices (Center for American Woman and Politics 2007). Women also have to contend with inequality in pay; they still earn only 77 cents for each dollar men earn, even when they have the same education level and are doing the same work (DeNavas-Walt et al. 2007).

Another challenge many women may face is on the other side of the shattered glass ceiling. That is, once some trailblazing women are granted access to senior positions, especially in organizations that have never had the experience of a female leader, they often contend with the difficulties of tokenism. Tokenism is the placement of a member from an underrepresented group (e.g., a woman or African American) within the work setting, the act being a symbolic gesture toward compliance with nondiscrimination policies rather than a genuine manifestation of an inclusive workplace (Anderson 2000). Given the inauthenticity of this practice, it is not surprising that such "token" women in male-dominated positions or environments often encounter marginalization and social isolation as well as an undermining of their authority. Their work lives may also be infused with stereotype threat, the anxiety that one feels when placed in a situation where they risk confirming negative stereotypes about them based on their membership in a particular demographic group (Bergeron et al. 2006; Brown and Pinel 2003; Steele 1997). This can result in women having to overcompensate by working harder and longer or being held to a higher standard of performance than males in the same position simply to prove they are capable and to dispel negative stereotypes (Anderson 2000; Goldenhar and Sweeney 1996; Spencer et al. 1999). Not surprisingly, women in these situations often experience poorer psychological and physical health, as well as adverse work outcomes (Bond et al. 2004; Goldenhar et al. 1998; Klonoff et al. 2000; Messing 2000).

As detailed in this section, the many ways in which gender discrimination manifests in the workplace (i.e., occupational segregation, sexual harassment, unequal pay, and the glass ceiling) not only illustrate how the workplace is more challenging for women than for men, but also point to the variety of work-related situations for which women are at risk for adverse impact. On a micro level, workplace discrimination threatens women's mental and physical health and damages work attitudes and performance. On a macro level, these discriminatory practices are first cousins of the more severe socioeconomic inequalities that relegate women from around the globe to conditions of poverty, violence, exploitation, and servitude. Yet our culture often does not witness the full extent of desperation facing some global women, often conceiving of their situations as irrelevant to our "civilized" way of life. However, the continuation of workplace practices, such as limiting women to low-wage, low-skill, low-status, emotionally burdensome jobs, emerges from and reproduces the same powerful system of injustice that spans history and geography, ensuring that women everywhere, at various levels of severity, remain perpetual victims of disempowerment, demoralization, and subjugation.

On a positive note, this also means that the workplace has a particularly influential role to play in transforming the existing socioeconomic system by instituting corrective action and policies that deliberately champion social justice regarding gender. If organizations were to engage in such an endeavor with the same effort and fervor with which they drive toward business results, the implications would most certainly be dramatic and far-reaching. As we shall see later in this chapter, some companies have begun to take such steps.

The Second Shift: Women's "Other" Work

In addition to the difficulties that manifest in the workplace because of gender discrimination, we must also consider that women and men can experience the workplace differently based on its design alone. It must be pointed out that the structure of today's workplace, originated during the industrial revolution, was created by men for a primarily male employee population that spent its workday engaged in repetitive physical tasks or operating mechanized equipment, while most of their wives stayed home with domestic and family-care responsibilities (Coontz 2001). Even though the world of work has evolved dramatically since that time, with women now constituting almost half of the workforce, dual-earner couples becoming the norm, and the nature of work being transformed by technology, this antiquated design remains the foundation for operating the contemporary workplace. As a result, this system poses difficulties for one group of employees whose needs were not considered when it was instituted: women. The workplace would have an entirely different configuration had it been designed by women with the intention of accommodating women's needs and lifestyles.

If women were to design the contemporary workplace "in their image," a major difference one might notice immediately would be a revised conceptualization of what "work" means. To most women, "work" is quantified by the entire range of work experiences in which they engage on a day-to-day basis, including both paid and unpaid work (i.e., housework and family carework). It has recently been acknowledged that the traditional conceptualization of work as a paid activity is based mainly on the previously mentioned outdated studies on working men, the findings of which cannot be assumed as thoroughly relevant to women (Tancred 1995; Thomas 1995). This bias toward the male perspective may also explain why unpaid labor, as "women's work," was a disregarded topic in early research on work. Its association with women, disempowered socially and economically throughout history, rendered domestic work invisible, as it was uncompensated, low-status, unacknowledged, with little opportunity for self-improvement (Doyal 1999): in essence, not "real" work. Yet, despite unpaid labor's clearly unappealing qualities, the misconceived male-centered perspective perpetuated the notion that women were naturally inclined toward housework and family carework, and moreover, that it was actually pleasurable and healthy for them to engage in such domestic activities (Doyal 1999; Lloyd 1999). More recent research over the past several decades has fortunately taken into account the perspectives of women in explaining their own work experiences, dispelling misconceptions, and now regarding the partitioning of paid and unpaid work as "artificial" (Hunt and Annandale 1993; Popay et al. 1993).

One of the main reasons why it is vital to consider women's unpaid work experiences is that they are a prominent feature in the lives of most women in a way that they are not for most men. This is a curious situation given that the twentieth century saw a dissolution of the tradition where the sexes inhabited "separate spheres," with men ruling the public domain of economics and politics in the work role, while women were relegated almost exclusively to the private domain and the home role, with its associated homemaking and family caretaking responsibilities. Despite the fact that the women have long since embraced the responsibility of the worker and financial provider roles and that men's roles have evolved to afford them more involvement with traditionally "female" activities such as housework and family nurturing, the tide has not quite turned. A preponderance of the research evidence shows that traditionally prescribed gender roles are still fairly intact on the home front. While women have adopted the market work role, there has not been a concomitant shedding of the traditional domestic role, and while men have maintained the work role, they have not yet fully adopted the home role, leaving working women in a situation where they carry a double workload, referred to in research as the "second shift" phenomenon (Hochschild 1989).

Women's double workload is exemplified in the vast body of research on the division of household labor which shows overwhelmingly that women spend more time in household chores and taking care of family than men. To illustrate, Robinson and Godbey (1997) found that from 1965 to 1985, even though there was a considerable decrease in the number of hours American women spent weekly on housework (from 24 to 16 hours) and an increase in the number of hours men spent weekly in housework (from 2 to 4 hours), women were still working 12 more hours per week than men; more recent research supports this (Coltrane 2000). Several studies have concluded that this inequitable division of household labor holds true regardless of the number of hours women spend in paid work (Kamo 1991; Shelton and John 1996). Marriage exacerbates the situation, with housework hours increasing substantially for women and decreasing for men when they marry (Gupta 1999; Waite and Gallagher 2000); the gap widens further still when couples become parents (Cowan and Cowan 1992; Johnson and Huston 1998; MacDermid et al. 1990; Shelton 1992). These disparities have been found among couples despite wives' education level or employment status (Hoffman 1978) and notwithstanding the couples' preparenthood division of household labor or beliefs about sex roles (Cowan et al. 1978; Stafford et al. 1977).

The unbalanced allocation of housework and family time and effort among the sexes is thought to be associated with the division of labor becoming increasingly more divided along traditional gender lines with the inception of marriage (South and Spitze 1994) and subsequently parenthood (Belsky et al. 1983; Cowan et al. 1978; Grossman et al. 1980). These life events seem to have a polarizing effect on women and men in terms of their participation in the home. Several studies have shown that many household and family-related tasks are characterized by gender (Coltrane 2000), not unlike the aforementioned occupational segregation in the workplace. Tasks such as cooking, cleaning, shopping, and laundry are frequently typed as "female" tasks (Antill et al. 1996; Blair and Lichter 1991; Orbuch and Eyster 1997; Presser 1994; Sanchez and Kane 1996; Starrels 1994), whereas home repair, yard work, and car maintenance are frequently typed as "male" tasks (Blair and Lichter 1991; Shelton 1992). In parenthood, husbands provide care for family by engaging in more "male" tasks (i.e., exterior home maintenance, finances), while wives engage in more "female" tasks (i.e., changing diapers, feeding; Cowan et al. 1978; Feldman et al. 1981; LaRossa and LaRossa 1981).

Studies have also noted that the nature of tasks typed as "female" and "male" is qualitatively different (Coltrane 2000). "Female" typed tasks are more time-consuming, require performance on an everyday basis, and are less optional than "male" typed tasks, which occur less routinely and more at one's own discretion. Moreover, "female" tasks have been characterized as unpleasant in comparison to "male" tasks (DeVault 1991; Robinson and Milkie 1997, 1998). Other distinctions are evident in the way the different genders enact home-work. For example, women are often considered "household managers" who initiates, delegates, oversees, and is ultimately accountable for home and family related tasks, whereas men play the more casual role of "helper" or "assistant" to their partners (Blain 1994; Coltrane 1996; Gunter and Gunter 1990; Hawkins et al. 1994; Mederer 1993; West and Fenstermaker 1993). Moreover, women are more likely to do behind-the-scenes work or family "shadow" work, such as making, scheduling, and coordinating medical appointments, childcare, holiday gatherings, and family meals (DeVault 1991; Hochschild 1989; Thompson and Walker 1989).

In addition to the social expectations that saddle women with qualitatively different, more onerous tasks than men, women have themselves been socialized to enact home-related work with an ethic of care (Gilligan 1982; Kroska 2003). That is, just as women's thoughts, feelings, and behaviors have been instilled with a pervasive sense of providing care for loved ones, so too do household and family tasks take on a relational and personalized meaning, rather than being strictly defined by the task alone. This can exacerbate women's workload by adding a dimension of emotional labor to tasks, influencing their self-concepts by pairing hard work with being a "good mother," and placing women at risk of sacrificing their own needs to show care for others (Henderson and Bialeschki 1991; Wearing 1984).

These differences in women's and men's roles in home-work and carework have been found to have detrimental effects for women. Research from several western, developed countries has found that the inequitable division of household labor is associated with depression and anxiety in women (Barnett and Shen 1997; Dennerstein et al. 1993; Desjarlais et al. 1995; Glass and Fujimoto 1994; Golding 1990; Larson et al. 1994). This may be related to the low-status nature of domestic work; many women report the perception that the care they provide is neither reciprocated nor appreciated and that they lack emotional and social support in carrying it out (Romito 1990). Similarly, as unpaid caregivers, women who provide care for elders or disabled people report decreased mental and physical health, financial concerns, and stress arising from their cumulative (i.e., work and home) workload, as well as exhaustion and depression resulting from feeling overwhelmed and undervalued in their work (Lloyd 1999).

The Intersection of Paid and Unpaid Work

It should be clear by now that the nature of women's and men's experiences of work and home life are very different and that these experiences have implications for personal well-being. Not surprisingly, research confirms that women and men do differ in their experiences of mental and physical health. For instance, women have more mental health concerns than men (Nelson and Burke 2002), reporting more psychophysiological symptoms including nervousness, increased heart rate, dizziness, nightmares, trembling, lack of motivation (Nelson and Burke 2002) and somatic symptoms associated with stress (i.e., headaches, backaches, insomnia, hypertension, and gastrointestinal problems). Also, women, when compared to men, use medical services more frequently, have more acute and chronic conditions, are issued more prescriptions, are more likely to abuse prescription medication, and are more prone to eating disorders (Anderson 2000; Nelson and Burke 2002). It is difficult to pinpoint the precise origins of women's and men's differences in well-being, given the variety of dissimilar life experiences that may act as contributing factors. Moreover, although research shows that the work and home domains can each have a particular impact on women's experiences of psychological and physical health, it shows that the interaction of work and home circumstances is a highly influential determinant in women's experiences of well-being.

The recent attention paid to the unique nature of women's dual workload (paid employment plus the "second shift") is both timely and needed because of the ways that it can manifest in stress. For instance, the cumulative responsibilities of work and home can lead women to role overload, which is the feeling of being overwhelmed by the amount of role responsibilities one has to accomplish (Daly 1996; Schor 1991; Ivancevich and Matteson 1980; Mattingly and Bianchi 2003; Reeves and Szafran 1996). Role overload is a potential stressor, since distress may manifest whenever people perceive that their personal resources (such as physical energy or mental attention) are drained or depleted (Hobfoll 1989). Not surprisingly, the resource drain posed by a heavy cumulative workload places many women at risk for role overload, which has been found to be associated with adverse behavioral, psychological, and physiological outcomes (Cartwright and Cooper 1997; Jex and Beehr 1991; Spector et al. 1988). Moreover, many women are so busy with their roles that they feel constantly pressed for time, an especially scarce resource; the stress of this "time-squeeze" can result in poorer mental health, physical health symptoms, and decreased life satisfaction (Hochschild 1989, 1997; LaRossa and LaRossa 1981; Leete and Schor 1994; Lehto 1998; Robinson and Godbey 1997; Schor 1991: Zuzanek 1998).

Distress can also arise when one feels pressured by work–family conflict. Work–family conflict is the experience of tension because the demands of one life domain are incompatible with demands of another life domain (Greenhaus and Beutell 1985). That is, the demands of work can interfere with family ("work-to-family conflict") and the demands of family can interfere with work ("family-to-work conflict"). Work–family conflict acts as a stressor especially for women, who are often pressured by the demands of multiple, simultaneously competing roles. Work–family conflict has been associated with poorer work outcomes (e.g., absenteeism, turnover, job satisfaction) and poorer personal outcomes (e.g., life and family satisfaction; Aryee 1992; Bedeian et al. 1988; Parasuraman et al. 1992; Perrewé et al. 1999; Rice et al. 1992; Thomas and Ganster 1995). In addition, it has been associated with emotional and physical difficulties including greater incidence of depression, anxiety, hostility, substance dependence disorders, physical health complaints, and hypertension (Beatty 1996; Frone 2000; Frone et al. 1993, 1996, 1997a).

As indicated, the stressors of role overload, time squeeze, and work–family conflict can adversely affect emotional and physical well-being (Frone et al. 1997a, b; Hobfoll 1989). Moreover, if such stressors persist for an extended period of time, as may be the case when one experiences work–family conflict while raising children over many years, chronic stress can result (Ivancevich and Matteson 1980). The reason this occurs is that if a person is unable to eliminate a perceived stressor, or does not have the opportunity to recover from exposure to the stressor, her or his psychobiological systems remain in a prolonged state of arousal; over time this causes physical and psychological wear and tear (Meijman and Mulder 1998; Sluiter et al. 1999; Ursin 1980). Opportunities for recovery (i.e., by ceasing exposure to role demands) are therefore essential for women in alleviating the pressure they feel from their double work duty, helping to restore well-being and preventing chronic conditions. Ironically, the same conditions that give rise to women's need for recovery also prevent it from taking place. That is, because of their great number of responsibilities and lack of personal free time (Bittman and Wajcman 2000; Henderson and Bialeschki 1991; Hochschild 1989; Searle and Jackson 1985; Shaw 1985, 1994; Shelton 1992), recovery opportunities for women are rare, placing them at increased risk of stress-related effects.

Even on those infrequent occasions when women can find time for relaxation, because of a perpetual awareness of their role-based obligations, they do not often experience true leisure as it is defined by unrestricted freedom and psychological disengagement (Bella 1990; Kelly and Godbey 1992). Rather, their leisure is more likely than men's to be combined with constraining activities such as looking after children and is more likely to be interrupted by family (Bittman and Wajcman 2000). This situation is exacerbated by the influence of social prescriptions dictating what it means to be a good mother, wife, homemaker: always making oneself accessible to family and sacrificing one's own needs to care for loved ones (Blair and Lichter 1991; Brown et al. 2000; Henderson et al. 1989; Wearing 1984). Unfortunately, this can give rise to feelings of emotional discomfort, guilt, or preoccupation when women are attempting to find the self-gratification, relaxation, and personal freedom that unfettered leisure time away from their obligations can grant them (Harrington and Dawson 1995; Henderson and Bialeschki 1991; Wearing 1990).

As well as allowing women recovery from their constant work roles, having personal free time also allows women to engage in activities that actively promote good physical, mental, and social health (Bianchi et al. 2000; Hochschild 1989; Nock and Kingston 1988). Research has shown that women with insufficient personal free time have inadequate opportunities for physical and mental health care, recreation, exercise, maintaining a healthy diet, social interaction, and quality time with their significant other (Gjerdingen et al. 2000; LaRossa and LaRossa 1981; McMurray 1999; Smith 1995). In fact, some studies have identified a relationship between women's heavy role responsibilities and riskier health behaviors, including substance use/abuse (i.e., tranquilizers, alcohol, and cigarettes), lack of physical exercise, and poor diet (Doyal 1999). By having some personal space outside of their cumulative roles (i.e., worker, mother, and wife), women may have the freedom and control to experience the fulfillment offered by self-care, self-expression, and self-improvement (Bianchi 2000).

As detailed in this section, the interaction between women's work and family roles, and the simultaneous demands it puts on their time and energy, can strongly impact their psychological and physical health. Looking at these difficulties faced by women since they made their historic migration out of the home and into the workplace, one might wonder if it was worth the resulting struggle, stress, and health effects. But it must be acknowledged that women enjoy a far better quality of life than was previously available to them when the only place for them was "the home." In spite of any difficulties arising from the dual demands of the work and home roles, paid work has been found to be a protective factor in terms of women's mental health (Arber and Lahelma 1993; Bromberger and Matthews 1994; Glass and Fujimoto 1994). Studies have shown that women who do paid work experience better health than those who do full-time unpaid work, and women in higher-status jobs (i.e., professional work) experience better health than women who have lower-status jobs (i.e., manual work; Arber 1991; Arber et al. 1985; Popay et al. 1993). Some research suggests that this can be explained by paid work offering a change of setting and social interaction (Jahoda 1982; Warr 1982), as social support is associated with a lower risk of depression and anxiety (Brown and Harris 1978, 1989).

Likewise the financial and social independence afforded by paid work (especially fairly paid, higher-status work), as well as a sense of purpose and control over one's life, cannot be underestimated in their ability to enhance quality of life, as men have always known.

Given that women are not only in the workplace to stay, but that it is beneficial for them to do so under the right conditions, we will next focus on some opportunities for employers to optimize women's experiences of well-being. Organizations can create an inclusive work environment, rectify long-standing discriminatory employment practices, maintain equal gender representation among jobs at all levels of pay and prestige, advocate the use of workplace social support, acknowledge and alleviate women's cumulative workload, redesign work to allow more flexibility and control, attend to women's mental and physical health concerns, and support their opportunities for relaxing leisure and active recreation. Some pioneering organizations have made a commitment to addressing these particular challenges in their workplaces by developing and encouraging the use of innovative policies, programs, and services. In the following section, the many efforts employers have made shall be detailed.

Workplace Services, Benefits, and Policies

The progressive companies that have recognized they can be instrumental in making work a more optimal experience for women, and indeed all employees, have engaged in a radical rethinking of the way work is conceptualized and structured. On their part, this required an initial acknowledgment that the original model for today's workplace is obsolete, based on a system that emerged with the first industrial sites in the late eighteenth and early nineteenth century. This outdated system, which has not evolved in step with a rapidly changing world, has been faulted for not being responsive to the dramatic social and technological shifts that make the world a very different place than it was even 30 years ago.

To be clear, let us engage in a brief, but concentrated, review of some of these changes. Today there are more women in the workplace than ever before (46% of the workforce are women; Toossi 2005), and their level of education has shown a remarkable improvement, from 18% college-educated (4 or more years) to 30% over the past 25 years (DiNatale and Boraas 2002). The age of first marriage and parenthood has increased, marriage rates are down, divorce rates are up, people are having fewer children, and dual-income couples have replaced the provider husband and stay-at-home mother duo. Family configurations have changed, too, as a result of more couples cohabitating, more families being headed by single mothers or fathers, lesbian and gay couples marrying and adopting children, remarriages creating blended families, and grandparents raising grandchildren. Technological advances and globalization have made the world a much smaller place, with geographic mobility becoming commonplace and long commutes and business travel a way of life. This has unfortunately resulted in families living farther distances from one another, having less time to spend together, and being less able to help one another. Economic and political changes have created a shrinking middle class, where the world's wealth has become more concentrated among the privileged few, while more people fall into poverty with fewer social services to assist them. A growing number of working families have also been affected by the lack of access to affordable healthcare and housing, the inability to financially provide for families even with two incomes, the high rate of poverty among women and children, the prohibitive cost of a college education, and the increasingly serious need to plan ahead for one's retirement.

Socially responsible organizations recognize that they are in a unique position to ameliorate some of these concerns facing their employees. Moreover, in the interest of self-preservation, insightful companies recognize that what harms their employees, harms the organization. That is, because the aforementioned realities provide the backdrop for the world workers are living in, and employees bring their whole selves and collective experiences with them to their jobs, employees' personal difficulties translate into a matter of concern for employers. Some businesses now pay serious attention to the research suggesting that not only women, but an increasing number of men, as well as members of Generations X and Y, place the greatest value on their personal and family lives, which they are unwilling to sacrifice for work (Families and Work Institute 2004). Among the business community, there is consensus that companies responsive to the personal needs of their employees are more attractive to and gain the commitment of the most creative and talented job candidates on the market, thereby having a leg up on the "war for talent" (Donlon 1999; McCracken 2000). By offering comprehensive programs and services to assist employees and their families with the range of concerns that affect them, as well as instituting progressive new modes of working that create a tailored fit between employees' work and personal lives, organizations can have happier, healthier workforces and more smoothly running, successful businesses.

There is an abundance of benefits, programs, and services that organizations utilize to meet the health and personal needs of their employees. The following section elaborates on the variety of approaches organizations are taking to meet these needs, whether by directly addressing the emotional and physical health concerns of employees, alleviating the burden of the dual workload, ensuring that women are treated equally in the workplace, or providing them access to satisfying jobs that provide a comfortable life for themselves and their families. Although it is difficult to quantify the prevalence of specific interventions across organizations, we do know that such practices have been instituted and are currently being utilized. It should also be noted that no one company offers the full range of policies and benefits discussed below, but some companies have a menu of services that features a variety of them. For more information about women-friendly companies and the specific services they offer, refer to *Working Mother* magazine, which annually publishes a list of the "100 Best Companies for Working Mothers."

Addressing Emotional and Physical Health Concerns

Probably the first solution one thinks of, in terms of how employers can address the well-being concerns of their workers, is the provision of health insurance. Given that health insurance in the USA is not provided universally through federal or state governments, and that the cost is often prohibitive for families to afford on their own, employer-sponsored health insurance plans are an integral part of the health-care delivery system. However, even when medical and mental health benefits are provided through one's employer, oftentimes there are restrictions on who and what services are covered, as well as which employees are eligible to receive coverage. One way some employers have remedied this problem is through the provision of affordable, comprehensive health benefits to all employees, regardless of how many hours one works. It is particularly advantageous for women, who are more likely to work part-time, to have access to full medical, mental health, dental, and retirement benefits without being forced into working full-time, especially when it may be to the detriment of self and family to do so. It also alleviates concerns when benefits are extended to domestic partners, as they are to spouses or children. Likewise, employers can pay special attention to providing comprehensive coverage for mental health and substance abuse treatment, which is not always adequate enough to meet the needs of those who have long-term emotional difficulties. Furthermore, employers can use their influence to be instrumental in supporting legislation for mental health parity, which requires health insurance plans to provide the same annual and lifetime dollar limits for mental health benefits as they do for medical benefits.

Employee Assistance Programs

A very popular workplace service for addressing employees' mental health needs is the employee assistance program (EAP); 67% of human resources (HR) professionals report having an EAP (Employee Assistance Professionals Association 2002). EAPs are viewed as being part of a comprehensive employee benefits package and also as part of the larger mental health delivery system. In short, EAPs are a free service designed to assist employees and their families in resolving personal difficulties, while maintaining their confidentiality. Originating after World War II in the USA as occupational alcoholism programs, in more recent years, EAPs have expanded to address a broad range of personal concerns, including emotional problems, stress, substance use/abuse, and marital or family difficulties (Employee Assistance Professionals Association 2003). Additionally, most EAPs offer referrals to legal and financial consultation services.

The core service of an EAP is some combination of professional assessment and short-term counseling or referral; EAPs are not intended for long-term treatment. Typically, the first EAP session involves an evaluation by a mental health professional. At the end of the evaluation, the counselor makes a recommendation to commence a short series of counseling sessions or offers a mental health referral, as is the case when clients have a long history of emotional difficulty or exhibit more severe symptoms. EAP cases in which brief counseling has been recommended typically last three to five sessions and have a solution-focused orientation. Specific client goals are set, usually in the second session; the subsequent sessions are used to help align the client's cognitions and behaviors with her or his identified goals. Although there is no standard qualification for EAP counselors, they are trained mental health professionals (e.g., licensed psychologist, clinical social worker, or professional counselor). Additionally, there is a professional certification (i.e., Certified Employee Assistance Professional or "CEAP") that may be obtained, but it is not required for practice.

EAPs have two main modes of service delivery. The original internal EAP model, rarely used in today's workplace, is based in-house, where the EAP consultant works exclusively for one organization and is a salaried employee of the organization. There usually is less formality regarding the number of sessions a client may receive, and often there is more visibility of EAP services to employees with this onsite model, which can be a concern to employees who want to maintain their privacy in utilizing EAP services. Another model that has increasingly grown popular is the external EAP which is based outside the organization (often a private EAP firm or community mental health center). These EAPs are much larger than internal EAPs, employing a full staff of EAP professionals and providing services for several organizations. Companies may either contract with the EAP for a negotiated number of sessions per employee per annum (e.g., $20 for three to four sessions per employee) or may operate on a fee-for-service basis, with a set charge for each session. Although most EAPs still offer services through conventional face-to-face sessions, some EAPs now offer telephone or internet-based counseling services and operate on a 24/7 basis to increase accessibility—important developments in the new global economy with a continuous workforce. Some EAPs offer support groups, workshops, and seminars on a variety of relevant topics (e.g., stress management, substance abuse, bereavement, domestic violence, time management) or assistance with professional development, through career counseling and executive coaching.

As well as helping employees and their families who voluntarily use the service to resolve personal difficulties, EAPs can be used as an organizational tool for consulting with managers on how to address employee emotional and behavioral issues that cause breakdowns in work performance, health, or organizational functioning (Employee Assistance Professionals Association 2003). For example, individuals classified as "heavy drinkers" comprise 12% of the workforce; 47% of industrial injuries and 40% of workplace deaths are linked to alcohol consumption (Atkinson 2001). Moreover, almost 14 million Americans use illegal drugs; as workers, they are four times more likely to be involved in an accident at work and five times more likely to file for workers' compensation benefits than nonusers (Nighswonger 2000). Therefore, EAPs can be instrumental in helping employees who have been referred because of alcohol and drug problems, an especially serious issue when they have safety sensitive jobs. Another difficulty that EAPs can assist with, which has gained increasing media attention, is domestic violence that spills over into the workplace, posing a risk not only to the targeted employee, but often resulting in a breach of security and a threat to the safety of other workers. This is particularly relevant for women, who are disproportionately affected by such violence.

EAPs are also useful in addressing organizational level concerns that affect employee well-being, including significant workplace change (i.e., organizational restructuring and downsizing) or traumatic workplace events (i.e., accidents, death, crime, and natural disasters), by offering management consultation, employee counseling, and critical incident stress debriefings (CISDs). For companies making positive changes in their work environments through the institution of new workplace policies (e.g., anti-harassment or discrimination, substance abuse/drug testing, zero tolerance for workplace violence), EAPs can provide relevant organizational consultation and manager/employee training.

As may be surmised, EAPs are highly useful to women for many reasons, and it is no surprise that women use EAPs more often than men (Blum and Roman 1992). One reason for this may be because women report mental health concerns more often than men and are more likely to seek help and social support. EAP counseling, support groups, and seminars can help women identify the sources of stress in their lives and develop strategies for coping with stressors (e.g., workplace discrimination, relationship issues, or work–family conflict). EAPs can provide psychoeducation to teach women how to set more reasonable expectations of themselves regarding their life roles and also provide strategies to decrease risk of overload (e.g., reducing workload, managing time, prioritizing responsibilities, asking for help, and delegating to others). In addition, EAPs can educate women on the need to communicate with their spouses and create a dialogue for sharing responsibility, or the need for them to take care of themselves as well as they do their families (e.g., through relaxation, social support, exercise, nutrition). Moreover, EAPs can provide women a safe forum for addressing alcohol or drug abuse, often considered more of a "man's problem."

Because EAPs are positioned to be highly accessible to workers, as evidenced by the newer 24/7, internet and telephonic models, they can be particularly helpful for women, given that they have scarce free time due to their cumulative workload. Additionally, because EAPs are free and available to employees' family members and women are more frequently the identified family caregivers, this service can be a valuable and trusted resource for helping them to find help for loved ones.

Some women also find EAPs a safe place to talk about encounters with work-related discrimination. Not only can EAPs offer social support and assistance in identifying emotional and active strategies for coping with discrimination, but for women who are uncomfortable with directly reporting discrimination to their employers, EAPs can provide an alternative place to address such concerns. EAPs can even assist women who need assistance in reporting; since counselors are often familiar with the workplace cultures and HR professionals of the organizations they provide services for, they can be instrumental in creating direct links between victimized employees and sources of help within the organization itself.

Health Promotion and Wellness Programs

In addition to directly addressing the mental health needs of employees, some employers offer health promotion and wellness programs to help employees with the physical health problems that sometimes give rise to, or result from, stress and poor emotional well-being. These programs may include onsite health screenings (i.e., hypertension, pulmonary functioning, cholesterol, diabetes, bone density, and cancer), immunizations (e.g., flu shots), consultation with a health or nutrition coach, or a 24-hour healthline staffed by registered nurses. Some offer smoking cessation or weight management programs (such as onsite Weight Watchers or "getting your body back" programs for new mothers). Other services can include discounts or reimbursement for membership at offsite health clubs. Alternatively, some companies have an onsite fitness or recreation center, which can include a range of amenities, including gym equipment, game courts, jogging tracks, rock-climbing walls, swimming pools, or whirlpools; some centers even offer free childcare. Some workplace campuses feature walking/running trails, bike paths, and sports fields. Other companies offer healthful and affordable cafeteria choices and ready-made take-home dinners, so that employees can have a convenient way to eat healthy at work and home.

Health promotion and wellness programs, like EAPs, are particularly advantageous to women because of their convenience. They are accessible (located at or near work), affordable (or free), and services can frequently be scheduled during the course of the workday (e.g., before or after work, during lunch hour, or on a work break). This is crucial for women, as it has been acknowledged that some women find it easier to find self-time within the work domain than the family domain (Hochschild 1997). In other words, when women do not find time to take care of their own concerns during the course of the workday, their needs often get disregarded, because once they get home from work, they are too consumed with the demands of home and family to care for themselves. Because of women's intense time commitments at work and home and their tendency to neglect self-care when it comes to proper exercise, diet, and leisure, health promotion and wellness programs can be invaluable for them. Not only do these programs help educate women on issues relevant to their health and well-being, but they also provide effective tools for addressing such concerns; weight management, fitness programs, and ready-made healthful meals are particularly relevant to addressing the health-related concerns identified by women.

Alleviating Women's Burden of the Dual Workload

The workplace services to be discussed in the following section, although they do not provide direct mental and physical healthcare, do benefit women greatly because of the instrumental support they provide. The role of instrumental support is an important determining factor in women's experiences regarding household labor, and therefore, the dual workload (Gerstel and Gallagher 2001; Starrels 1994). Unlike social support, which is emotionally based, instrumental support has to do with the amount of actual help one receives in carrying out households tasks. Research has revealed that instrumental support is very beneficial to women. When men share in routine housework such as cleaning, meal preparation, and laundry, their female partners report experiencing a reduced workload, a feeling of fairness in the relationship, and less depression (Coltrane 2000). Marital satisfaction is higher when married couples have a more equitable division of housework (Biernat and Wortman 1991; Erickson 1993; Orbuch and Eyster 1997; Pina and Bengtson 1993). Also, when male partners share in domestic labor, women have better emotional and physical health than when they carry the burden by themselves (Arber et al. 1985).

Lamentably, though partners are the most apropos and readily available resource for providing instrumental support, women are not always able to secure such support from their male partners. For this reason many women have compensated by finding alternate sources of help with housework and childcare, including family of origin, extended family, children, kin networks, and neighbors (Gallagher 1994; Gerstel and Gallagher 1994, 2001; Padgett 1997). Paid services have also gained in popularity among those who can afford them, with people increasingly paying for childcare, prepared meals, and house cleaning (Bergen 1991; Cohen 1998; Oropesa 1993; Presser 1994).

The services discussed in the next section fall under the umbrella of employee compensation and benefits, as well as HR policies. They are indispensable to the women who use them, as they provide access to convenient and/or affordable sources of instrumental help and grant women the control they need to effectively and efficiently manage the many demands of their lives. This can result in the direct alleviation of stress and prevent adverse impact on well-being. The provision of these benefits and services has been associated with more "family-friendly" organizations, so called because of their dedication to reducing the work–family conflict experienced when the competing worlds of work and family collide. In recent years "work–family" benefits have moved away from their exclusive focus on family and evolved into comprehensive suites of "work–life" services that address a broader range of personal needs relevant to employees' lives. To reiterate, no one company offers the full breadth of services detailed below, though some companies offer a wide range of them.

Childcare Services

When people think "work-life," the service they probably think of most often is dependent care, especially childcare, although there has been increasing focus on care for the elderly and school-age children. When women are the ones primarily responsible for the care of children, it is clear that for working mothers, childcare is an absolute necessity, and there are a range of services employers can offer to make finding affordable, conveniently located, high-quality childcare easier for parents. Because it can be prohibitively expensive, some employers make it more affordable by offering reimbursement or subsidies for center-based or in-home childcare (e.g., at the rate of 33, 65, or even 90%). Employers may also provide pretax flexible spending accounts to pay for childcare or offer discounts at national or regional childcare chains.

For convenience, some employers offer an onsite childcare center or have a secured number of slots at company-sponsored childcare centers near the office. The close proximity of childcare is important as it cuts down on pick-up and drop-off time, making parents more accessible to children during the day (whether for a parent–child visit, or in case the child is ill). Organizations often utilize local child-care resource and referral networks, giving employees the opportunity to have a telephone conversation with a consultant who will help them identify their particular childcare needs, the range of care options (e.g., daycare centers, in-home care, family care providers, nursery schools), and help them find accredited, quality childcare. Companies can also address the gaps in childcare; for example, they can provide options for what to do when the regular daycare falls through or when children are sick and are not able (or allowed) to attend daycare. In these cases, companies can provide access to backup care or sick-child care, either in-home or center-based; some companies even allow up to 25 free days of backup care at a national childcare chain. Other services include daycare that is open 7 days a week, has extended hours, or offers occasional night time care so that parents can enjoy an adults-only evening.

In addition to just offering childcare services for preschool children, some companies go a step further by providing a full range of programs for children spanning the lifestages of birth to college. There are a variety of services for employees even in the planning stages of parenthood. For example, companies may offer reimbursement for in vitro fertilization procedures or access to adoption consultation and/or reimbursement. For pregnant employees in their third trimester, some companies offer a valet parking program. For nursing mothers, lactation programs can provide access to private workplace lactation rooms, free pumps at work, subsidies to purchase pumps for home, or 24-hour hotlines for education and support from a lactation consultant.

Parents also have particular needs regarding school-age children (Kindergarten through 12th grade). They must contend with the arrangement of care for school-age children who would otherwise spend every afternoon alone, during the time gap between when children get out of school in the afternoon and when parents return home from work in the evening. This same scenario applies to parents who leave for work earlier than their children leave for school. Because unsupervised children are at increased risk of obesity, exposure to violence through TV and videogames, loitering, sexual activity, substance abuse, and victimization (Barnett and Gareis 2006a, b; Cohen et al. 2002; Kurz 2002), it is no surprise that parents who are highly concerned about their children's after-school care report lower well-being (Barnett and Gareis 2006a, b). To alleviate parents' concerns, some employers offer to fill this time gap with before- and after-school programs. Seasonal schedule changes (e.g., school vacations and holidays, snow days, and summertime) also pose challenges for which parents must arrange care for school-age children. To make things easier, companies may offer access to school holiday care, snow day backup care, or summer camps.

Some companies offer onsite services for school-aged children (i.e., young children, tweens, and teens) such as an educational center (e.g., offering classes in nutrition, self-defense, art, music, foreign language) or summer camps (e.g., sports, science, academic). Additionally, they may offer tutoring services or a free homework helpline. They may provide assistance for children with learning difficulties or special needs, including resource and referral programs, support groups, behavioral therapy, advocates, and medical specialists. For teens, companies can coordinate community service or volunteer programs and safe driver programs. They may offer onsite summer internships, assistance with college applications, discounted SAT test preparation, and scholarships for employees' children.

Elder Care Services

It is increasingly being recognized that in addition to caring for children, more and more people are providing care for elderly family members or other disabled adults. These caregivers may even be "sandwiched" between two or three generations needing care (i.e., children, aging parents, and/or grandchildren) which can interfere with one's work schedule, and at worst, one's work performance. Elder care responsibilities can be a particular challenge as they often are needed at a time when individuals have just finished the caregiving responsibilities that come with parenting children, but unlike caring for children, the need to provide eldercare may not be anticipated and can become increasingly demanding over time (Azarnoff and Scharlach 1988). Contrary to popular belief, most long-term eldercare is not provided by residential programs or social agencies, but by informal caregivers including friends and family. Women in particular tend to be the ones providing care for elders, not necessarily providing direct care but acting as the care manager (similar to the previously mentioned role of "household manager"), even for far-away relatives: making telephone calls, scheduling appointments, and providing transportation (Piercy and Blieszner 1999). It must be noted that many of these activities necessarily take place during business hours (i.e., doctor appointments, banking, insurance, and Medicare consultations), when women are working. For these reasons, some companies offer eldercare programs and services which provide help in choosing a physician or health specialist or making decisions about care, whether at home or in a residential setting. They may also provide referrals to other services including home health aids or adult daycare, assisted living or skilled nursing facilities, geriatric case management, or hospice. In tandem with these services, companies may offer an eldercare resource and referral service (usually provided by local Area Agencies on Aging), which provide employees the opportunity to have a telephone consultation with a professional who will help identify their dependant elder's needs and local options for providing them care or assistance (e.g., home-delivered meals, recreation, volunteer opportunities).

Convenience Services

In recognition that the little details and errands of employees' lives can add up and consume a great deal of their time and energy, companies may alleviate these daily hassles by offering onsite services providing employees access to a range of services. Such services include take-home meals, laundry or dry cleaning, car repair/oil change, car wash/detailing, massage therapy, spa services, hair and nail salon services, dental care, postal services, photo development, and banking. When car trouble strikes or someone misses the train to work, some companies offer emergency transportation programs, paying for a cab or rental car. In addition to these onsite services, an increasingly popular employee offering is personal assistance through convenience or "concierge" services. By calling a toll-free number or logging onto a website, employees gain access to free services that can take care of almost anything on one's "to-do" list. For instance, it can help employees find someone to pick up dry cleaning, deliver groceries, feed or walk pets, ship packages, find a plumber or electrician, and even wait for the cable man. These services can also help with travel, entertainment, and reservations, including planning a child's birthday, hiring a wedding planner, researching airfares, car rental, moving services, or getting concert tickets. An additional benefit employers may offer is access to discounted services in the community, increasing the affordability of financial counselors, local retailers, or recreational activities (e.g., movie tickets, theatre productions, zoo, aquarium, sports events).

In addition to these services, some companies internally coordinate onsite seminars, emails, newsletters, or support groups for the purposes of providing employees with information, education, and available resources, regarding a variety of matters that concern them. Whether the topic is parenting, work stress, time management, or wellness, helping employees become aware of important life issues, giving them a means for getting assistance, and providing a forum for sharing concerns with one another makes their lives less stressful and more satisfying. Such steps toward creating work environments that foster the integration of employees' personal and professional lives can be augmented by instituting similar policy (i.e., casual dress, take your daughter/son to work day, allowing employees to bring dogs to the office), mandating manager training on work–life balance and lifestyle diversity, or establishing employee resource networks (e.g., supper clubs where employees take turns making dinner for one another).

The work–life benefits detailed in this section are highly valuable for women in particular. For example, because women are more likely than men to be engaged in either providing or coordinating care for family members, childcare and elder-care benefits can be especially helpful for them. Not only do such affordable and accessible services permit caregivers the physical freedom to work outside the home, but assurances of good quality dependent care allow women the psychological freedom to work knowing that their loved ones are safe and happy. And because women do so much of the home-related work, convenience services are particularly helpful in alleviating the burden associated with their most time-consuming routine tasks (i.e., through the identification of services to outsource clothes laundering, grocery delivery, meal preparation, and house cleaning). Women, because of their role as behind-the-scenes family coordinator and household manager, also find concierge services helpful, especially for assistance with planning family events (Blain 1994; Coltrane 1996; DeVault 1991; Gunter and Gunter 1990; Hawkins et al. 1994; Hochschild 1989; Mederer 1993; Thompson and Walker 1989; West and Fenstermaker 1993). As stated previously, although such dependent care and convenience services do not directly address mental and physical health, they can help reduce strain associated with role overload and work–life conflict, as well as potentially provide women with some much-needed free time.

Flexible Work Arrangements

When it comes to managing the simultaneous and constant demands of work and family, having the option of flexible work arrangements can be a godsend. Companies that offer such options typically allow for employee discretion in terms of work time and work location, provided that such arrangements do not negatively impact work performance. Additionally, such personal-life oriented policies explicitly state that their use by employees must not jeopardize career advancement in the organization. "Flex time" allows employees to select their preferred start and stop times, for example, working from 7 a.m. to 3 p.m., rather than 9 a.m. to 5 p.m. Compressed workweeks allow employees to work their weekly hours in a condensed format, for example, working a 40-hour week in four days rather than five. Another flexible option includes working reduced hours. Some companies offer alternatives to working full-time, such as part-time work or the ability to switch from full-time to part-time when needed. Job-sharing is another option that allows two people to share one position, dividing the hours and pay accordingly. In the summertime, some employees enjoy their company's policy of reduced hours, or "summer hours" which allows employees to leave work early on Fridays. Setting one's own work hours has a variety of benefits, including missing the daily commute, allowing one to spend time with family or run errands, and potentially providing more opportunities for self-care (e.g., medical appointments, going to the gym).

Another flexible arrangement has to do with the employee not being required to report to an office every day. "Telecommuting" allows an employee to work from a remote location, whether from home, a satellite office closer to home, or any location convenient for the employee. Some companies support this option by providing the necessary technology to make sure that working between home and the office is seamless, whether by providing employees an allowance to set up a home office (i.e., to purchase a computer and furniture), or by directly providing them the technology (e.g., laptops, BlackBerrys, high-speed internet access, wireless services, conference calling, cell phones, phone cards). Offices can complement these home-based services by utilizing technology such as videoconferencing and webcasts to ensure that employees do not miss important office-based meetings or special events when they are offsite. Employees especially enjoy the side-benefits of working remotely as they do not have to get dressed up for work, do not have to struggle through the commute, and many report that they can get much more done when working from home because they do not have to contend with office distractions.

The establishment of these flexible work arrangements allows employees to have a greater sense of control over their time, work, and personal lives, providing them a much needed buffer against the stress and adverse health outcomes brought on by life demands (Ganster 1991; Halpern 2005; Karasek 1979; Karasek and Theorell 1990). It is an acknowledgment by employers that employees have to contend with unique personal life circumstances and are in a better position of deciding which options work best for them, rather than mandating a rigid policy that may or may not work well for every employee. Companies now see that as long as employees can meet their job requirements, work hours, and perform well, the when and where of the work is not always of utmost importance.

Work Leave

Another strategy to help employees integrate their work and family lives is to allow employees to have time away from their employment for various personal reasons, without putting their job in jeopardy. The Family Medical Leave Act of 1993 (FMLA) allows eligible employees to take up to 12 weeks of job-protected, unpaid leave either because of the employee's own serious health problem or to take care of a family member. Although a step in the right direction, the USA lags far behind other industrialized nations in terms of providing suitable work leave policies for its employees. The relatively new FMLA legislation has been criticized because it only allows short-term, unpaid leave for a subset of legally eligible workers (i.e., it specifies permanent workers, not seasonal or temporary, who work in an organization with more than 50 employees). Moreover, it is restrictive because it utilizes a narrow family definition. Women and men can take leave to care for a child (i.e., newborn, adopted, or foster child) or sick family member (i.e., spouse, or elderly parent), but FMLA does not cover the range of family members needing care: unmarried partners (either lesbian/gay or heterosexual), siblings, grandparents, aunts/uncles, in-laws, or nonblood kin. The fact that it is unpaid poses challenges to those who need to take work leave, as many employees cannot afford to go without a paycheck or have to cut their leave time short because of financial concerns (Waldfogel 2001). This is particularly relevant for women, as they are more likely to take work leave than men; this may explain why many women quit work when a baby is born. FMLA legislation also favors those who have greater financial resources and traditional family configurations (i.e., white, wealthy, and married individuals; Gerstel and McGonagle 1999). Some progressive employers have responded to this need by offering paid and/or extended leave, sometimes offering fully or partially paid extra time off to new mothers, fathers, or adoptive parents, sometimes up to three months. Other companies additionally offer paid "pre-maternity leave" (up to four weeks) for mothers preparing to give birth.

Because the USA does not have a minimum number of sick and vacation days that employers must provide by law, it is up to companies to provide for employees in this way (Heymann et al. 2004). Some companies offer a generous amount of paid time off in the form of sick days, vacation time, or personal days. In addition, some companies support their employees' efforts to volunteer or participate in community service programs by offering them paid time off for just this purpose (sometimes up to 40 hours per year). Other companies allow employees with a certain number of years in tenure to take paid sabbaticals (e.g., six months) or give them the option to take a career break with their job guaranteed for five years.

The availability of flexible work arrangements and job-protected paid work leave is especially relevant for women given their role as family caretaker. Flextime and telecommuting are helpful for women who have many cumulative role demands and a finite amount of time in which to accomplish them. These tools allow them to find a better fit between their work and home roles, gaining an increased sense of control over their lives. Generous work leave policies likewise benefit women because as caretakers they are more likely to take extended time off from work or reduce working hours to care for family. Good work leave policy can alleviate worries for women while they are away, knowing that their jobs are secure. For companies that offer leave with pay, it provides an additional dimension of security because it alleviates financial concerns, especially for single parents and women who do not want to feel financially dependent on a spouse while out of work. Paid work leave also allows people to have more control regarding when to return to work, rather than the choice being dictated by financial necessity. Again, as with work–life services, these policies cannot directly address mental and physical health concerns, but they may be invaluable in helping employees to manage situations that give rise to everyday stress or to respond effectively to occasional life crises.

Ensuring that Women are Treated Fairly in the Workplace

Making a commitment to fair employment practices can be especially meaningful to women, as they have historically been discriminated against in the workplace. Policies against sexual harassment, coupled with relevant management and employee training, offer protection to women who have been affected by sexism ranging from hostile work environments to outright sexual aggression. In addition, some employers set explicit policies regarding equal employment and nondiscrimination, including affirmative action policy, which provides women with opportunities to move into occupations or positions traditionally held by men, and fair pay (or "comparable worth") policy which brings women's wages on par with men's for jobs requiring equivalent skills and experience (i.e., by offering equitable salaries at the time of hire and by monitoring and auditing compensation systems to verify that pay is maintained at equitable levels).

There are many ways in which employers create opportunities for women's advancement. One opportunity comes in the form of direct assistance through career development programs, career counseling, and coaching. Another is for employers to offer access to training and education to their female employees, whether through formal education opportunities like tuition reimbursement or scholarships for undergraduate or graduate programs, educational leave of absence to pursue a degree or certification, or onsite MBA programs (i.e., the company acts as a satellite campus for a local university). Other companies offer their own in-house professional development curricula, such as a "corporate university," or leadership training programs to groom women for leadership roles. Women can also find opportunities for leadership in companies that have programs designed for placing women into traditionally male professions (e.g., engineering, technology, hard sciences), executive succession programs targeted at women, and women's mentoring programs where senior leaders coach more junior staff members. In an acknowledgment that many careers have benefited by having friends in high places (i.e., "the old boys' network"), having the opportunity to connect with "people resources" can be invaluable. For this reason, some employers sponsor forums for women's networking (e.g., panels of female leaders, employee affiliation/resource groups, business lunches, conferences, workshops, or lectures).

Another organizational strategy supportive of women's career development directly targets a challenge most frequently faced by women: how to handle returning to work after a career leave taken to provide care for children or family members. Some women who have been away from the workplace for caregiving find that when they return to work they are given less responsibility, fewer challenging assignments, and restricted travel opportunity. Moreover, they may have fewer developmental opportunities, less pay, and fewer benefits (Nelson and Burke 2002). Some employers have tried to ease the difficulty for returning caregivers by providing re-entry programs for women who have been on extended leave, educating them about new technology or policies that they may not be familiar with. There are also programs for phasing back new parents which allow primary caregivers to work reduced hours for a period of time before returning fully to work.

The policies and programs detailed in this section all attempt to correct long-standing gender inequality in the workplace and establish inclusive environments. These initiatives are particularly meaningful for women. Career and leadership development, mentoring programs, and employee affiliation networks can create a "level playing field" by bringing women's formal and informal access to work opportunities, education, information, and social resources more in line with men's. Additionally, return-to-work strategies are beneficial to women in particular because of their role of family caretaker. Such practices can ease the difficulties associated with taking a career break (i.e., having work experience gaps in their resume, losing touch with professional networks, technological updates, and marketplace trends) and facilitate their ability to re-engage with the work world. Finally, fair treatment initiatives in the workplace have an obvious benefit for women's psychosocial health, improving perceptions of justice and self-efficacy. Moreover, companies that ensure equal compensation for equal work and access to leadership positions can help improve women's status on a societal and even global level, helping to create a fairer distribution of resources such as wealth and power among the genders.

Implications for Women's Mental Health

This chapter has examined the variety of ways in which women's experiences of work (paid, unpaid, and combined) influence their well-being and quality of life. It has also addressed the opportunities available to organizations for improving these aspects of women's lives on multiple levels. First, employers can ensure that they have inclusive and affirming workplace cultures where all employees are treated with the same dignity and respect and offered equal access to jobs and wages. Second, organizations can adopt policies and benefits such as work–life services and flexible work arrangements to alleviate women's dual workload and find a more comfortable fit between their work, family, and leisure roles. Third, companies can directly address employees' mental health and medical needs when they do arise through the provision of comprehensive insurance policies, EAPs, health promotion, and wellness programs. Addressing women's concerns at these three levels of intervention constitutes a systems-based approach and can help in creating "psychologically healthy" organizations for women (Cynkar 2007).

As we have seen throughout this chapter, these interventions have implications not only for individuals and organizations, but also for the larger mental health community. The provision of mental health and related services within the workplace is not only an effective way to serve the estimated 26.2% of American adults who are affected yearly by a diagnosable mental disorder (National Institute of Mental Health (NIMH) 2006), but it legitimizes such treatment. Providing supportive services to high-functioning, working people who seek assistance with emotional or stress-related difficulties helps to break the taboo that only "crazy" people require psychological help. Such services raise awareness about mental health issues, which are often invisible but fairly common, cutting across all populations of people regardless of employment status, gender, ethnicity, age, or socioeconomic status. Moreover, offering mental health and related services at work lends another layer of support to the existing mental health delivery system. In addition to helping organizational leaders be more aware and supportive of the psychological issues that affect their employees, mental health professionals in the community can refer clients to free and convenient sources of help by being aware of the workplace services available to employees.

Before concluding, it must be mentioned that, for the sake of maintaining focus on the identified topic, several related issues have gone unaddressed but are nonetheless critical in telling a fuller story. For example, although this chapter focused exclusively on the workplace as a site for change in addressing and remedying issues of gender-based inequality and women's well-being, it must be pointed out that there are other vital agents of change. One very critical source of change is men, who, as a group, continue to hold an inequitable share of social power and economic resources, both in society and on the homefront. By becoming aware of the ways in which they participate in everyday inequalities and making personal commitments to the betterment of women's lives, men are perhaps the most effective source of change toward dramatically improving the circumstances and health of the women in their lives and their society. However, this topic is immense and beyond the scope of this chapter. Likewise, this chapter did not address the challenges faced by women who contend with social inequalities beyond those based on gender. Women who face compound forms of prejudice and discrimination include those who are non-white, older, poor, lesbian, physically disabled, mentally ill, overweight, uneducated, and foreign born. The critical importance of these topics merit their own dedicated chapters.

In conclusion, although the intersection of work and mental health is clearly changing for the better for women, there is still quite a way to go. For a full understanding of how far women have come, one needs only to look at the statistics detailing women's social and economic status today as compared to 30 years ago. To see how much farther women have to climb to reach true equality, however, one must take a look at the statistics detailing their social and economic status today as compared to that of men. The discrepancy is clear and sobering.

References

Anderson, M. (2000). *Thinking about women: Sociological perspectives on sex and gender* (5th ed.). Boston: Allyn and Bacon.

Antill, J. K., Goodnow, J. J., Russell, G., & Cotton, S. (1996). The influence of parents and family context on children's involvement in household tasks. *Sex Roles, 34,* 215–236.

Arber, S. (1991). Revealing women's health. In H. Roberts (Ed.), *Women's health counts*. London: Routledge.

Arber, S., Dale, A., & Gilbert, G. N. (1985). Paid employment and women's health: A benefit or source of role strain? *Sociology of Health and Illness, 7*(3), 375–400.

Arber, S., & Lahelma, E. (1993). Inequalities in women's and men's ill health: Britain and Finland compared. *Social Science and Medicine, 37*(8), 1055–1068.

Armstrong, P., & Armstrong, H. (1990). *Theorizing women's work*. Toronto: Garamound Press.

Aryee, S. (1992). Antecedents and outcomes of work-family conflict among married professional women: Evidence from Singapore. *Human Relations, 45,* 813–837.

Atkinson, W. (2001). EAPs: Investments, not costs. *Textile World, 151*(5), 42–44.

Azarnoff, R., & Scharlach, A. (1988). Can employees carry the eldercare burden? *Personnel Journal, 67,* 60–69.

Barling, J., Kelloway, E. K., & Frone, M. (Eds.). (2005). *Handbook of work stress*. Thousand Oaks, CA: Sage Publications.

Barnett, R. C., & Gareis, K. C. (2006a). Antecedents and correlates of parental after-school concern: Exploring a newly identified work-family stressor. *American Behavioral Scientist, 49*(10), 1382–1399.

Barnett, R. C., & Gareis, K. C. (2006b). Parental after-school stress and psychological well-being. *Journal of Marriage and Family, 68,* 101–108.

Barnett, R. C., & Shen, Y. C. (1997). Gender, high and low schedule control housework tasks and psychological distress: A study of dual-earner couples. *Journal of Family Issues, 18*(4), 403–428.

Beatty, C. A. (1996). The stress of managerial and professional women: Is the price too high? *Journal of Organizational Behavior, 17,* 233–251.

Bedeian, A. G., Burke, B. G., & Moffett, R. G. (1988). Outcomes of work-family conflict among married male and female professionals. *Journal of Management, 14,* 475–491.

Bella, L. (1990). Women and leisure: Beyond androcentrism. In E. Jackson & T. Burton (Eds.), *Understanding leisure and recreation: Mapping the past, charting the future* (pp. 151–180). State College, PA: Venture Publishing Co.

Belsky, J., Spanier, G. B., & Rovine, M. (1983). Stability and change in marriage across the transition to parenthood. *Journal of Marriage and the Family, 45,* 553–556.

Berdahl, J. L. (2007). Harassment based on sex: Protecting social status in the context of gender hierarchy. *Academy of Management Review, 22,* 641–658.

Bergen, E. (1991). The economic context of labor allocation: Implications for gender stratification. *Journal of Family Issues, 12,* 140–157.

Bergeron, D. M., Block, C. J., & Echtenkamp, B. A. (2006). Disabling the able: Stereotype and women's work performance. *Human Performance, 19*(2), 133–158.

Bianchi, S. M. (2000). Maternal employment and time with children: Dramatic change or surprising continuity? *Demography, 37*(4), 401–414.

Bianchi, S. M., Milkie, M. A., Sayer, L. C., & Robinson, J. P. (2000). Is anyone doing the housework? Trends in the gender division of household labor. *Social Forces, 79,* 191–228.

Biernat, M., & Wortman, C. B. (1991). Sharing of home responsibilities between professionally employed women and their husbands. *Journal of Personality and Social Psychology, 60,* 844–860.

Bittman, M., & Wajcman, J. (2000). The rush hour: The character of leisure time and gender equity. *Social Forces, 79,* 165–189.

Blain, J. (1994). Discourses of agency and domestic labor: Family discourse and gendered practice in dual earner families. *Journal of Family Issues, 15,* 515–549.

Blair, S. L., & Lichter, D. T. (1991). Measuring the division of household labor: Gender segregation of housework among American couples. *Journal of Family Issues, 12,* 91–113.

Blum, T. C., & Roman, P. M. (1992). A description of clients using employee assistance programs. *Alcohol Health & Research World, 16*(2), 120–128.

Bond, M. A., Punnett, L., Pyle, J. L., Cazeca, D., & Cooperman, M. (2004). Gendered work conditions, health, and work outcomes. *Journal of Occupational Health Psychology, 9*(1), 28–45.

Bromberger, J. T., & Matthews, K. A. (1994). Employment status and depressive symptoms in middle age women: A longitudinal investigation. *American Journal of Public Health, 84*(2), 202–206.

Brown, G., & Harris, T. (1978). *Social origins of depression*. London: Tavistock.

Brown, G., & Harris, T. (1989). *Life events and illness*. New York, NY: Guilford Press.

Brown, R. P., & Pinel, E. C. (2003). Stigma on my mind: Individual differences in the experience of stereotype threat. *Journal of Experimental Social Psychology, 39,* 626–633.

Brown, W. J., Mishra, G., Lee, C., & Bauman, A. (2000). Leisure time physical activity in Australian women: Relationship with well-being and symptoms. *Research Quarterly for Exercise and Sport, 71*(3), 206–216.

Bruk-Lee, V., & Spector, P. E. (2006). The social stressors-counterproductive work behaviors link: Are conflicts with supervisors and coworkers the same? *Journal of Occupational Health Psychology, 11,* 145–156.

Buunk, B. P., de Jonge, J., Ybema, J. F., & de Wolff, C. J. (1998). Psychological aspects of occupational stress. In P. J. D. Drenth, H. Thierry, & C. J. de Wolff (Eds.), *Handbook of work and organizational psychology* (Vol. 2, pp. 145–182). East Sussex: Psychology Press.

Cartwright, S., & Cooper, C. L. (1997). *Managing workplace stress*. Thousand Oaks, CA: Sage Publications.

Catalyst. (2006a). *2005 Catalyst Census of Women Board Directors of the Fortune 500*. Retrieved August 3, 2007, from http://www.catalyst.org/files/full/2005%20WBD.pdf

Catalyst. (2006b). *2005 Catalyst Census of Women Corporate Officers and Top Earners of the Fortune 500*. Retrieved August 3, 2007, from http://www.catalyst.org/files/full/2005%20COTE.pdf

Center for American Woman and Politics. (2005). *Sex Differences in voter turnout.* Rutgers, NJ. Retrieved August 3, 2007, from http://www.cawp.rutgers.edu/Facts/sexdiff.pdf

Center for American Woman and Politics. (2007). *Women in elective office 2007.* Rutgers, NJ. Retrieved August 3, 2007, from http://www.cawp.rutgers.edu/Facts/Officeholders/elective.pdf

Cleveland, J. N., Stockdale, M., & Murphy, K. R. (2000). *Women and men in organizations: Sex and gender issues at work.* Mahwah, NJ: Lawrence Erlbaum Associates.

Cohen, D. A., Farley, T. A., Taylor, S. N., Martin, D. H., & Schuster, M. A. (2002). When and where do youths have sex? The potential role of adult supervision. *Pediatrics, 110,* 66.

Cohen, P. N. (1998). Replacing housework in the service economy: Gender, class, and race-ethnicity in service spending. *Gender and Society, 12*(2), 219–231.

Coltrane, S. (1996). *Family man: Fatherhood, housework, and gender equality.* New York, NY: Oxford University Press.

Coltrane, S. (2000). Research on household labor: Modeling and measuring the social embeddedness of routine family work. *Journal of Marriage and the Family, 62,* 1208–1233.

Coontz, S. (2001). What we really miss about the 1950s. In A. S. Skolnick & J. H. Skolnick (Eds.), *Family in transition* (11th ed.). Boston, MA: Allyn and Bacon.

Cowan, C. E., Cowan, P. A., Coie, L., & Coie, J. (1978). Becoming a family: The impact of a first child's birth on the couple's relationship. In L. Newman & W. Miller (Eds.), *The first child and family formation.* Chapel Hill, NC: Carolina Population Center.

Cowan, C. P., & Cowan, P. A. (1992). *When partners become parents: The big life change for couples.* New York, NY: Basic Books.

Cynkar, A. (2007). Whole workplace health. *APA Monitor, 38*(3), 28–31.

Daly, K. J. (1996). Spending time with kids: Meanings of family time for fathers. *Family Relations, 45,* 466–476.

Davidson, M. J., & Fielden, S. (1999). Stress and the working woman. In G. Powell (Ed.), *Handbook of gender and work* (pp. 413–426). Thousand Oaks, CA: Sage Publications.

DeNavas-Walt, C., Proctor, B., & Smith, J. (2007). *Income, poverty, and health insurance coverage in the United States: 2006.* Washington, DC: U.S. Census Bureau. Retrieved August 3, 2007, from http://www.census.gov/prod/2007pubs/p60-233.pdf

Dennerstein, L., Asbury, J., & Morse, C. (1993). *Psychosocial and mental health aspects of women's health.* Geneva, Switzerland: World Health Organization.

Desjarlais, R., Kleinman, A., Eisenberg, L., & Good, B. (Eds.). (1995). *World mental health: Problems, priorities, and responses in low-income countries.* London: Oxford University Press.

DeVault, M. (1991). *Feeding the family: The social organization of caring and gendered work.* Chicago, IL: University of Chicago Press.

DiNatale, M., & Boraas, S. (2002). The labor force experience of women from "Generation X." *Monthly Labor Review, 125*(3), 3–15.

Donlon, J. P. (1999). The war for talent. *Chief Executive, 146,* 68–75.

Doyal, L. (1999). Women and domestic labor: Setting a research agenda. In N. Daykin & L. Doyal (Eds.), *Health and work: Critical perspectives* (pp. 21–34). New York, NY: St. Martin's Press.

Employee Assistance Professionals Association. (2002). *Recent EAP cost/benefit statistics/research 2000 – present.* Arlington, VA. Retrieved August 3, 2007, from http://www.eapassn.org/public/articles/EAPcostbenefitstats.pdf

Employee Assistance Professionals Association. (2003). *EAPA standards and professional guidelines for employee assistance programs.* Arlington, VA. Retrieved August 3, 2007, from http://www.eapassn.org/public/articles/EAPA_STANDARDS_web0303.pdf

Erickson, R. J. (1993). Reconceptualizing family work: The effect of emotion work on perceptions of marital quality. *Journal of Marriage and the Family, 55,* 888–900.

Families and Work Institute. (2004). *Generation & gender in the workplace.* Watertown, MA: American Business Collaboration.

Feldman, S. S., Biringer, Z. C., & Nash, S. C. (1981). Fluctuations of sex-related self-attributions as a function of stage of family life cycle. *Developmental Psychology, 17,* 24–35.

Fitzgerald, L. F., Drasgow, F., Hulin, C. L., Gelfand, M. J., & Magley, V. J. (1997). Antecedents and consequences of sexual harassment in organizations: A test of an integrated model. *Journal of Applied Psychology, 82*(4), 578–589.

Fitzgerald, L. F., Shullman, S., Bailey, N., Richards, M., Swecker, J., Gold, A., et al. (1988). The incidence and dimensions of sexual harassment in academia and the workplace. *Journal of Vocational Behavior, 32,* 152–175.

Frone, M. R. (2000). Work-family conflict and employee psychiatric disorders: The national comorbidity survey. *Journal of Applied Psychology, 85,* 888–895.

Frone, M. R., Russell, M., & Barnes, G. M. (1996). Work-family conflict, gender, and health-related outcomes: A study of employed parents in two community samples. *Journal of Occupational Health Psychology, 1*(1), 57–69.

Frone, M. R., Russell, M., & Cooper, M. L. (1993). Relationship of work-family conflict, gender and alcohol expectancies to alcohol use/abuse. *Journal of Organizational Behavior, 14,* 545–558.

Frone, M. R., Russell, M., & Cooper, M. L. (1997a). Relation of work-family conflict to health outcomes: A four-year longitudinal study of employed parents. *Journal of Occupational and Organizational Psychology, 70,* 325–335.

Frone, M. R., Yardley, J. K., & Markel, K. S. (1997b). Developing and testing an integrative model of work-family interface. *Journal of Vocational Behavior, 50,* 145–67.

Gallagher, S. K. (1994). Doing their share—comparing patterns of help given by older and younger adults. *Journal of Marriage and the Family, 56,* 567–578.

Ganster, D. C. (1991). The effects of job demands and control on employee attendance and satisfaction. *Journal of Organizational Behavior, 12,* 595–608.

Gerstel, N., & Gallagher, S. (1994). Caring for kith and kin: Gender, employment, and the privatization of care. *Social Problems, 41,* 519–539.

Gerstel, N., & Gallagher, S. K. (2001). Men's caregiving: Gender and the contingent character of care. *Gender & Society, 15,* 197–217.

Gerstel, N., & McGonagle, K. (1999). Job leaves and the limits of the family and medical leave act. *Work and Occupations, 26*(4), 510–534.

Gilligan, C. (1982). *In a different voice.* Cambridge, MA: Harvard University Press.

Gjerdingen, D., McGovern, P., Bekker, M., Lundberg, U., & Willemsen, T. (2000). Women's work roles and their impact on health, well-being, and career: Comparisons between the United States, Sweden, and The Netherlands. *Women and Health, 31*(4), 1–20.

Glass, J., & Fujimoto, T. (1994). Housework, paid work, and depression among husbands and wives. *Journal of Health and Social Behavior, 35,* 179–191.

Glomb, T. M., Munson, L. J., Hulin, C. L., Bergman, M. E., & Drasgow, F. (1999). Structural equation models of sexual harassment: Longitudinal explorations and cross-sectional generalizations. *Journal of Applied Psychology, 84*(1), 14–28.

Goldenhar, L. M., & Sweeney, M. H. (1996). Tradeswomen's perspectives on occupational health and safety: A qualitative investigation. *American Journal of Industrial Medicine, 29,* 516–520.

Goldenhar, L. M., Swanson, N. G., Hurrell, J. J., Ruder, A., & Deddens, J. (1998). Stressors and adverse outcomes for female construction workers. *Journal of Occupational Health Psychology, 3*(1), 19–32.

Golding, J. M. (1990). Division of household labor, strain, and depressive symptoms among Mexican Americans and non-Hispanic Whites. *Psychology of Women Quarterly, 14,* 103–117.

Greenhaus, J. H., & Beutell, N. J. (1985). Sources of conflict between work and family roles. *Academy of Management Review, 10,* 76–88.

Grossman, E., Eichler, L., & Winickoff, S. (1980). *Pregnancy, birth, and parenthood.* San Francisco, CA: Jossey-Bass.

Gunter, N. C., & Gunter, B. G. (1990). Domestic division of labor among working couples: Does androgyny make a difference. *Psychology of Women Quarterly, 14,* 355–370.

Gupta, S. (1999). The effects of marital status transitions on men's housework performance. *Journal of Marriage and the Family, 61,* 700–711.

Guy, M. E., & Newman, M. A. (2004). Women's jobs, men's jobs: Sex segregation and emotional labor. *Public Administration Review, 64*(3), 262–271.

Halpern, D. F. (2005). How time-flexible work policies can reduce stress, improve health, and save money. *Stress and Health, 21,* 157–168.

Harrington, M. & Dawson, D. (1995). Who has it best? Women's labor force participation, perceptions of leisure, and constraints to enjoyment of leisure. *Journal of Leisure Research, 27,* 4–24.

Hawkins, A. J., Roberts, T. A., Christiansen, S. L., & Marshall, C. M. (1994). An evaluation of a program to help dual-earner couples share the second shift. *Family Relations, 43,* 213–220.

Henderson, K. A., & Bialeschki, M. D. (1991). A sense of entitlement to leisure as constraint and empowerment for women. *Leisure Sciences, 13,* 51–65.

Henderson, K. A., Bialeschki, M. D., Shaw, S. M., & Freysinger, V. J. (1989). *A leisure of one's own.* State College, PA: Venture.

Heymann, J., Earle, A., Simmons, S., Breslow, S. M., & Kuehnhoff, A. (2004). *The work, family, and equity index: Where does the United States stand globally?* Boston, MA: Project on Global Working Families, Harvard School of Public Health.

Hobfoll, S. E. (1989). Conservation of resources: A new attempt at conceptualizing stress. *American Psychologist, 44,* 513–524.

Hochschild, A. (1989). *The second shift.* New York, NY: Avon.

Hochschild, A. R. (1997). *The time bind: When work becomes home and home becomes work.* New York, NY: Metropolitan Books.

Hoffman, L. W. (1978). Effects of the first child on the woman's role. In W. B. Miller & L. F. Newman (Eds.), *The first child and family formation* (pp. 340–367). Chapel Hill, NC: Carolina Population Center.

Hunt, K., & Annandale, E. (1993). Just the job? Is the relationship between health and domestic and paid work gender-specific? *Sociology of Health and Illness, 15*(5), 632–664.

Hyde, J. S. (2005). The gender similarities hypothesis. *American Psychologist, 60*(6), 581–592.

Ivancevich, J. M., & Matteson, M. T. (1980). *Stress and work: A managerial perspective.* Glenview, IL: Scott, Foresman, & Company.

Jahoda, M. (1982). *Employment and unemployment: A social-psychological analysis.* Cambridge: Cambridge University Press.

Jex, S., & Beehr, T. (1991). Emerging theoretical and methodological issues in the study of work-related stress. *Research in Personnel and Human Resource Management, 9,* 311–365.

Johnson, E. M., & Huston, T. L. (1998). The perils of love, or why wives adapt to husbands during the transition to parenthood. *Journal of Marriage and the Family, 60,* 195–204.

Kahn, R. L., & Byosiere, P. H. R. (1992) Stress in organizations. In M. D. Dunette & L. M. Hough (Eds.), *Handbook of industrial and organizational psychology* (2nd ed., Vol. 3, pp. 571–650). Palo Alto, CA: Consulting Psychologists Press.

Kamo, Y. (1991). A non-linear effect of the number of children on the division of household labor. *Sociological Perspectives, 34,* 205–218.

Karasek, R. (1979). Job demands, job decision latitude and mental strain: Implications for job redesign. *Administrative Science Quarterly, 24,* 285–306.

Karasek, R., & Theorell, T. (1990). *Healthy work: Stress, productivity and the reconstruction of working life.* New York, NY: Basic Books.

Kelly, J. R., & Godbey, G. (1992). *The sociology of leisure.* State College, PA: Venture Publishing.

Klonoff, E. A., Landrine, H., & Campbell, R. (2000). Sexist discrimination may account for well-known gender differences in psychiatric symptoms. *Psychology of Women Quarterly, 24,* 93–99.

Kouvonen, A., Kivimaki, M., Vaananen, A., Heponiemi, T., Elovainio, M., Ala-Mursula, L., et al. (2007). Job strain and adverse health behaviors: The finnish public sector study. *Journal of Occupational & Environmental Medicine, 49*(1), 68–74.

Kroska, A. (2003). Investigating gender differences in the meaning of household chores and child care. *Journal of Marriage and the Family, 65*(2), 456–473.

Kurz, D. (2002). Caring for teenage children. *Journal of Family Issues, 23,* 748–767.

LaRossa, R., & LaRossa, M. M. (1981). *Transition to parenthood: How infants change families.* Beverly Hills, CA: Sage Publications.

Larson, R. W., Richards, M. H., & Perry-Jenkins, M. (1994). Divergent worlds: The daily emotional experience of mothers and fathers in the domestic and public spheres. *Journal of Personality and Social Psychology, 67,* 1034–1046.

Lazarus, R. S., & Folkman, S. (1984). *Stress, appraisal and coping.* New York, NY: Springer.

Leete, L., &. Schor, J. B. (1994). Assessing the time-squeeze hypothesis: Hours worked in the United States, 1969–89. *Industrial Relations, 33,* 25–43.

Lehto, A. M. (1998). Time pressure as a stress factor. *Society and Leisure, 21*(2), 491–511.

Lloyd, L. (1999). The well-being of carers: An occupational health concern. In N. Daykin & L. Doyal (Eds.), *Health and work: Critical perspectives* (pp. 54–70). New York, NY: St. Martin's Press.

Lovallo, W. R. (2005). *Stress and health: Biological and psychological interactions.* Thousand Oaks, CA: Sage Publications.

MacDermid, S. M., Huston, T. L., & McHale, S. M. (1990). Changes in marriage associated with the transition to parenthood: Individual differences as a function of sex-role attitudes and changes in the division of household labor. *Journal of Marriage and the Family, 52,* 475–486.

Mattingly, M. J., & Bianchi, S. M. (2003). Gender differences in the quantity and quality of free time: The U.S. experience. *Social Forces, 81,* 999–1029.

McCracken, D. M. (2000). Winning the talent war for women: Sometimes it takes a revolution. *Harvard Business Review, 78*(6), 159–167.

McMurray, A. (1999). *Community health and wellness: A sociological approach.* Sydney: Mosby.

Mederer, H. J. (1993). Division of labor in two-earner homes: Task accomplishment versus household maintenance as critical variables in perceptions about family work. *Journal of Marriage and the Family, 55,* 133–145.

Meijman, T. F., & Mulder, G. (1998). Psychological aspects of workload. In P. J. D. Drenth & H. Thierry (Eds.), *Handbook of work and organizational psychology* (Vol. 2, pp. 5–33). Hove, England: Psychology Press.

Messing, K. (2000). Multiple roles and complex exposures: Hard-to-pin-down risks for working women. In M. B. Goldman & M. Hatch (Eds.), *Women and health* (pp. 455–462). San Diego, CA: Academic Press.

Morris, J. A., & Feldman, D. C. (1997). Managing emotions in the workplace. *Journal of Managerial Issues, 9*(3), 257–274.

Munson, L. J., Hulin, C., & Drasgow, F. (2000). Longitudinal analysis of dispositional influences and sexual harassment: Effects on job and psychological outcomes. *Personnel Psychology, 53*(1), 21–46.

National Institute of Mental Health. (2006). *The numbers count: Mental disorders in America* (NIH Publication No. 06-4584). Retrieved August 3, 2007, from http://www.nimh.nih.gov/health/publications/the-numbers-count-mental-disorders-in-america.shtml

National Institute of Occupational Safety and Health. (1999). *Stress...at work.* Retrieved August 3, 2007, from http://www.cdc.gov/niosh/stresswk.html

Nelson, D. L., & Burke, R. J. (Eds.). (2002). *Gender, work stress, and health: Current research issues.* Washington, DC: American Psychological Association.

Nighswonger, T. (2000). Just say yes to preventing substance abuse. *Occupational Hazards, 62*(4), 39–42.

Nock, S. L., & Kingston, P. W. (1988). Time with children: The impact of couples' work-tome commitments. *Social Forces, 67*(1), 59–85.

Orbuch, T. L., & Eyster, S. L. (1997). Division of house-hold labor among Black couples and White couples. *Social Forces, 76,* 301–332.

Oropesa, R. S. (1993). Using the service economy to relieve the double burden: Female labor force participation and service purchases. *Journal of Family Issues, 14,* 438–473.

Padgett, D. L. (1997). The contribution of support networks to household labor in African American families. *Journal of Family Issues, 18,* 227–250.

Parasuraman, S., Greenhaus, J. H., & Granrose, C. S. (1992). Role stressors, social support, and well-being among two-career couples. *Journal of Organizational Behavior, 13,* 339–356.

Perrewé, P., Hochwarter, W., & Kiewitz, C. (1999). Value attainment: An explanation for the negative effects of work/family conflict on job and life satisfaction. *Journal of Occupational Health Psychology, 4*(4), 318–326.

Piercy, K. W., & Blieszner, R. (1999). Balancing family life: How adult children link eldercare responsibility to service utilization. *Journal of Applied Gerontology, 18*(4), 440–459.

Pina, D. L., & Bengtson, V. L. (1993). The division of household labor and wives' happiness—ideology, employment, and perceptions of support. *Journal of Marriage and the Family, 55,* 901–912.

Popay, J., Bartley, M., & Owen, C. (1993). Gender inequalities in health: Social position, affective disorders and minor physical morbidity. *Social Science and Medicine, 36*(1), 21–32.

Presser, H. B. (1994). Employment schedules among dual-earner spouses and the division of household labor by gender. *American Sociological Review, 59,* 348–364.

Reeves, J. B., & Szafran, R. F. (1996). For what and for whom do you need more time? *Time & Society, 5,* 237–251.

Rice, R. W., Frone, M. R., & McFarlin, D. B. (1992). Work-nonwork conflict and the perceived quality of life. *Journal of Organizational Behavior, 13,* 155–168.

Robinson, J. P., & Godbey, G. (1997). *Time for life: The surprising ways that Americans use time.* University Park, IL: Pennsylvania State University Press.

Robinson, J. P., & Milkie, M. (1997). Dances with dust bunnies: Housecleaning in America. *American Demographics, 59,* 37–40.

Robinson, J. P., & Milkie, M. A. (1998). Back to the basics: Trends in and role determinants of women's attitudes toward housework. *Journal of Marriage and the Family, 60,* 205–218.

Romito, P. (1990). Postpartum depression and the experience of motherhood. *Acta Obstetricia Gynecoligica Scandinavica, 69,* 1–37.

Rubenstein, M. (1989). Preventing sexual harassment at work. *Industrial Relations Journal, 20*(3), 226–236.

Rubenstein, M. (1992). *Preventing and remedying sexual harassment at work: A resource manual* (2nd ed.). London: Eclipse Group.

Sanchez, L., & Kane, E. W. (1996). Women's and men's constructions of perceptions of housework fairness. *Journal of Family Issues, 17,* 358–387

Schneider, K. T., Swan, S., & Fitzgerald, L. F. (1997). Job-related and psychological effects of sexual harassment in the workplace: Empirical evidence from two organizations. *Journal of Applied Psychology, 82*(3), 401–415.

Schor, J. (1991). *The overworked American: The unexpected decline of leisure.* New York, NY: Basic Books.

Searle, M. S., & Jackson, E. L. (1985). Socioeconomic variations in perceived barriers to recreation participation among would-be participants. *Leisure Sciences, 7,* 227–249.

Shaw, S. M. (1985). Gender and leisure: Inequality in the distribution of leisure time. *Journal of Leisure Research, 17*(4), 266–282.

Shaw, S. M. (1994). Gender, leisure, and constraint: Towards a framework for the analysis of women's leisure. *Journal of Leisure Sciences, 26*(1), 8–22.

Shelton, B. A. (1992). *Women, men and time: Gender differences in paid work, housework and leisure.* New York, NY: Greenwood Press.

Shelton, B. A., & John, D. (1996). The division of household labor. *Annual Review of Sociology, 22,* 299–322.

Sluiter, J. K., Van Der Beek, A. J., & Frings-Dresen, M. H. W. (1999). The influence of work characteristics on the need for recovery and experienced health: A study on coach drivers. *Ergonomics, 42*(2), 573–583.

Smith, A. (1995). An analysis of altruism: A concept of caring. *Journal of Advanced Nursing, 22,* 785–790.

South, S. J., & Spitze, G. (1994). Housework in marital and nonmarital households. *American Sociological Review, 59,* 327–347.

Spector, P. E., Dwyer, D. J., & Jex, S. M. (1988). Relation of job stressors to affective, health, and performance outcomes: A comparison of multiple data sources. *Journal of Applied Psychology, 73,* 11–19.

Spencer, S. J., Steele, C. M., & Quinn, D. M. (1999). Stereotype threat and women's math performance. *Journal of Experimental Social Psychology, 35,* 4–28.

Spraggins, R. E. (2005). *We the people: Women and men in the United States: Census 2000 special reports*. Washington, DC: U.S. Census Bureau. Retrieved August 3, 2007, from http://www.census.gov/prod/2005pubs/censr-20.pdf

Stafford, R., Bachman, E., & diBona, P. (1977). The division of labor among cohabitating and married couples. *Journal of Marriage and the Family, 39,* 43–57.

Starrels, M. E. (1994). Husbands' involvement in female gender-typed household chores. *Sex Roles, 31,* 473–491.

Steele, C. M. (1997). A threat in the air: How stereotypes shape intellectual identity and performance. *American Psychologist, 52,* 613–629.

Tancred, P. (1995) Women's work: A challenge to the sociology of work. *Gender, Work, and Organizations, 2*(1), 11–19.

Thomas, C. (1995). Domestic labor and health: Bringing it all back home. *Sociology of Health and Illness, 17*(3), 328–352.

Thomas, L. T., & Ganster, D. C. (1995). Impact of family-supportive work variables on work-family conflict and strain: A control perspective. *Journal of Applied Psychology, 80*(1), 6–15.

Thompson, L., & Walker, A. J. (1989). Gender in families: Women and men in marriage, work, and parenthood. *Journal of Marriage and the Family, 51,* 845–871.

Toossi, M. (2005). Labor force projections to 2014: Retiring boomers. *Monthly Labor Review, 128*(11), 25–44. Retrieved August 3, 2007, from http://www.bls.gov/opub/mlr/2005/11/art3full.pdf

Ursin, H. (1980). Personality, activation and somatic health. A new psychosomatic theory. In S. Levine & H. Ursin (Eds.), *Coping and health* (pp. 259–279). New York, NY: Plenum Press.

Waite, L. J., & Gallagher, M. (2000). *The case for marriage: Why married people are happier, healthier, and better off financially*. New York, NY: Doubleday.

Waldfogel, J. (2001). Family and medical leave: Evidence from the 2000 surveys. *Monthly Labor Review, 124*(9), 17–23.

Warr, P. B. (1982). *Work, unemployment and mental health.* Oxford: Oxford University Press.

Wearing, B. (1984). *The ideology of motherhood.* Sydney: George Allen and Unwin.

Wearing, B. (1990). Beyond the ideology of motherhood: Leisure as resistance. *Australian and New Zealand Journal of Sociology, 26,* 36–58.

West, C., & Fenstermaker, S. (1993). Power and the accomplishment of gender. In P. England (Ed.), *Theory on gender/feminism on theory* (pp. 151–174). New York, NY: Aldine deGruyter.

Willness, C. R., Steel, P., & Lee, K. (2007). A meta-analysis of the antecedents and consequences of workplace sexual harassment. *Personnel Psychology, 60*(1), 127–162.

Zuzanek, J. (1998). Time use, time pressure, personal stress, mental health, and life satisfaction from a life cycle perspective. *Journal of Occupational Science, 5,* 26–39.

Chapter 15
Organizational Stress and Trauma-Informed Services

Sandra L. Bloom

Introduction

Frequently, we think of service delivery in an abstract way, as if human emotions and human life experiences play little if any role in the "delivery" of services. The words themselves give rise to images of help being sent through a mail slot or dropped down the chimney like the legendary stork carrying a new baby. But clearly that is a rationalization we use, perhaps to protect our discourse from the messiness of all-too-human emotions.

In reality, services are delivered by people, and the people who deliver these services may be, at any point in time, experiencing stressful events in their own lives. Furthermore, a majority of them, given the results from large epidemiological studies, will experience at least one traumatic event in their lifetime. This is compounded by the fact that public mental health delivery systems are seriously underfunded and struggle to meet an ever increasing demand for services (New Freedom Commission on Mental Health 2003).

It is the contention of this chapter that as a result of widespread exposure to acute and chronic stressors, there are organizational processes that run in parallel to the destructive processes that so influence the lives of the clients that these organizations serve. These parallel processes in individual organizations then interfere significantly with the ability of current mental health systems to address the actual needs of women with mental health and substance abuse problems, most of whom are likely to have also been exposed to childhood adversity and adult trauma (Bloom 2002; Edwards et al. 2003; Goodman et al. 1997; Kessler et al. 1995).

This chapter discusses the dynamics of organizational stress using a paradigm derived from the study of traumatized and chronically stressed individuals and from the organizational development literature focused largely on the business community (Bloom 1997, 2006). The chapter concludes with ideas about

S. L. Bloom (✉)
Health Management and Policy, Drexel University School of Public Health,
1505 Race Street, Bellet Building, 11th Floor, PA 19102, Philadelphia, USA

B. L. Levin, M. A. Becker (eds.), *A Public Health Perspective of Women's Mental Health*,
DOI 10.1007/978-1-4419-1526-9_15, © Springer Science+Business Media LLC 2010

the implications of this paradigm for changes in services delivery for vulnerable (female) populations.

Trauma-Organized Systems

We know from epidemiological studies (Dube et al. 2001; Felitti et al. 1998), including the Adverse Experiences Study, that it is likely that large segments of the population will have significant encounters with maltreatment, dysfunction, loss, and violence as children and as adults (Felitti et al. 1998). As an illustration, in a recent training experience that involved staff members from residential programs for children, juvenile justice programs, community-based workers, public health professionals, and other clinicians working in the mental healthcare industry, participants did an anonymous activity calculating the group Adverse Childhood Experiences Score. Out of 78 people working in these health and social services, 33 had experienced psychological abuse at the hands of parents, 24 had been physically abused by parents, 22 had been sexually abused by someone as children, 33 had been emotionally neglected, 8 had been physically neglected, 32 had lived as a child with a household member who was a substance abuser, 29 had experienced parental separation, 20 of them witnessed domestic violence directed at their mothers, and 14 of them had lived with a household member who was imprisoned.

These professionals are the very same vulnerable human beings who come together to form organizations. As human beings combine their collective conscious and unconscious energies, a complex adaptive system emerges that has its own unique and often perplexing characteristics that cannot be understood or explained by understanding the individuals who comprise that organization (Senge 1990). Organizations, like individuals, are vulnerable to the impact of repetitive or chronic stress and are vulnerable to the traumatic experiences that occur to and within institutions. When an individual becomes part of a group, his or her identity is expanded to include a group identity. As a result, there is an ongoing and interactive challenge of productively managing stress between the individuals within the organization and within an organization as a whole (Carr 2001; Ettin et al. 1995).

Although there is an extensive body of knowledge in the organizational development and business management literature about the impact of stress on individuals and organizations, this impact has not been well described in the literature pertaining to social service or mental health services delivery (Bloom 2006). Yet the sources of stress within organizations that serve the health, mental health, and social service needs of women are extensive. Numerous reports have declared that the system is now in a state of chronic crisis (Appelbaum 2002; Bazelon Center for Mental Health Law 2001; President's New Freedom Commission on Mental Health 2003). These reports document that "the overall infrastructure is under stress, and access to all levels of behavioral health care is affected" (National Association of Psychiatric Health Systems 2003, p. 4).

Just as the lives of people exposed to repetitive and chronic trauma, abuse, and maltreatment become organized around the traumatic experience, so too can entire systems become organized around the recurrent and severe stresses that accompany delivering behavioral health services to women, especially when there still exists vast social denial about the posttraumatic origins of so many mental health, substance abuse, and social problems (Bentovim 1992). As a result, complex interactions, which we refer to as "parallel processes," often occur between traumatized clients, stressed staff, frustrated administrators, and pressured organizations that result in services delivery that often recapitulates the very experiences that have proven to be so toxic for the people we are treating.

Parallel Process

The idea of parallel process has its origin in the psychoanalytic concept of transference and was developed conceptually by Searles in 1955, when he noted that the "relationship between patient and therapist is often reflected in the relationship between therapist and supervisor" (Searles 1955, p. 135). At an organizational level, the idea of "collective disturbance," a specific form of parallel process, was first explored by early sociological studies of mental hospitals (Caudill 1958; Stanton and Schwartz 1954). Since then, it has become more widely recognized that conflicts belonging at one location in a system are often displaced and enacted elsewhere because of a parallelism between the conflicts at the place of origin and the place of expression. As one investigator described it, "When two or more systems—whether these consist of individuals, groups, or organizations—have significant relationships with one another, they tend to develop similar effects, cognition, and behaviors, which are defined as parallel processes" (Smith et al. 1989, p. 13).

This largely unconscious process sets up an interactive dynamic with results that are uncanny and disturbing. The clients bring their past history of traumatic experience into the mental health and social service sectors, consciously aware of certain specific goals but unconsciously struggling to defend against the pain, terror, and loss of the past. They are greeted by individual service providers, subject to their own personal life experiences, who are embedded in entire systems that are under significant stress. Given what we know about exposure to childhood adversity and other forms of traumatic experience, the majority of service providers have experiences in their background that may be quite similar to the life histories of their clients.

Parallel Processes Between Clients and Staff

For many institutions, the end result of this complex, interactive, and largely unconscious process is that the clients, children and adults, enter the systems of care feeling unsafe and often engaging in behaviors that are dangerous to themselves or others. They are likely to have difficulty managing anger and aggression. They may feel hopeless and act helpless, even when they can make choices that will effectively change their situations, while at the same time this chronic *learned helplessness* may drive them to exert methods of control that become pathological. They are likely to be chronically hyperaroused, and although they try to control their bodies and minds, the methods used (such as substance use) are often problematic. They may have significant memory problems and may be chronically dissociating their memories and/or feelings, even under minor stress. They are likely, therefore, to have fragmented mental functions. These clients are not likely to have learned good communication skills, nor can they easily engage in conflict management because of chronic difficulties with emotional management. They often feel overwhelmed, confused, and depressed and have poor self-esteem. Their problems have emerged in the context of disrupted attachment, and they may not know how to make and sustain healthy relationships, nor is it likely that they know how to grieve for all that has been lost. Instead, they have an increased vulnerability to revictimization or the victimization of others, and in doing so, may repetitively reenact their past terror and loss.

Likewise, in chronically stressed organizations, individual staff members, many of whom have a past history of exposure to traumatic and abusive experiences, do not feel particularly safe with their clients, with management, or even with each other. They are chronically frustrated and angry, and their feelings may be vented on the clients and emerge as escalations in punitive measures and counteraggressive behavior. They feel helpless in the face of the enormity of the problems confronting them, their own individual problems, and the pressures from management for better performance. As they become increasingly stressed, the measures they take to "treat" the clients may backfire, and they become hopeless about the capacity of either the clients or the organization to change. The escalating levels of uncertainty, danger, and threat that seem to originate on the one hand from the clients, and on the other hand from "the system," create in the staff a chronic level of hyperarousal as the environment becomes increasingly crisis-oriented. Members of the staff who are most disturbed by the hyperarousal and rising levels of anxiety implement additional control measures, resulting in an increase in aggression, counteraggression, dependence on both physical and biological restraints, and punitive measures directed at clients and each other. Key team members, colleagues, and friends leave the setting and take with them key aspects of the memory of what worked and what did not work, and team learning becomes impaired. Communication breaks down between staff members; interpersonal conflicts increase and are not resolved. Team functioning becomes increasingly fragmented. As this happens, staff members are likely to feel overwhelmed, confused, and depressed, while emotional exhaustion, cynicism, and a loss of personal effectiveness lead to demoralization and burnout.

Parallel Processes at the Organizational Level

The staff members of service delivery organizations are frequently caught between the demands of the system and the needs of the clients. Unable to see beyond the crises that present each day, staff members are apt to lose continuity between the past and the present, while lacking the energy and enthusiasm to plan for the future. It is not unusual to hear bewildered mental health professionals and other social service employees wonder how it is possible that their organizations can be so dysfunctional, when, taken individually, most of their colleagues seem reasonable, caring, and committed. Efforts to create change often appear to confound the very process of change, and as that happens, staff demoralization escalates. It is possible then to see the parallel processes just described at the organizational level.

Over the past few decades, a large body of knowledge has been accumulating about organizational function at a conscious and unconscious level, mostly in the world of business. Although many mental health organizations have been significantly stressed by the indiscriminate application of business models to service professions, the transfer of knowledge about organizations has not been adopted by behavioral health and social service organizations. The remainder of this chapter endeavors to define what the barriers to knowledge transfer are for these organizations. As we have learned from our traumatized clients, recovery begins with a new understanding of the problem.

The Organizational Impact of Chronic Stress

Chronic Stressors and Collective Trauma

Mental health systems, and virtually every other health and social service component that interacts with mental health systems, have been, and continue to be, under conditions of chronic stress. Many systems have individually and collectively experienced repetitive trauma, and they are functioning within an overall social and political environment that is complacent about, if not overtly hostile to, the aims of recovery. It is a "system under siege."

The sources of this chronic stress are wide-ranging and multiple, including excessive paperwork; increased demands for productivity that ignore the client's demands for time and empathic regard; competition for workers, undereducated workers, inadequate time for supervision, case consultation, and collaboration; constant ethical conflicts resulting from the needs of clients as they conflict with the requirements of a managed environment; adapting to new technology; staff turnover; downsizing, leading to everything from loss of basic safety to the loss of friendship patterns, peer support, and organizational memory; and confusion about the underlying premises of mental health systems—diagnoses, nature vs. nurture, mind/body dichotomy, and stabilization vs. recovery. In addition, there are the traumatic events that can accompany working with a very vulnerable group of people in less than ideal times: suicides, homicides, client injuries, staff injuries, scandals, media attacks, and lawsuits.

Mental health systems, taken as a whole, have undergone such radical change in the past several decades that it is possible to consider the use of terms, such as "collective trauma" and "collective disaster" to describe the results. Kai Erikson has used both of these terms in his poignant descriptions of communities that have been struck by natural and man-made disasters. He sees collective trauma as

> a blow to the basic tissues of social life that damages the bonds attaching people together and impairs the prevailing sense of communality. The collective trauma works its way slowly and even insidiously into the awareness of those who suffer from it, so it does not have the quality of suddenness normally associated with 'trauma'. But it is a form of shock all the same, a gradual realization that the community no longer exists as an effective source of support and that an important part of the self has disappeared … 'I' continue to exist, though damaged and maybe even permanently changed. 'You' continue to exist, though distant and hard to relate to. But 'we' no longer exist as a connected pair or as linked cells in a larger communal body (Erikson 1994, p. 233).

Lack of Basic Safety

As a result of these combinations of acute and chronic stress, in many helping organizations, neither the staff nor the administrators feel particularly safe with their clients or even with each other. This lack of safety may present as a lack of basic physical safety. After law enforcement, persons employed in the mental health sector have the highest rates of all occupations of being physically victimized while at work or on duty. Nonfatal assaults occur nearly four times more often in the healthcare sector than in all private sector industries combined (Clements et al. 2005). The Department of Justice's (DOJ) National Crime Victimization Survey (for 1993–1999) lists average annual rates of nonfatal violent crime by occupation. The average annual rate for nonfatal violent crime for all occupations is 12.6 per 1,000 workers. But the average annual rate for mental health professionals is 68.2 per 1,000, and for mental health custodial workers it is 69 per 1,000 (Occupational Safety and Health Administration (OSHA) 2004). Despite this, over 70% of workplaces in the USA do not have a formal program or policy that addresses workplace violence (Bureau of Labor Statistics 2006).

According to OSHA, the actual number of incidents is probably much higher than reported because incidents of violence are likely to be underreported, largely because of the persistent perception within the healthcare industry that assaults are part of the job (OSHA 2004). Underreporting may reflect a lack of institutional reporting policies, employee beliefs that reporting will not benefit them, or employee fears that employers may deem assaults the result of employee negligence or poor job performance.

As dramatic as the statistics on physical violence are, they do not reflect the other forms of violence to which mental health and social service workers are routinely exposed in their workplace. Mental health environments are not immune to bullying, harassment, and other forms of psychological violence. Emotional abuse is defined by the World Health Organization as "the intentional use of power, including threat of physical force, against another person or group that can result in harm to physical, mental, spiritual, moral or social development, and includes verbal abuse, bullying/mobbing, harassment, and threats" (World Health Organization 2002, p. 4). According to a recent workplace study, approximately 35–50% of US workers experience one negative act at least weekly in any 6–12 month period, and nearly 30% frequently experience at least two types of negativity (Lutgen-Sandvik et al. 2007). In another survey, 44% of American workers said they have worked for a supervisor or employer whom they consider abusive, while over half have been the victim of, or heard about, supervisors/employers behaving abusively by making sarcastic jokes/teasing remarks, rudely interrupting, publicly criticizing, giving dirty looks, yelling at subordinates, or ignoring them as if they were invisible (Employment Law Alliance 2007).

Trust is the basis for all positive social relationships. The erosion of trust in the workplace has become a major barrier to instituting trauma-informed care and significantly interferes with the provision of adequate health and mental healthcare to women. In failing to ask about women's trauma histories and thus failing to incorporate the information into ongoing treatment planning, the traumatic experiences of women are denied and/or forgotten. In failing to recognize that most of the staff also have been subjected to childhood adversity and may have significant difficulties managing their own emotions and reactions that get triggered in the therapeutic environment, organizational managers inadvertently support the ongoing denial of the traumatic origins of their clients' problems. Workers do not trust that responding to the past traumatic experience of their female clients and empowering women to make decisions for themselves will enable the workers to feel safe. At the same time, administrators may not trust that the decisions they make about the well-being of their institutions will be respected by their superiors or by funding sources.

Loss of Emotional Management

Organizations manage emotions through regular and productive meetings, retreats, and an atmosphere of participatory management, all of which are likely to cease under the influence of chronic stress. At the organizational level, the failure to cope with workplace emotions and conflict may promote a situation that covertly supports substance abuse, harassment, bullying, and sexual misconduct in the workplace. As one group of investigators illustrated,

> … affect permeates organizations …. Affective processes (more commonly known as emotions) create and sustain work motivation. They lurk behind political behavior; they animate our decisions; they are essential to leadership. Strong affective feelings are present at any time we confront work issues that matter to us and our organizational performance. (Barsade and Gibson 2007, p. 36).

Exposure to recurrent, systemic violence and chronic stress creates an atmosphere of recurrent or constant crisis, which severely constrains the ability of staff to involve all levels of staff in decision-making processes, constructively confront problems, engage in complex problem-solving, or even talk to each other. Team meetings become ritualized, severely attenuated, or cancelled altogether. Under the pressures for increased productivity, informal conversations diminish. Atmospheres of chronic stress and fear contribute negatively to poor services. Organizations that are crisis-driven become hypersensitive to even minor threats and, if there are a sufficient number of crises, may become chronically hyperaroused. Under these circumstances, it is not unusual for staff members within caregiving systems to become counteraggressive, failing to de-escalate and, instead, escalating tension within their clients. This can result in more injuries to staff and clients and increases the use of coercive practices, leading to further decreases in safety and increases in the level of fear in the environment.

Dissociation, Amnesia, and Fragmentation of Function

Organizational learning is both a cognitive and a social process that involves capturing, storing, and diffusing knowledge within the organization. Organizational learning results in organizational adaptation to changing environments (Othman and Hashim 2004). Organizational learning depends on a constant flow of information, but under conditions of chronic stress, communication networks tend to break down. As people are laid off, key employees leave and long-time leaders retire or move out of the organization. Explicit knowledge may be retained because it is in tangible form: policies, paperwork, and records. But the critically important implicit knowledge, which is experiential, intuitive, and most effectively communicated in face-to-face encounters, is lost (Conklin 2001; Crossen et al. 1999; Lahaie 2005; Othman and Hashim 2004). In this way, organizational memory is lost; organizational amnesia affects function; and service delivery becomes increasingly fragmented.

Like clients who have a dissociative disorder, such chronically stressed systems of care engage in faulty and inadequate problem-solving under stress, usually reverting to old ways of doing things even if old ways no longer work, and therefore they are unable to adapt well to changing circumstances. Without a shared memory and lacking a systematic shared theoretical framework, organizations begin to look more and more dissociative as the "right hand" knows less and less about what the "left hand" is doing.

When a company loses its medium and long-term memory, it repeats its past mistakes, fails to learn from past successes and often forfeits its identity …. Hard-won and expensively acquired organizational memory walks out the door every time an employee retires, quits, or is downsized (Kransdorrf 1997, p. 35).

Today, in behavioral health and social service organizations, identity confusion in organizations is evident in the recurrent conflicts between theory and practice, various professional groups, management and workers, and clients and staff. These conflicts represent a failure to "get on the same page," to engage in processes that increase the likelihood of synthesis, convergence, integration, and creative emergence. "Even though organizations do not have a biological existence, they can still act in ways that suggest they have forgotten key lessons previously learned. Lessons learned and knowledge previously generated are sometimes lost and forgotten" (Othman and Hashim 2004, p. 273).

Systematic Error

When organizational amnesia and multiple breakdowns in the communication networks occur, so too do the feedback loops that are necessary for consistent and timely error correction (Kanter and Stein 1992). This is particularly noticeable when a repetitive crisis occurs. Under stress, the communication network within caregiving organizations tends to break down. Formal lines of communication become more rigid and convey less information, while the slack is picked up by the grapevine which may or may not convey accurate information.

Stressed organizations frequently respond to a fear of impending chaos by becoming more structured. Unfortunately, an increase in structure can easily lead to a system that is too rigid and inflexible. When this occurs, rule-making and rule-enforcement become substitutes for process discussions, resulting in fixed expectations and consequences that punish clients for the problems that bring them into treatment in the first place and that punish staff for errors that should create opportunities for organizational learning. Organizational boundaries may become so rigid and overstructured that no useful feedback information gets utilized at all.

Alternately, stressed organizations can become so befuddled about boundaries that they do not have clear role definitions or expectations for behavior. As a result, interpersonal and intraorganizational boundaries become confused and overly permeable. This diffused permeability may lead to a significant increase in interpersonal conflict.

Increased Authoritarianism

As communication breaks down, errors compound and the situation feels increasingly out of control; organizational leaders attempt to correct the problems but in doing so, they frequently adopt measures that are both controlling and authoritarian (Kanter and Stein 1992; Weick 2001). On the other hand, authoritarian responses to crises can be extremely helpful, as the group pulls together to respond to the direction of a single leader in charge. However, chronic authoritarian responses minimize the critical thinking of everyone lower in the hierarchy and diminish the possibility of organizational learning (Altemeyer 1996). Under these circumstances, workplace bullying is likely to increase at all levels. In the worst cases, authoritarian leaders may become petty tyrants (Ashforth 1994). As mentioned earlier, over 44% of American workers report that they have worked for a supervisor or employer who they consider abusive, and repetitive crises can turn otherwise fair and participatory leaders into potential abusers (Employment Law Alliance 2007).

Impaired Cognition and Silencing of Dissent

As decision making becomes increasingly nonparticipatory and problem solving more reactive, an increasing number of short-sighted policy decisions are made that appear to compound existing problems. Organizational democratic processes are eroded, and accompanying this loss is an escalating inability to deal with complexity. Dissent is silenced, leading to simplistic decisions and lowered morale (Kassing 1997; Morrison and Milliken 2000).

Chronically stressed systems are more likely to make poor judgments, particularly when dissent is silenced and alternative points of view cannot be properly aired (Mellers et al. 1998). Whenever participatory processes are minimized or eliminated, organizational thought processes are likely to become oversimplified, extremist, and reactive. As stress increases and participatory processes are eliminated, both individual and group decision making are likely to become progressively compromised (Sunstein 2003).

Impoverished Relationships

In an organization where lines of communication are broken and people are becoming afraid of each other, interpersonal conflicts increase and are not resolved because the system lacks the capacity for adequate conflict resolution. Under these circumstances, unresolved and pre-existing interpersonal, intradepartmental, and interdepartmental conflicts are likely to increase. Measures that should be taken to adequately manage and dissolve those conflicts do not occur. There is an inverse relationship between interpersonal conflict in the workplace and the ability to engage in constructive conflict over specific tasks. The greater the interpersonal conflict, the less likely it is that members of the organization will be able to engage in the kind of conflict that leads to creative and innovative approaches to new problems. At the same time, interorganizational conflicts are likely to increase. The organizational conflict culture becomes rigid and inflexible; hierarchies become more fixed, with one conflict management style dominating the rest (Amason 1996; Jehn 1995; Jehn et al. 1999).

The chronic failure of communication and conflict resolution in the system may emerge as a "collective disturbance" that flows down from the original source of unspoken conflict and manifests in problematic behavior, first in the staff and later in the clients. In organizations, "collective disturbance" represents the separation of cognitive and emotional content of an experience (Caudill 1958; Stanton and Schwartz 1954). Problems cannot be honestly, openly, and safely discussed. Secrets exist at many levels, or at least an air of secrecy, and a lack of transparency is felt by everyone. Little differentiation is made between privacy and secrecy, so secrets may be kept while privacy is invaded. Conflicts at the level of the administration or the staff are then unconsciously projected upon the clients who act out the emotional elements of the conflict. Meanwhile, no one understands or grapples with the cognitive content. In this way, an acute collective disturbance easily becomes a chronic unresolved conflict and a source of further stress.

Organizations that cannot explore, resolve, and transform conflict cannot learn from experience and are likely to make the same mistakes over and over again.

> Call it escalation of commitment, organizational defensiveness, learning disability—or even more bluntly—executive blindness. It is a phenomenon of behavior in organizations that has been widely recognized. Organizational members become committed to a pattern of behavior. They escalate their commitment to that pattern out of self-justification. In a desire to avoid embarrassment and threat, few if any challenges are made to the wisdom and viability of these behaviors. They persist even when rapid and fundamental shifts in the competitive environment render these patterns of behavior obsolete and destructive to the well-being of the organization (Beer and Spector 1993, p. 642).

Disempowerment and Helplessness

As the organization becomes more hierarchical and autocratic, there is a progressive and simultaneous isolation of leaders and a "dumbing down" of staff, with an accompanying "learned helplessness" and loss of critical thinking skills.

Chronically threatened organizations become extremely risk avoidant in trying to control clients' risky behavior and, in doing so, may virtually eliminate the expectation that clients need to take risks in order to change. Since all change involves risk, the more risk-avoidant the environment, the less likely it is that anything, including the clients, will change.

While this depleting spiral is operating, the staff in chronically stressed organizations and service delivery systems may become increasingly helpless about the possibility of change in their clients, their organizations, or service delivery systems. When challenged to empower themselves, they may helplessly wait for someone else to "tell them what to do" (McGrath 1994).

Increased Aggression

Stressed systems and organizations may fail to see the larger issues that are clouding vision and impairing performance, and instead attempting to address the problems using a system of rewards and punishment that does not address the core issues. Staff respond to the perceived punitive measures and the escalation of conflict by acting out and engaging in a wide variety of passive–aggressive behaviors. Rumors fly and nasty forms of gossip increase as do absenteeism, poor performance, errors, and counteraggression (Baker and Jones 1996).

Unresolved Grief

Caregiving organizations under stress may become oblivious to the most obvious question, "Is what we are doing working?" Instead, quality assurance issues will focus on the more mundane aspects of the environment, such as completed paperwork and adequate fire alarms, while neglecting the most vital aspects of quality care: catalyzing positive change in clients, staff, and the living system as a whole. Meanwhile, a chronic organizational disaster is unfolding. Erikson (1994) has defined a "chronic disaster" as one that:

> … gathers force slowly and insidiously, creeping around one's defenses rather than smashing through them. People are unable to mobilize their normal defenses against the threat, sometimes because they have elected consciously or unconsciously to ignore it, sometimes because they have been misinformed about it, and sometimes because they cannot do anything to avoid it in any case. In individuals this manifests as a numbness of spirit, a susceptibility to anxiety and rage and depression, a sense of helplessness, an inability to concentrate, a loss of various motor skills, a heightened apprehension about the physical and social environment, a preoccupation with death, a retreat into dependency, and a general loss of ego functions (Erikson 1994, p. 21).

Friends and colleagues leave or are laid off, leaders depart, programs close or are greatly diminished, and clients do not respond to interventions in satisfactory ways. Everyone in the system experiences losses that no one is permitted to fully address. When leaders fail to pay attention to the effects of these losses on their subordinates, they convey the attitude that there is nothing to be gained by working through loss, so no one does. As a result, loss is compounded upon loss, further contributing to the atmosphere of demoralization and depression (Jeffreys 2005).

Chronically stressed organizations tend to have significantly lowered abilities for creative change, instead mirroring the clients' reenactment behavior by reenacting failed treatment strategies and policies that do not work while remaining unaware of the repetitive nature of their interventions. In a system, constant reenactment is a sign of unresolved grief (Bloom 2007a). The result may be failure of the purported organizational mission.

Loss of Meaning and Demoralization

In chronically stressed organizations, staff often become progressively hopeless, helpless, and demoralized about the work they are doing and the possibility of seeing significant change in the clients, failing to recognize that much of their hopelessness and helplessness is related not to the clients but to the larger systems within which they are all embedded. Chronically stressed organizations may be controlled top-to-bottom by people who are "burned out"—emotionally exhausted, cynical about their clients, doubting any personal efficacy (Angerer 2003; Cordes and Dougherty 1993). Over time, leaders and staff lose sight of the essential purpose of their work together and derive less and less satisfaction and meaning from the work. This foreshortened sense of future in organizations presents as a loss of vision of true purpose, as well as a loss of hope that the organization and all of the staff together can play a significant role in helping people to recover.

Implications for Women's Mental Health

Judging from the extent of exposure to childhood adversity, it is no longer acceptable to believe that we can consign some special treatment programs to the alleviation of trauma-related problems. Every mental health service agency, every educational institution, and every workplace needs to be trauma-informed and trauma-sensitive. It must be possible for injured women and children to enter any mental health or social service environment and have experiences that are potentially healing, rather than experiences that compound their injuries as so often happens today.

As has been detailed in the previous sections, the results of complex and interactive stress-related problems plaguing our service delivery systems and negatively impacting the treatment of women and children can readily be compared to the complex problems of chronically maltreated clients. At this point, our social service network can be viewed as a "trauma-organized system" (Bentovim 1992), still largely unaware of the multiple ways in which its adaptation to chronic stress has created a state of dysfunction that in some cases virtually prohibits the recovery of the individual clients who are the source of its underlying and original mission and damages many of the people who work within it. While reading this chapter, you may have recognized some or all of the ways in which your own organization is functioning. Therefore, how can you help be an agent of positive change?

It is useful to think about parallel processes of recovery, because in reality we cannot stop mental health delivery systems from functioning in order to fix what is broken. The flow of clients who need services has not and will not stop in any world that we can realistically anticipate today. So we have to mend our broken organizations and systems at the same time that we are providing services to the people who need them. As daunting a process as this may seem, it is consistent with both the recovery movement and the drive for trauma-informed care. What needs to be added is a heightened awareness of the interconnected, living nature of all of our systems and a recognition that significant changes in one part of the corporate "body" can only occur if the whole body changes as well.

The total-systems approach that we have designed to help organizations reverse the stress-related trends described in this chapter is called "The Sanctuary Model." Based on more than 20 years of experience in responding to the needs of traumatized individuals, Sanctuary® is a repackaging of an enormous amount of tacit clinical wisdom that has been slowly increasingly missing from the health, mental health, and social service systems, while integrating within it the new trauma-informed knowledge that is so vital if we are to make progress in improving women's mental health.

The Sanctuary Model expands the idea of "trauma-informed" care to include the individual staff members of our systems of care as well as each organization and the system-as-a-whole. It offers one possible model of services that could respond to women with mental health problems.

The Sanctuary Model is based on the parallel process notion that analogous relationships exist between each organizational level, and therefore the maximum gain and the potential for true transformation lie in instituting individual and systemic change simultaneously.

It is not a trauma intervention by itself, or a trauma-specific treatment. It represents the necessary framework of the "house": the roof, the ceiling, and the frame within which must be built an array of treatment methods, approaches, policies, and procedures that represent the rooms of the "house" and the "furniture" in the rooms. Like the homes we live in, every program must have its own unique identity, its own character and personality, and its own methods for accomplishing its mission. But every program must bear the characteristics of the total system.

Sanctuary is what can emerge when groups of people come together, create a community, engage in authentic behavior, share common values and a common language, and make seven specific cultural commitments: (1) commitment to nonviolence; (2) commitment to emotional intelligence; (3) commitment to social learning; (4) commitment to open communication; (5) commitment to democracy; (6) commitment to social responsibility; and (7) commitment to growth and change (Bloom 2005, 2007b).

In Sanctuary, we are endeavoring to describe and model what it means for a system to be alive: growing, changing, learning, and even reproducing. As a network of programs, we are together discovering the day-to-day "technology" that is necessary to maximize systemic health (see www.sanctuary.com). The only way to effectively remove barriers to trauma-informed care delivered to individual trauma survivors is to become "trauma-sensitive" to the ways in which managers, staff, organizations, and systems are impacted by individual and collective exposure to overwhelming stress. Ultimately, the goals of the Sanctuary Model are to improve clinical outcomes, increase staff satisfaction and health, increase leadership competence, and develop a technology for creating and sustaining healthier systems that can develop and deliver optimal mental health services for women.

References

Altemeyer, B. (1996). *The authoritarian specter*. Cambridge, MA: Harvard University Press.

Amason, A. C. (1996). Distinguishing the effects of functional and dysfunctional conflict on strategic decision making: Resolving a paradox for top management teams. *Academy of Management Journal, 39*, 123–148.

Angerer, J. M. (2003). Job burnout. *Journal of Employment Counseling, 40*(3), 98.

Appelbaum, P. S. (2002). Starving in the midst of plenty: The mental health care crisis in America. *Psychiatric Services, 53*(10), 1247–1248.

Ashforth, B. (1994). Petty tyranny in organizations. *Human Relations, 47*(7), 755–778.

Baker, J. S., & Jones, M. A. (1996). The poison grapevine: How destructive are gossip and rumor in the workplace? *Human Resource Development Quarterly, 7*(1), 75.

Barsade, S. G., & Gibson, D. E. (2007). Why does affect matter in organizations? *Academy of Management Perspectives, 21*(1), 36–59.

Bazelon Center for Mental Health Law. (2001). *Disintegrating systems: The state of states' public mental health systems.* Washington, DC: Bazelon Center for Mental Health Law.

Beer, M., & Spector, B. (1993). Organizational diagnosis: Its role in organizational learning. *Journal of Counseling and Development, 71,* 642–650.

Bentovim, A. (1992). *Trauma-organized systems: Physical and sexual abuse in families.* London: Karnac Books.

Bloom, S. L. (1997). *Creating sanctuary: Toward the evolution of sane societies.* New York, NY: Routledge.

Bloom, S. L. (2002). *The PVS disaster: Poverty, violence and substance abuse in the lives of women and children. A literature review.* Philadelphia, PA: Women's Law Project.

Bloom, S. L. (2005). The sanctuary model of organizational change for children's residential treatment. *Therapeutic Community: The International Journal for Therapeutic and Supportive Organizations, 26*(1), 65–81.

Bloom, S. L. (2006). *Organizational Stress as a Barrier to Trauma-Sensitive Change and System Transformation, White Paper for the National Technical Assistance Center for State Mental Health Planning (NTAC), National Association of State Mental Health Program Directors.* http://www.nasmhpd.org/publications.cfm

Bloom, S. L. (2007a). Loss in human service organizations. In A. L. Vargas & S. L. Bloom (Eds.), *Loss, hurt and hope: The complex issues of bereavement and trauma in children* (pp. 142–206). Newcastle, UK: Cambridge Scholars Publishing.

Bloom, S. L. (2007b). The sanctuary model of trauma-informed organizational change. *The Source: The National Abandoned Infants Assistance Resource Center, 16*(1), 12–14, 16.

Bureau of Labor Statistics. (2006). *News – Survey of Workplace Violence Prevention, 2005* (http://www.bls.gov/iif/oshwc/osnr0026.pdf ed. Vol. October 27). Washington, DC: United States Department of Labor.

Carr, A. (2001). Understanding emotion and emotionality in a process of change. *Journal of Organizational Change Management, 14*(5), 421–434.

Caudill, W. (1958). *The psychiatric hospital as a small society.* Cambridge, MA: Harvard University Press.

Clements, P. T., DeRanieri, J. T., Clark, K., Manno, M. S., & Kuhn, D. W. (2005). Workplace violence and corporate policy for health care settings. *Nursing Economics, 23*(3), 119–124.

Conklin, J. E. (2001). *Designing organizational memory: Preserving Intellectual Assets in a Knowledge Economy,* http://www.impactalliance.org/file_download.php?location=S_U&filename=10383541181Touchstone_Tools_and_Resources.htm. Washington, DC: Touchstone Consulting.

Cordes, C. L., & Dougherty, T. W. (1993). A review and an integration of research on job burnout. *Academy of Management. The Academy of Management Review, 18*(4), 621.

Crossen, M. M., Lane, H. W., & White, R. E. (1999). An organizational learning framework: From intuition to institution. *Academy of Management Review, 24*(3), 522–537.

Dube, S. R., Anda, R. F., Felitti, V. J., Chapman, D. P., Williamson, D. F., & Giles, W. H. (2001). Childhood abuse, household dysfunction, and the risk of attempted suicide throughout the lifespan. *Journal of the American Medical Association, 286,* 3089–3096.

Edwards, V. J., Holden, G. W., Felitti, V. J., & Anda, R. F. (2003). Relationship between multiple forms of childhood maltreatment and adult mental health in community respondents: Results from the Adverse Childhood Experiences Study. *American Journal of Psychiatry, 160*(8), 1453–1460.

Employment Law Alliance. (2007). *Nearly 45% of U.S. Workers Say They've Worked for an Abusive Boss.* Employment Law Alliance. Retrieved 2007 from the World Wide Web: http://www.employmentlawalliance.com/node/1810

Erikson, K. (1994). *A new species of trouble: The human experience of modern disasters.* New York, NY: W.W. Norton.

Ettin, M. F., Fidler, J. W., & Cohen, B. D. (Eds.). (1995). *Group process and political dynamics.* Madison, CT: International Universities Press.

Felitti, V. J., Anda, R. F., Nordenberg, D., Williamson, D. F., Spitz, A. M., Edwards, V., et al. (1998). Relationship of childhood abuse and household dysfunction to many of the leading causes of death in adults. The Adverse Childhood Experiences (ACE) Study. *American Journal of Preventive Medicine, 14*(4), 245–258.

Goodman, L. A., Rosenberg, S. D., Mueser, K. T., & Drake, R. E. (1997). Physical and sexual assault history in women with serious mental illness: Prevalence, correlates, treatment, and future research directions. *Schizophrenia Bulletin, 23*(4), 685–696.

Jeffreys, J. S. (2005). *Coping with workplace grief: Dealing with loss, trauma, and change, Revised Edition.* Boston, MA: Thomson Course Technology.

Jehn, K. A. (1995). A multimethod examination of the benefits and detriments of intragroup conflict. *Administrative Science Quarterly, 40*(2), 256.

Jehn, K. A., Northcraft, G. B., & Neale, M. A. (1999). Why differences make a difference: A field study of diversity, conflict, and performance in workgroups. *Administrative Science Quarterly, 44*(4), 741.

Kanter, R. M., & Stein, B. A. (1992). *The challenge of organizational change: How companies experience it and leaders guide it.* New York, NY: The Free Press.

Kassing, J. W. (1997). Articulating, antagonizing, and displacing: A model of employee dissent. *Communication Studies, 48*(4), 311.

Kessler, R. C., Sonnega, A., Bromet, E., Hughes, M., & Nelson, C. B. (1995). Posttraumatic stress disorder in the National Comorbidity Survey. *Archives of General Psychiatry, 52*(12), 1048–1060.

Kransdorrf, A. (1997). Fight organizational memory lapse. *Workforce, 76*(9), 34–39.

Lahaie, D. (2005). The impact of corporate memory loss: What happens when a senior executive leaves? *Leadership in Health Services, 18*(3), 35–47.

Lutgen-Sandvik, P., Tracy, S. J., & Alberts, J. K. (2007). Burned by bullying in the American workplace: Prevalence, perception, degree and impact. *Journal of Management Studies, 44*(6), 837–862.

McGrath, R. (1994, April). Organizationally induced helplessness: The antithesis of employment. *Quality Progress, 27,* 89–92.

Mellers, B. A., Schwartz, A., & Cooke, A. D. J. (1998). Judgment and decision making. *Annual Review of Psychology, 49,* 447.

Morrison, E. W., & Milliken, F. J. (2000). Organizational silence: A barrier to change and development in a pluralistic world. *The Academy of Management Review, 25*(4), 706.

National Association of Psychiatric Health Systems. (2003). *Challenges facing behavioral health care: The pressures on essential behavioral healthcare services.* Washington, DC: National Association of Psychiatric Health Systems.

New Freedom Commission on Mental Health. (2003). *Achieving the Promise: Transforming Mental Health Care in America. Final Report* (DHHS Publication No. SMA-03-3832). Rockville, MD: New Freedom Commission on Mental Health.

Occupational Safety and Health Administration. (2004). *Guidelines for preventing workplace violence for health care & social service workers.* Washington, DC: United States Department of Labor.

Othman, R., & Hashim, N. A. (2004). Typologizing organizational amnesia. *The Learning Organization, 11*(2/3), 273–284.

President's New Freedom Commission on Mental Health. (2003). *Achieving the promise: Transforming mental health care in America.* Rockville, MD: New Freedom Commission on Mental Health.

Searles, H. (1955). The informational value of the supervisor's emotional experience. *Psychiatry, 18,* 135–146.

Senge, P. (1990). *The fifth discipline: The art and practice of the learning organization.* New York, NY: Doubleday.

Smith, K. K., Simmons, V. M., & Thames, T. B. (1989). "Fix the Women": An intervention into an organizational conflict based on parallel process thinking. *The Journal of Applied Behavioral Science, 25*(1), 11–29.

Stanton, A. H., & Schwartz, M. S. (1954). *The mental hospital: A study of institutional participation in psychiatric illness and treatment*. New York, NY: Basic Books.

Sunstein, C. R. (2003). *Why societies need dissent*. Cambridge, MA: Harvard University Press.

Weick, K. E. (2001). *Making sense of the organization*. Malden, MA: Blackwell.

World Health Organization. (2002). *Framework guidelines for addressing workplace violence in the health sector*. Geneva, Switzerland: International Labour Office.

Chapter 16
Services in Rural Areas

Pamela L. Mulder, Robert Jackson and Sarah Jarvis

Introduction

The need for interdisciplinary collaboration and the open exchange of information among professionals in public health, medicine, the ministry, and various mental health and social services disciplines is clearly demonstrated when mental health issues affecting women are viewed in the context of rurality. This is particularly true when these mental health issues are considered in terms of the broader perspective of behavioral health as recommended by the American Psychological Association (Mulder et al. 2000). Many of the most critical mental health and substance abuse concerns of rural women are shared by urban and suburban women. However, cultural, social, economic, and geographic factors commonly associated with rural residence frequently result in unique behavioral presentations that require culturally appropriate, multidimensional, and interdisciplinary responses that cover practice, policy making, and the setting of future research agendas.

Although the issues and concerns themselves can be readily listed, their unique manifestations and the equally specialized approaches required to address the issues can only be understood in context. A single chapter can provide only a general overview of behavioral health issues that commonly affect rural women in the USA, the unique sociocultural environment in which these concerns arise, and the need to design and implement solutions that are culturally sensitive and locally sustainable. To provide this overview, the authors begin this chapter by presenting many of the common characteristics that define rural communities. After the reader has the opportunity to become familiar with the context of rurality, the authors describe the most significant and prevalent mental health concerns confronting women in many rural communities. These mental health issues include specific mental illnesses such as depression (affective disorders) and anxiety (and related disorders) as well as additional behavioral health concerns such as substance abuse and obesity. As

P. L. Mulder (✉)
Department of Psychology, Marshall University,
1 John Marshall Drive, Huntington, WV 25755, USA

B. L. Levin, M. A. Becker (eds.), *A Public Health Perspective of Women's Mental Health*,
DOI 10.1007/978-1-4419-1526-9_16, © Springer Science+Business Media LLC 2010

is true in urban and suburban settings, many of these disorders are co-occurring in rural communities (a more complete discussion of co-occurring mental and physical disorders is provided in Chap. 5 of this text). To illustrate the importance of considering the impact of rural residence when attempting to address these mental health and substance abuse concerns, the authors also describe many of the unique social, cultural, geographic, and economic barriers to effective services delivery in rural communities.

The chapter concludes with a discussion of implications for the field of women's mental health with regard to policy, research, and practice. Perhaps the single most important implication is the need for interdisciplinary collaboration to design, develop, implement, and evaluate services and interventions that are effective, culturally informed, and regionally sustainable. Several examples of approaches that have real or potential efficacy in rural communities are described. The final section of this chapter is not intended to present a final conclusion to the issues raised. Rather, the authors hope that readers will recognize the challenges and calls for action integrated throughout this chapter and be inspired to apply their own areas of expertise to address concerns of a population that has been overlooked for far too long.

Rural Areas

Communities and land areas are usually defined as being rural and/or frontier on the basis of their significantly lower population density in comparison with urban, suburban, and metropolitan types of residence. Rural areas are found in every state in the USA. Frontier areas, which have the lowest population densities, are found in about one-third of the states. Ninety-five percent of the nation's land mass qualifies as rural under one or more of the many currently used definitions. These rural areas are home to 27–30% of the US population (Fisher 2005).

It is important to note that, although common characteristics of rural life can be identified, rural people are not a homogenous population. Thus, rural communities are not all alike. Included among ruralites are representatives of every ethnic/cultural background, every national origin, every occupation, and every socioeconomic status. Rural communities include isolated, sparsely populated conclaves comprised of a few families as well as seasonally popular resorts, parks, and reserves. The rural designation can be applied to reservations, to large working ranches, dairies and farms, and also to areas famous for large privately owned estates. This diversity also means that not all rural women are at high risk for the development of behavioral health problems. Nevertheless, a great many rural women do experience significant psychological and emotional distress. The prevalence of many behavioral health problems in rural communities equals or exceeds that which is observed in more urban communities (Wagenfeld et al. 1993; Wagenfeld 2003), but the resources available to address these problems are very different from those which are commonly accessed in larger population centers.

Common Elements of Rural Residence

There are common elements which characterize rural communities and their residents. These elements can be initially perceived as either positive (psychologically protective) or negative (psychologically damaging). However, the critical and creative reader will quickly note that most of these elements have the potential to be both protective and damaging depending on perspective and purpose. Making informed decisions about categorizing these defining characteristics is important, both for identifying issues and concerns and for developing culturally appropriate and sustainable solutions.

Some of the common elements which characterize rural communities include low population density, geographical distance from large metropolitan centers, and challenging terrain. The low population density can result in isolation, a limited tax base to fund needed services, and catchment area approaches to service provision (a system which bases the location and number of service providers on the number of people to be served rather than on the actual amount of land area to be covered). These characteristics are associated with loss of economic and educational opportunities and limited manpower resources despite relatively high demand for services.

As an example, a single volunteer fire department or a single sheriff's deputy may have the daunting task of covering several large counties at significantly greater cost and with far less effectiveness than would be required to achieve the same ratio of emergency responders to residents in more densely populated communities. Similarly, to meet the cost of staffing and equipping a single rural school, students may have to ride school buses for hours at a time in rural areas. Patients may have to travel significant distances over roads that the small community cannot afford to repair. These factors often limit the extent to which national leaders attend to the needs of rural communities and deprive these sparsely populated communities of political power. Alternatively, these factors can also mean that the local mayor and various regionally elected government officials are well known in the communities to which they are accountable. Similarly, there may be few activities for young community members outside school hours. This can be cause for alarm over the possibility that bored youngsters will engage in mischief, or these young residents can be viewed as a valuable volunteer workforce, a potentially significant community resource.

In spite of the low population density, rural communities often have very dense social networks composed of large, extended family groups that have frequently resided in a given community for generations. Common attitudes and values favor traditionalism, self-reliance, and respect for local authorities combined with a sense of separation from more distant sources of oversight and governance. In addition, these attitudes and values favor close kinship ties and interdependence of family members, a resistance to change, tremendous interpersonal familiarity among locals, and a distrust of those considered to be "outsiders." These conditions have been discussed in terms of problems with anonymity, confidentiality, stigma, provider objectivity, lack of privacy, and deeply enmeshed families which may prevent personal development and maintain pathological patterns of behavior and interaction.

As examples of how these factors may be psychologically protective, ruralites commonly work together to help one another and to look out for one another. Extended families share financial and childcare burdens, traditions provide meaning and stability, and familiarity means that people can interact with one another as individuals, neighbors, and fellow stakeholders in the community. Alternatively, these factors may mean that the emergency responder who shows up in response to a call for help from a battered wife is a friend or relative of the batterer, that the newly sexually active unmarried teenager who would have preferred to practice safe sex cannot obtain condoms or birth control at the local pharmacy because the pharmacist is a friend of their family, or that everyone will know who is seeking help from the local mental health provider simply by recognizing the cars parked in certain places.

Rural women are more likely than urban women to be married, to have children, and to have begun having their children at an earlier age. They are less likely to be employed full time outside the home and, on average, have fewer years of formal education and earn lower wages than their urban counterparts (Schoenberg et al. 2005). Rural women are also more likely to be caregivers for members of their immediate and extended families and are often involved in helping to provide care for other members of the community. In fact, rural women have expressed a significant preference for receiving care from persons known to them (Bushy 1993; Mulder et al. 2000).

Not all of the common rural factors are as readily amenable to changes in connotation or perspective. Rural communities tend to have higher percentages of uninsured or underinsured residents. In general, there is a much greater reliance on Medicare and Medicaid funding even though rural residents are less likely to be aware of their eligibility for these programs (Simmons et al. 2008a). Rural communities have disproportionately large populations of elderly women and women with disabilities, women who report chronic illnesses, and women living in poverty (Baca et al. 2007; DeLeon et al. 1989; Mulder et al. 2000).

More than 800 rural counties have unusually high rates of persistent (generational) poverty and the majority of impoverished counties in the USA are located in nonmetropolitan areas of the nation. Nearly 70% of the substandard housing in the USA is found in rural areas (DeLeon et al. 1989). Fifty-three percent of the nation's poor reside in the rural southeast (Rowland and Lyons 1989). Poverty rates among rural minorities are much higher than those of rural Caucasians and substantially higher than those of minorities residing in urban centers, although nearly two-thirds of the rural poor were non-Hispanic Caucasians, a factor largely attributable to the large Caucasian majority in the rural population. Poverty rates are highest for rural

African-Americans, followed by Native Americans and Hispanics. Rural families headed by women, rural women living alone, and those who are elderly and/or have disabilities experience the highest poverty rates of all family types (United States Department of Agriculture 1998).

Specific Mental Health and Substance Abuse Concerns in Rural Communities

The survey which eventually led to the development of *Rural Healthy People, 2010* (Gamm et al. 2003) identified several mental and behavioral healthcare issues as being among the top 10 areas of concern in rural communities. Mental health/mental disorders were determined to have the fourth highest priority, with suicide, depression, and anxiety disorders being the most commonly cited areas of concern in rural communities. Among those concerns that have strong behavioral health components amenable to preventive interventions, heart disease and strokes (respectively the first and third leading causes of death in the USA and the most frequent causes of hospitalization for rural elders) were tied with diabetes for second place. Tobacco use and substance abuse were tied for sixth place on the priority list, and nutrition/obesity was tied with cancer and maternal/infant/adolescent health in the tenth position.

Depression

Depression is the most commonly studied and the most prevalent mental disorder in rural areas (Mulder et al. 2000; United States Department of Health and Human Services (HHS) 2000). Research suggests that depression is more prevalent in rural areas than in urban centers and that depression among rural women is a major public health concern (Probst et al. 2006; Simmons et al. 2008b). Rural women at highest risk for depression include those who are younger and who perceive themselves as lacking in social support networks and social attachments (Hillemeier et al. 2007). Rural women with disabilities and those who are experiencing chronic illness and/or pain are also at high risk for depression (Bushy 1993; Gamm et al. 2003).

Despite the high prevalence rates for depression in rural communities, and in spite of the fact that psychological complaints account for more than 40% of all patient visits to rural family practitioners, on average, rural family practice physicians detect 50% less depression in their patients than do their urban counterparts (Rost et al. 1995a). Depressed rural women frequently present in primary care settings with psychosomatic symptoms such as headaches, backaches, insomnia, fatigue, and abdominal pain, which may obscure underlining mental health conditions. However, a nationwide survey showed that as many as 50% of physicians working in primary care settings intentionally misdiagnosed depression. The reasons given include uncertainty about the diagnosis, concerns that reimbursement for services will be delayed if a diagnosis of depression is given, and fear that the patient may not be able to obtain health insurance in the future (Jameson and Blank 2007).

Moreover, although research has shown that the best outcomes are achieved with combined medication and psychotherapy (National Institutes of Mental Health 2005), when rural providers diagnose depression in their female patients, medication is frequently the only treatment option offered. Reasons given for limiting the treatment approach vary, but often include the lack of mental health professionals in rural areas to whom referrals can be made, cost of services, and an unwillingness among rural women to be perceived as needing mental health care. However, even when mental health professionals were available near physicians' offices, only 5% of the depressed patients received any form of mental health care. Research shows that it is not unusual for more than two-thirds of depressed patients initially seen by family practitioners in rural primary care settings to meet the criteria for major depression 5 months later (Rost et al. 1992, 1995b). For additional information on depression, see Chap. 6 in this volume.

Depression and Disability

Women with disabilities constitute approximately 8% of the total US population, but approximately 26% of all rural women have significant disabilities. Disabled rural women tend to be poorer and less educated than their urban counterparts. They are more likely to be unemployed, to have poorer overall health, to lack access to providers who are trained to address their specific disabilities, and to be more dependent on government social service programs (Mulder et al. 2000). In general, rural women who report higher levels of subjective depression also reported a higher percentage of other physical complaints (Simmons et al. 2007) compared to their urban counterparts.

Depression and Anxiety

The prevalence of anxiety disorders in general is about the same in rural and urban settings. However, rural women face many stressors which are associated with both anxiety and depression and which differ qualitatively from those that are commonly experienced in more urban settings. It was previously noted that rural women serve as caregivers for immediate and extended families and for members of their community. Although it is not unlikely that urban women also face the stress of caring for others, the added burdens of poverty, limited access to professional assistance and opportunities for respite, and the traditionalist, patriarchal attitudes that are common in rural areas impact rural women differently than women who live in urban areas (Mulder et al. 2000). Gallagher and Delworth (1993) first described the "third shift" as a significant stressor for rural women. They noted that rural women often do seek employment outside the home, on either a full- or part-time basis. After completing the duties of employment, the rural woman is likely to have significant responsibilities as a homemaker and mother.

Finally, to make ends meet, many rural women face yet a third job or shift as a result of involvement with a family-operated business. Cottage industry businesses, farming, maintaining large gardens, canning, caring for livestock, and keeping associate financial records are all common "third shift" responsibilities that can significantly increase the stress of daily life for rural women.

In contrast to these findings, both Bushy (1993) and Hillemeier et al. (2007), using samples of elderly rural women and women of reproductive age, respectively, found that activities such as volunteering, being active in one's community, being able to care for loved ones, and being a part of an operation (such as a family farm) correlated negatively with self-reported stress, depression, and anxiety. Some research has suggested that rural women who report lower levels of depression have had a child in the past 3 years (Simmons et al. 2007). It is likely that stress for rural women is similar to that of women in general, with a poor match between perceived environmental demands and one's perceptions of available resources being the critical factor in determining the impact of life challenges upon rural women.

Suicide

Suicide rates are higher in rural areas than in urban and suburban communities, particularly in rural regions of western states where young women are three times more likely to commit suicide than young women who live in urban and suburban communities (Suicide Prevention Resource Center 2008). Violence in the form of both homicide and suicide is disproportionately high among young Native Americans living in rural areas, and there are many more nonfatal injuries that are tied to suicide attempts among these young people (Carmona 2005).

Rural women are more likely to use a firearm to commit suicide than their urban counterparts. However, in the event that any question as to the cause of death may exist, it is not unusual for rural physicians, acting as coroners, to accede to family requests that another cause be listed (Mulder et al. 2000; Suicide Prevention Resource Center 2008). This has probably led to the underreporting of suicide rates in rural areas.

Violence Against Rural Women

Violence against women in all forms is no less prevalent and problematic in rural areas than in urban and metropolitan settings. The incidence of spousal abuse does not differ significantly across these residential environments (United States Department of Justice 1997). Approximately half of the homeless women in the USA are without shelter because they are fleeing from spousal abuse (Mulder et al. 2000). Women in rural areas are more likely to be married to an abusive male partner than are women in an urban area, and the battered rural woman tends to have remained with the perpetrator for a longer period of time (an average of 10 years for rural women versus 5 years for women in more metropolitan settings). There are other differences in the manifestation of spousal violence in rural and urban settings. For example, about 25% of rural victims report that her partner has attempted to run her over with a car, and a larger proportion of rural victims report having been threatened with weapons (Roenker 2003).

Rural women frequently have more difficulty obtaining protective orders. Many rural counties impose fees for protective orders in spite of ordinances which prohibit this. Moreover, in some rural communities, the names of the victims are published in local newspapers (Roenker 2003). Practices of this kind discourage reporting and increase problems related to stigma. Leaving the area to escape violence may deprive the rural victim of the sources of interpersonal and family support she has depended on throughout her lifetime. In some cases, choosing to escape by leaving the area may actually violate local customs in a manner that results in alienation and censure of the rural victim, often casting her in the role of the "home wrecker" (Mulder et al. 2000; Rural Womyn Zone 2008).

Rural women who try to escape from violent situations, possibly trying to reach a safe shelter, face difficulties that are not commonly encountered by victims in more metropolitan settings. Rural women who have responsibilities in a family business or on a family farm are often indispensable partners in these operations, meaning that leaving the home may entail economic losses that can never be recouped (Mulder et al. 2000; Rural Womyn Zone 2008). Rural women are often emotionally bound to their lands and without continued care, precious livestock may be endangered (Mulder et al. 2000). Any available domestic violence shelters may be so far from the woman's home or work location that escape would equate to the abandonment of a job or a childcare placement in an area where these resources are extremely scarce (Mulder et al. 2000; Rural Womyn Zone 2008).

Poverty and other socioeconomic circumstances which correlate significantly and positively with rurality impact the incidence of violence against women. Single women and women heads-of-household with total incomes that fall below the poverty line are approximately five times more likely to be victims of violence (United States Department of Justice 1997). Although metropolitan rates for attempted rapes per 1,000 women are approximately twice as high as that reported for rural residents, the incidence of completed rape does not differ between settings (Donnermeyer 1995). Stranger rape is not common in rural areas; rape victims in rural areas are more likely to be attacked by someone they know, which alters the psychological experience of reporting the crime.

Victims who do report violent assaults are likely to discover that services are substandard or entirely unavailable. Few rural hospital emergency rooms have rape kits or personnel who are trained to examine and interview rape victims (Mulder et al. 2000).

Substance Abuse

Information about substance abuse in rural communities is difficult to find, and many of the studies which have been conducted have yielded contradictory results (Mulder et al. 2000). It is also apparent that regional patterns of substance abuse are changing rapidly. These changes appear to be occurring over time as national educational efforts have been increased and information has become more readily available to women in all parts of the world as a result of the World Wide Web (Baca et al. 2007).

Alcohol Abuse

Rural and urban residents report similar rates of alcohol use overall, but the drinking patterns and outcomes vary. Rural residents who are "problem drinkers" tend to have worse problems with alcohol than their urban counterparts (Baca et al. 2007; Hayes et al. 2002). Rural women are more likely to report frequent, even regular, binge-drinking episodes, and they continue to be less likely than urban women to significantly reduce their rates of alcohol use during pregnancy (Hayes et al. 2002). Patterns of alcohol use by rural women appear to be strongly correlated with family histories of alcohol abuse and with the use of alcohol by male peers, partners, and spouses. Rural women are more likely to abuse alcohol if the significant other in her life is also doing so (Hayes et al. 2002).

Other Substances

Tobacco use continues to be disproportionately high among rural populations. Women in many of the most rural counties are more likely to smoke than those in urban communities (Gamm et al. 2003).

Previous studies have suggested that rural versus urban samples have similar rates of marijuana use. Women in rural areas were initially found to be less likely to use cocaine, opiates, and amphetamines (Hayes et al. 2002; Mulder et al. 2000). Recently, however, rural residents have faced an influx of drugs, as drug dealers from larger metropolitan centers have targeted the smaller communities as new markets. Moreover, some ruralites have become drug producers themselves. The isolation available in rural regions and the ease with which methamphetamine can be manufactured using readily accessible ingredients has resulted in large numbers of hidden labs and the increased availability of methamphetamine in both rural and urban communities (Clay 2007).

Nationwide, admission rates for abuse of narcotic painkillers increased 230% between 1992 and 2005. This increase was smallest in large central metropolitan areas (103%) and greatest in the most rural areas (between 440 and 462% depending on the distance from a city; Cline 2007). Roenker (2003) reports that rural women are more likely than their urban counterparts to abuse prescription medications.

Concerns About Substance Abuse Treatment

Treatment options for rural residents are limited, and the nearest facility may be several hundred miles away from a woman's home. This means that rural women who do seek treatment face many of the same problems that are encountered by women seeking shelter from violence. As of the late 1990s, only approximately 10% of rural hospitals offered any kind of substance abuse treatment services in comparison to 25% of metropolitan hospitals (Dempsey et al. 1999), and there do not appear to be significant gains in the meantime. Treatment facilities in rural areas continue to lack the staff, the expertise and the resources they need to address substance abuse. In many cases, available treatment programs focused almost exclusively on alcoholism and had very little experience treating other forms of substance abuse (Clay 2007).

Prevention efforts and support programs for substance abusers and their families are also scarce. Although programs such as Alcoholics Anonymous (AA) may exist in rural areas, meetings may take place only once a week in contrast to more highly populated areas where the AA motto suggests that there are accessible meetings going on 24 hours a day, every day (Clay 2007). Moreover, given the lack of anonymity in rural communities, even the best of programs is unlikely to offer the participants truly anonymous options. For additional information on substance abuse and women, see Chap. 9 in this volume.

Obesity and Exercise

The prevalence of obesity among all American women has increased rapidly in recent years. In the 5 year span from 1976–1980, 17% of American women 20–74 years old were obese. This figure jumped to 26% by 1994 and to 34% in 2000 (Bove and Olson 2006). Currently, rural women have, on average, higher body mass indexes (BMIs), and they are more likely to report weight-related chronic conditions (Doyle et al. 2006). Women living in suburban communities or in "fringe counties" near large metropolitan areas (commuter communities, not commonly plagued by poverty) have the lowest age-adjusted prevalence of self-reported obesity, whereas those residing in the most rural counties have the highest rates of obesity (Bove and Olson 2006).

Bove and Olson (2006) conducted a multivariate analysis of national data from the 1970s and 1980s and found that the difference between urban and rural Caucasian women who were obese (with the latter usually being significantly more overweight) decreased when age and education were controlled in the analysis. This strongly suggests that at least some of the rural–urban weight differences among white women may be due, in large part, to demographic differences. For example, body weight is inversely related to socioeconomic status (SES) in women in the USA and other industrialized countries. Low SES in childhood increases the risk of obesity for adult women; low SES in adulthood increases the risk of weight gain during adulthood for white women.

Bove and Olson (2006) also found that overweight and obesity are more prevalent among "food-insecure women" than among "food-secure women" in national cross-sectional studies. They also demonstrated that "food insecurity" correlates strongly with low SES. "Food insecurity" is defined as the result of perceptions that the availability of nutritionally adequate and safe food, or the ability to acquire acceptable foods in socially acceptable ways, is limited or uncertain. Studies on food-insecure women indicate that mothers restrict their own intakes when they perceive that the household food supply is either low or threatened so that they can ensure food for their children. These mothers perceived they went hungry when financial constraints compelled them to change their eating habits. Olson and Strawderman (2008) found that women who were obese early in life and women who were raised in lower SES families were at significantly greater risk for becoming food insecure and for continued obesity.

Rural women are more likely to express preferences for culturally developed food choices and less likely to engage in healthy lifestyle activities such as regular physical exercise and activity. With regard to food choices, the preferred diet of farmers who worked from dawn to dusk and survived on what they raised included significant amounts of animal fats, fried foods, and starchy vegetables. This diet is still preferred in many rural communities, particularly where residents still rely on being able to produce much of what they consume.

In suburban settings, walking is considered to be an excellent form of regular exercise for most women, and young mothers are often encouraged to include their children in these walks. Surveys suggest that rural women are less likely than their urban counterparts to have walked a continuous mile in the past month (Doyle et al. 2006). Rural homes are often located along highways and roadways without sidewalks or streetlights. Many rural roads are unpaved, often muddy in spring from rain and icy or snow-covered in winter. It is more difficult in general to walk under these conditions, especially if one has any impairment of mobility. In addition, pushing a stroller on these tertiary roads is nearly impossible even when the roads are dry (Bove and Olson 2006).

A number of studies have found that residents are more likely to walk if they have ready access to locations where there are more street intersections and shorter blocks. Perceived safety is particularly important to women in rural communities. In fact, one clear illustration of the interactions among a variety of demographic factors involves findings that residing in environments where safety is perceived as being low, or where there are high rates of crime, may be more detrimental to women's health than to men's health, particularly with respect to walking, obesity and related health factors such as diabetes and hypertension, and respondents' self-rated health (Doyle et al. 2006). For additional information on eating disorders, see Chap. 7 in this volume.

Serious Mental Illness

Although the prevalence rates for serious mental illness (SMI) are approximately equal across residence types, the manifestation is somewhat different. Individuals with SMI are more likely to be cared for by their families in rural areas and are less likely to appear to be homeless even if they are actually residing in largely abandoned, substandard housing. The primary caregivers for individuals with SMI who live in rural areas are generally mothers and other female family members who, as previously noted, may fulfill these duties at the expense of their own physical and emotional well-being. The stress of caring for others is made even more difficult because of the lack of available services that can be used to support home care, the distances that often must be traveled to obtain services, and financial difficulties (Mulder et al. 2000).

Therefore, it is not surprising to find that rural residents with chronic mental illnesses employ crisis services more frequently. Rural residents are less likely than their urban counterparts to have access to inpatient mental health services. In many isolated rural counties, inpatient psychiatric services are almost nonexistent (Wagenfeld et al. 1993). The public/community mental health system is often the only provider in rural areas, and they primarily serve persons with SMI. There are many who believe, however, that these community mental health centers, given the underfunding and reliance on many of the least well trained providers, are not up to the task (Mulder et al. 2000).

Accidents and Traumatic Injuries

Rural women are susceptible to injury as a result of accidents. Many injuries are related to the nature of rural employment, which is frequently physically demanding. Rural employment often involves the use of heavy equipment in farming, logging, mining, and fishing. Injuries may arise from accidental exposure to farm and garden chemicals. Additionally, injuries occur as a result of having to travel long distances on secondary and tertiary roads where the geography, terrain, or weather conditions may make such travel unusually treacherous. Not only are traumatic injuries more common in rural areas, injured ruralites face worse outcomes and higher risks of death than urban patients. Some of the reasons for these poorer outcomes include any of a number of transportation problems and a lack of advanced life support training for emergency medical personnel (Agency for Health Care Policy and Research 1996).

Other Chronic Conditions

Overall, research suggests that rural residents have a higher prevalence of smoking, obesity, physical inactivity, and chronic physical illnesses (Simmons et al. 2008a). Rural women are beset with a number of health concerns, often to a greater extent than rural men and urban residents in general. When compared to urbanites, ruralites suffer from higher incidences of chronic illness and experience more disability and morbidity related to diabetes, cancer, hypertension, heart disease, stroke, and lung disease. This may partially be due to ruralites' lack of knowledge about early detection and prevention measures or the inability to access preventive and screening services (Mulder et al. 2000).

Rural women are less likely than urban and suburban women to have had mammograms and Pap tests on a regular basis. Many rural women, particularly those who do not have health insurance, cite cost as a key barrier to obtaining this coverage. Interestingly, these women are also likely to overestimate the cost of these services (McAlearney et al. 2007).

In some cases, traditional attitudes may prevent rural women from openly disclosing their concerns with physicians. Many have stated that because they smoked or were overweight, they anticipated negative reactions and avoided seeking any kind of medical care, particularly for such intimate examinations as annual Pap tests (Schoenberg et al. 2005). Because of cultural attitudes favoring modesty, many rural women will refuse to be physically examined by male physicians. Many elderly rural women and rural women who are not sexually active have reported that they did not believe that these preventative and screening procedures continued to be necessary (Schoenberg et al. 2005). As a result of the underuse of these health services, rural women are often first diagnosed with a serious illness later in the course of an illness than urban women, resulting in poorer prognoses and often requiring more invasive and more costly medical intervention (Mulder et al. 2000).

Special Populations

Issues of distrust, lack of cultural awareness, and language barriers have made it very difficult to obtain health data for immigrant and migrant women. However, many issues and concerns have been repeatedly raised. In 2003, female immigrants, women without US citizenship, and women living in the rural border communities of the southwestern United States were among the most likely to lack access to primary healthcare and to lack health insurance coverage.

This trend was more evident among certain racial and ethnic groups, with the greatest disparities being experienced by non-Hispanic Black and Hispanic women who had been in the USA for less than 5 years. More than one-third of families in the border region of the USA have incomes at or below the Federal poverty level. The quality of the air, water, and soil in this region is an issue of particular concern.

A very large percentage of households are not connected to sources of clean water. High levels of industry and agriculture in this region expose residents to harmful pesticides and other chemicals. Infectious diseases, including tuberculosis and both hepatitis A and B, are significantly more prevalent in individuals living in the border region than in the general US population (Singh and Siahpush 2002).

Barriers to Service Delivery in Rural Areas

Many of the key barriers to services utilization, including lack of health insurance, cost of services, isolation, and distance from available providers, have already been mentioned in the previous section. Overall, socioeconomic issues are probably the most critical factors underlying the barriers to services delivery in rural areas (Simmons et al. 2008a).

Access to care is one of the 10 leading health indicators identified by the U.S. Department of Health and Human Services. The team responsible for developing the *Rural Healthy People, 2010* (RHP 2010; Gamm et al. 2005) reports surveyed local and state level leaders working in rural public health agencies, in hospitals, and in rural health clinics to determine the access to care issues that would be given priority by these leaders and also to determine the priority that these experts would assign to a variety of important public health issues. The most highly prioritized barriers to accessing care included, in order:

- the lack of access to insurance, particularly for ruralites 65 years and older, and for residents of rural communities which rely on a poorly paid workforce primarily employed by small businesses;
- the lack of access to primary care in rural areas;
- the lack of access to mental health care;
- the lack of access to oral health care; and
- the lack of access to emergency medical services (EMS).

Professional mental health providers tend to be concentrated in urban areas. Rural areas have serious shortages of trained mental health professionals (Gamm et al. 2005). This often means that rural residents who do seek mental health services are most often seen by primary care physicians who may be poorly prepared to recognize and treat individuals with mental disorders. Moreover, in the absence of trained mental health providers, or because of cultural preference, rural individuals often seek mental health services from the "*de facto* mental health system" which is made up of a variety of paraprofessionals, members of the clergy, and culturally appropriate healers (Mulder et al. 2000).

Access issues are not restricted to the unavailability of various individual and organizational providers. The lack of coordination, collaboration, and integration among providers (even to the point of "turf wars") are serious problems in rural areas where resources for provider survival are also limited. Concerns about provider objectivity, confidentiality, cultural sensitivity, and even language barriers all contribute to the lack of access to quality care for rural women. Stigma, lack of anonymity, and cultural attitudes which favor self-reliance and distrust of outsiders all impede services delivery in rural communities. Even when treatment facilities are available, concerns about the lack of privacy and anonymity may prevent women from seeking mental health treatment in small rural communities where knowledge of clients and their families outside of the therapeutic relationship is common and dual relationships are not easily avoided (Baca et al. 2007).

Additional barriers include the fact that public transportation is virtually nonexistent in rural communities, and many rural residents lack reliable personal transportation or the means to cover the costs of upkeep and fuel (Schoenberg et al. 2005). Lack of childcare and limited employment options combined with inflexible provider schedules that do not include evening and weekend hours further impede access to care (Fisher 2005; Jameson and Blank 2007; Mulder 2002).

Importantly, rural communities lack "wraparound" services and efforts to design communities in ways that would maximize opportunities for developing healthy lifestyles (Doyle et al. 2006; Mulder 2002). Providers in urban and suburban communities rely, intentionally or otherwise, on a variety of services that promote healthier lifestyles and provide support for their patients. Among these services are public transportation, specialized assistance for persons with disabilities, specialized educational programs in public schools, housing assistance, vocational training, job counseling, free or low-cost legal clinics, parenting classes, community colleges, libraries, after school activities, and recreational facilities such as parks, bicycle paths, and simple sidewalks.

Implications for Women's Mental Health: Developing, Assessing, and Implementing Effective Approaches and Interventions

Attention to rural mental health and substance abuse concerns has increased over the past two decades. Prior to the 1980s, there were very few articles, papers, or texts which mentioned the social, emotional, or behavioral health issues in rural areas. During the past two decades, some very significant policy changes have taken place, but few of these have been sufficient. For example, in recognition of the importance of diversity in research, agencies such as the National Institutes of Health/Mental Health (NIH/NIMH) and the Substance Abuse and Mental Health Services Administration (SAMHSA) now mandate the inclusion of rural residents in government-funded projects. Other federal and state policies have been implemented to ensure that small hospitals and rural healthcare providers have access to Medicare and other funding sources, but there are still tremendous disparities in reimbursement rates between urban and rural settings. Legislation intended to establish reimbursement parity for mental health and substance abuse treatment has been passed. However, because private insurers are not required to offer mental health coverage, they can avoid compliance with parity laws merely by dropping mental health coverage. Graduate Medical Education policies and practices intended to fund higher education and provide student loan repayment options for health professionals have been extended to include mental health and substance abuse. This funding has helped to support training focused on identifying and addressing the needs of underserved populations, including rural and frontier residents. However, these programs do not provide equivalent coverage for physical and mental health conditions. Financial support for educating those entering the medical and nursing fields far exceeds that which is made available for all mental health professions combined.

To overcome these disparities and to provide quality mental health and substance abuse services to rural women, healthcare providers representing every discipline will need to work together and support one another. It is important for us to set aside the "turf wars" and become advocates for policies and practices that encourage collaboration and holistic approaches to health and wellness. Interdisciplinary collaboration is more effective and also more professionally fulfilling when the service providers have trained together and are familiar with one another's scope of practice and areas of expertise. One current area of professional contention is prescription privileges. As has been stated, research clearly shows that protocols which combine pharmaceutical and psychotherapy interventions are vital for treating many mental health disorders. The shortage of psychiatrists (and other specialists) in rural areas, the underdiagnosis of many mental health conditions by general medical practitioners, and the fact that medical education does not include significant training in psychotherapy are significant barriers to some of the most appropriate and effective interventions. Resolving this problem will require medical and mental health professionals to work together toward a solution that will benefit rural women and their families. As another example, service providers must be able to support themselves and their own families in communities where resources are limited, where there are few referral and consultation options, and where significant sociocultural barriers (such as stigma and distrust of strangers) hamper effective service delivery. Pooling resources and establishing interdisciplinary practices are ways of addressing these shortcomings.

Recruitment, training, and retention of all kinds of health professionals are problematic for rural areas. Professionals who were initially residents of rural communities and/or have received special educational preparation for working in rural communities are more likely to remain and practice successfully than those professionals who have not had similar exposure to the challenges involved. However, there are fewer than 10 training programs which specialize in preparing doctoral level mental health providers for practice in rural communities. Recruitment and retention difficulties are also likely to be compounded by issues related to gender and cultural diversity. More female medical and mental health practitioners are needed to help address some of the sociocultural norms which may prevent rural women from receiving the best care available.

Regardless of profession or field of study, to successfully address the mental health and substance abuse needs of women living in rural communities, providers and researchers must acknowledge that solutions and approaches that have demonstrated efficacy in metropolitan, urban, and suburban settings do not automatically transfer to rural and frontier situations. As a result, we must develop creative and innovative approaches and programs that can successfully address rural mental health concerns, critically evaluate and refine our responses, disseminate our findings, and train future professionals to make use of what has been learned.

With these goals in mind, the team which created the RHP 2010 (Gamm et al. 2005) reports was tasked with gathering, assessing, and disseminating information about possible solutions or approaches that states, communities, and service providers could use to address the identified issues. In recognition of the fact that urban solutions do not always translate well into successful rural interventions, the RHP 2010 team distinguished between *best practices, model programs*, and *models for practice*. These distinctions recognize the importance of developing and implementing procedures which are robustly evidence-based while also allowing for the development and assessment of new procedures which are innovative, locally sustainable, and culturally appropriate.

The RHP 2010 reports use the terms *best practices* and *evidence-based practices* interchangeably. These are techniques and methods which demonstrate reliability in replications, often across a variety of different settings.

Model Programs are those which have demonstrated effectiveness over time and which have been innovative and problem-focused with efforts employing new approaches and technologies, establishing new coalitions of providers, and often involving radical changes to existing practices. These programs are experimental in nature and still require ongoing assessment of their effectiveness.

Finally, the RHP 2010 team proposed the term *Models for Practice* to refer to approaches that combine conceptual elements underlying both the *best practices* and *model programs* in the development of approaches that are true to the collaborative perspectives of public health, community health, and mental health disciplines. The resulting document defines *models for practice*, in part, as those which can move successfully from pilot to implementation, address one or more of the high priority rural health focus areas, are community based, include the residents of the area as partners and stakeholders, and depend on their *buy-in*.

Acknowledgment of the need for model practices and programs has allowed rural providers to propose and test many innovative approaches. Over the past decade, many of these practices have become accepted as being evidence-based. Because rural women experiencing mental and emotional distress often turn to informal sources of care (including friends, family, spouses, and religious organizations), indigenous paraprofessionals are often more readily accepted than professionals who are viewed as unknowns or newcomers. Many innovations have focused on identifying, mobilizing, and strengthening local support systems that rural women are readily able to access. Specially trained paraprofessionals indigenous to the region can help to bridge cultural or linguistic gaps, lessening the impact of stigma. Rural providers are learning to respect and work with other healers, even nontraditional healers, and to make use of the "*de facto* mental healthcare system" (Jameson and Blank 2007).

There is a growing awareness of "rural" versus "urban" knowledge, which includes the recognition that most rural residents have learned how to meet the challenges of rural life and that the knowledge they have gained over the generations is no less worthy of our attention than the knowledge which has arisen in more urban settings. To make use of this knowledge base, rural mental health providers are more likely than their urban counterparts to include extended family members in the treatment processes. This inclusion allows for increased social support, makes use of the cultural norms of providing care for family members in the home, and treats the patient in her environment. Similarly, to decrease stigma and distance, providers are being encouraged to make their practices more homelike, even serving refreshments and engaging in small talk with patients to align their own approaches with cultural norms. Other provider changes include keeping more flexible hours to include evening and weekend appointments, traveling to alternative treatment sites including the patients' homes, and locating their offices in buildings where there are many varied businesses to lessen "parking lot stigma." Reliance on alternative treatment sites, such as schools and churches, is becoming common in small communities. Schools and churches can provide usable space, and they are often centrally located and easy to access, making them valuable locations for self-help groups and other meetings. Schools often serve as primary care sites, and many children receive most of their medical and mental health care from school nurses and counselors.

Rural mental health providers are also finding that they need to be accepted as members of the community. They need to be seen as stakeholders in the success of the community rather than as outsiders trying to import change. As a part of this effort, providers have begun serving as local experts on grant writing and community organizing to help community residents access needed wraparound/ancillary services, fund safe areas for recreation and social gatherings, and make other positive changes in the local environment. Providers are expanding their perspectives on "mental and behavioral health" to include helping residents create healthier communities rather than focusing on providing one-to-one mental health services. Successful mental health programs now incorporate grassroots efforts to address the mental health needs of women in rural communities. Local citizens have begun their own "shelters" for victims of domestic violence by using private homes. Even more common are the growing number of private homes that have become live-in and/or daycare options for ill or elderly rural residents, in the same mold as those homes where young parents provide childcare for other children while staying home with their own children. Shared "homeschooling" duties are becoming common options for parents who find that small rural schools do not meet their needs or for parents who prefer not to send their children on long bus rides. All of these innovations make use of the rural environment in the design of interventions to improve mental health options for women.

Access to technology is also expanding options for services delivery in rural communities. These technologies can help to overcome geographic barriers and often lessen patient concerns about confidentiality and stigma (not always accurately, depending on the level of technology and the steps that providers have taken to ensure privacy of electronic communications). Access to technology may provide increased opportunities for rural women in terms of education and employment.

Additionally, technology can broaden their social support networks and improve responses when help is needed.

Service providers have made increasing use of synchronous communications allowing immediate transmission of the message and the response (text messaging, scheduled online chat or email sessions, telephone and televideo sessions) and asynchronous methods (unscheduled email, fax and forum style messaging). These technologies have been shown to be effective for diagnosis and follow-up, for increasing the patient's and caregiver's perceived levels of social support through opportunities to interact with various others, for providing online patient education and reminders about appointments, and even for monitoring addicts and alcoholics in recovery. Providers are also benefiting from new technologies when they are used to obtain cost-effective continuing education credits and professional consultations. There are also indications that provider burnout is lessened as a result of enhanced opportunities for communication (Baca et al. 2007).

In conclusion, addressing rural women's mental health and substance abuse concerns is a goal that cannot be accomplished by professionals in any single discipline. To address these needs, the seats at the table need to be filled by healthcare specialists, businesspeople, experts in technology and community planning, healers and community leaders from many backgrounds, social scientists, and rural women themselves. Solutions will require the design, implementation, and assessment of innovative treatment models in addition to using best practices. Rural service providers must be familiar with and respect the diversity and special needs of the local residents, open to new ideas, and willing to pay attention to the years of accumulated wisdom that rural residents have already amassed.

These problems cannot be addressed by providers who are intent upon maintaining the face to face "50 Minute Hour" in their private offices or by those who cling to beliefs in dualities, either that a mind can be treated apart from a body or that people can be treated apart from their environment and culture. There is little use for providers who persist in "turf wars," who refuse to become stakeholders in the communities they seek to serve, or who cannot become a part of a team in partnership with patients and with both traditional and nontraditional caregivers.

References

Agency for Health Care Policy and Research (AKA Agency for Healthcare Research and Quality). (1996). Improving health care for rural populations. Research in action fact sheet agency for health care policy and research (AHCPR Publication No. 96-P040). Rockville, MD: Author.

Baca, C. T., Alverson, D. C., Manuel, J. K., & Blackwell, G. L. (2007). Telecounseling in rural areas for alcohol problems. *Alcoholism Treatment Quarterly, 25*(4), 31–45.

Bove, C. F., & Olson, C. M. (2006). Obesity in low-income rural women: Qualitative insights about physical activity and eating patterns. *Women & Health, 44*(1), 57–78.

Bushy, A. (1993). Rural women: Lifestyles and health status. *Nursing Clinics of North America, 28*(1), 187–197.

Carmona, R. H. (2005, June 15). Comments on suicide prevention among native American youth. Testimony given before the Indian affairs committee of the United States Senate. Retrieved January 20, 2009, from http://www.hhs.gov/asl/testify/t050615.html

Clay, R. A. (2007). Rural substance abuse: Overcoming barriers to prevention and treatment. *SAMHSA News, 16*(4). Retrieved January 20, 2009, from http://www.samhsa.gov/SAMHSA_news/VolumeXV_4/article1.htm

Cline, T. L. (2007). From the administrator: Putting rural substance abuse "On the Map". *SAMHSA News, 16*(4). Retrieved January 29, 2009, from http://www.samhsa.gov/SAMHSA_news/VolumeXV_4/article4.htm

DeLeon, P. H., Wakefield, M., Schultz, A. J., Williams, J., & VandenBos, G. R. (1989). Rural America: Unique opportunities for health care delivery and health services research. *American Psychologist, 44*(10), 1298–1306.

Dempsey, P., Bird, D. C., & Hartley, D. (1999). Rural mental health and substance abuse. In T. C. Ricketts (Ed.), *Rural health in the United States* (pp. 159–178). New York, NY: Oxford University Press.

Donnermeyer, F. (1995) Crime and violence in rural communities. In S. M. Blaser, J. Blaser, & K. Pantoja (Eds.), *Perspectives on violence and substance use in rural America* (pp. 27–63). Oakbrook, IL: North Central Regional Educational Laboratory.

Doyle, S., Kelly-Schwartz, A., Schlossberg, M., & Stockard, J. (2006, Winter). Active community environments and health. *Journal of the American Planning Association, 71*(1), 19–31.

Fisher, V. M. (2005). *Help-seeking for Depression in Rural Women: A Community Portrait.* Unpublished doctoral dissertation, Virginia Commonwealth University, Richmond.

Gallagher, E., & Delworth, U. (1993). The third shift: Juggling employment, family, and the farm. *Journal of Rural Community Psychology, 12,* 21–36.

Gamm, L. D., Hutchison, L. L., Dabney, B. J., & Dorsey, A. M. (Eds.). (2003). *Rural healthy people 2010: A companion document to healthy people 2010* (Vol. 1). College Station, TX: The Texas A&M University System Health Science Center, School of Rural Public Health, Southwest Rural Health Research Center.

Gamm, L. D., Hutchison, L. L., Dabney, B. J., & Dorsey, A. M. (Eds.). (2005). *Rural healthypeople 2010: A companion document to healthy people 2010* (Vol. 3). College Station, TX: The Texas A&M University System Health Science Center, School of Rural Public Health, Southwest Rural Health Research Center.

Hayes, M. J., Brown, E., Hofmaster, P. A., Davare, A., Parker, K. G., & Raczek, J. (2002). Prenatal alcohol intake in a rural, caucasian clinic. *Family Medicine, 34*(2), 120–125.

Hillemeier, M. M., Weisman, C. S., Chase, G. A., & Dyer, A. M. (2007) Individual and community predictors of preterm birth and low birthweight along the rural-urban continuum in Central Pennsylvania. *Journal of Rural Health, 23*(1), 42–48.

Jameson, J. P., & Blank, M. B. (2007). The role of clinical psychology in rural mental health services: Defining problems and developing solutions. *Clinical Psychology: Science and Practice, 14*(3), 283–298.

McAlearney, A. S., Reeves, K. W., Tatum, C., & Paskett, E. D. (2007). Cost as a barrier to screening mammography among underserved women. *Ethnicity and Health, 12*(2), 189–203.

Mulder, P. L. (2002). Rural communities lack ancillary services. *The Family Psychologist, 18*(1), 7–9.

Mulder, P. L., Kenkel, M. B., Shellenberger, S., Constantine, M., Streiegel, R., Sears, S. F., et al. (2000). *Behavioral health care needs of rural women.* Washington, DC: American Psychological Association, Committee on Rural Health. Retrieved February 3, 2009, from http://www.apa.org/rural/ruralwomen.pdf

National Institute of Mental Health. (2005). *Depression.* NIMH Information Center. Retrieved April 16, 2009, from http://www.nimh.nih.gov/health/publications/depression/nimhdepression.pdf

Olson, C., & Strawderman, M. (2008). The relationship between food insecurity and obesity in rural childbearing women. *The Journal of Rural Health, 24*(1), 60–66.

Probst, J. C., Laditka, S. B., Moore, C. G., Harun, N., Powell, M. P., & Baxley, E.G. (2006). Rural-urban differences in depression prevalence: Implications for family medicine. *Family Medicine, 38*(9), 653–660.

Roenker, R. (2003). Domestic violence: Fighting back. *Odyssey of the University of Kentucky, Office of the Vice President for Research.* Retrieved February 7, 2009, from http://www.research.uky.edu/odyssey/fall03/domesticviolence.html

Rost, K., Wherry, J., Williams, C., & Smith, G. R. Jr., (1992). *De pression in rural primary care practices: Treatment and outcome.* National Institute of Mental Health mental health research conference on mental health problems in the general health care sector. Washington, DC: National Institute of Mental Health.

Rost, K., Williams, C., Wherry, J., & Smith, G. R. Jr., (1995a). The process and outcomes of care for major depression in rural family practice settings. *The Journal of Rural Health, 11*(2), 114–121.

Rost, K., Zhang, M., & Fortney, J. C. (1995b). *One year outcomes among untreated depressed individuals: Implications for outreach efforts.* National Institute of Mental Health mental health services research conference. Washington, DC: National Institute of Mental Health.

Rowland, D., & Lyons, B. (1989). Triple jeopardy: Rural, poor, and uninsured. *Health Services Research, 23,* 975–1004.

Rural Womyn Zone. (2008). Violence against rural women, What is different? Retrieved February 10, 2009, from http://www.ruralwomyn.net/

Schoenberg, N. E., Hopenhayn, C., Christian, A., Knight, E. A., & Rubio, A. (2005). An in-depth and updated perspective on determinants of cervical cancer screening among central Appalachian women. *Women & Health, 42*(2), 89–105.

Simmons, L., Anderson, E., & Braun, B. (2008a). Health needs and health utilization among rural, low-income women. *Women and Health, 47*(4), 53–68.

Simmons, L., Braun, B., Charnigo, R., Havens, J., & Wright, D. (2008b). Depression and poverty among rural women: A relationship of social causation or social selection? *The Journal of Rural Health: Official Journal of the American Rural Health Association and the National Rural Health Care Association, 24*(3), 292–298.

Simmons, L., Huddleston-Casas, C., & Berry, A. (2007). Low-income rural women and depression: Factors associated with self-reporting. *American Journal of Health Behavior, 31*(6), 657–666.

Singh, G. K., & Siahpush, M. (2002). Ethnic-Immigrant differentials in health behaviors, morbidity, and cause-specific mortality in the United States: An analysis of two national data bases. *Human Biology, 74*(1), 83–109.

Suicide Prevention Resource Center. (2008). *Preventing youth suicide in rural America: Recommendations to states.* Retrieved February 11, 2009, from http://www.sprc.org/library/ruralyouth.pdf

United States Department of Agriculture. (1998). *Metro and nonmetro income data based on census information.* Retrieved February 12, 2009, from http://www.usda.gov/news/pubs/fbook98/ch4e.htm

United States Department of Health and Human Services. (2000). *Healthy people 2010.* Washington, DC: U.S. Department of Health and Human Services. Available from http://www.healthypeople.gov/document/html/objectives/18-09.htm

United States Department of Justice, Violence Against Women Grants Office. (1997). Domestic violence and stalking: The second annual report to congress under the violence against women act. Washington, DC: Office of Justice Programs – United States Department of Justice.

Wagenfeld, M. O. (2003). A snapshot of rural and frontier America. In B. Hudnall Stamm (Ed.), *Rural behavioral health care: An interdisciplinary guide* (pp. 33–40). Washington, DC: American Psychological Association.

Wagenfeld, M. O., Murray, J. D., Mohatt, D. F., & DeBruyn, J. C. (1993). *Mental health and rural America: 1980–1993*. Washington, DC: Office of Rural Health Policy.

Chapter 17
Social and Community Contexts

Jane K. Burke-Miller

Introduction

Social context is increasingly thought to be as important as individual characteristics in determining mental health outcomes. Therefore, mental health service providers, researchers, and policy-makers need to give equal consideration to women's social contexts in order to deliver effective services. Such services are especially important for women, whose mental health is influenced by their vulnerable social status, unique social roles, and overrepresentation among the urban poor. This chapter will describe the use of social epidemiology in studying the contexts of women's mental health, the effect of social contexts on women's mental health, and implications for women's mental health prevention and treatment programs at the community level.

Social Epidemiology and Mental Health

In the late twentieth century, research into social inequalities in health grew into the field of social epidemiology, which sought to draw focus away from decontextualized individual characteristics and toward their social or ecological context. McKinlay and Marceau (2000) describe this as the philosophies of collectivism and a holistic view of health. Contextual research in social epidemiology is guided by frameworks that incorporate multiple levels of influence on individual health, including a focus on the role of place, often neighborhood, in the social production of health and health disparities (Kawachi and Berkman 2003; Krieger 2002; Mays et al. 2007). In addition, social epidemiology focuses on theories and constructs useful for analyzing social inequalities in health related to gender, class, race/ethnicity, sexuality, and disability (Krieger 2004).

J. K. Burke-Miller (✉)
Department of Psychiatry, University of Illinois at Chicago,
1601 West Taylor Street, Chicago, IL 60612, USA

B. L. Levin, M. A. Becker (eds.), *A Public Health Perspective of Women's Mental Health*,
DOI 10.1007/978-1-4419-1526-9_17, © Springer Science+Business Media LLC 2010

Although women as a group experience higher rates of affective disorders and psychological distress than men (Kessler 2003; United States Department of Health and Human Services (USDHHS) 1999), there is considerable heterogeneity among women. Explanations of this gender inequality and heterogeneity in mental health often focus on individual biochemical and psychosocial risk factors (Chen et al. 2005). However, rather than construing these aspects of experiences of inequality as solely a matter of personal identities and behaviors, practitioners of social epidemiology consider the social, political, and economic contexts in which women live their lives. These contexts are social determinants and are important considerations in understanding women's mental health and the development of community mental health services for women.

Social Class, Gender, Race, and Mental Health

The consistent relationship between lower social class (as measured by education, occupation, and economic resources) and psychological distress is well established in mental health research and psychiatric epidemiology (Eaton 2001; McLeod and Kessler 1990; Mirowsky and Ross 2003). Lower social class is thought to directly influence women's mental health by increasing deleterious exposures and limiting access to health enhancing resources throughout the lifecourse, from prenatal and childhood conditions through adulthood (Lynch and Kaplan 2000).

In addition to the deprivation of poverty, the relative nature of social class is an important mental health risk factor (Marmot and Wilkinson 2001; Murali and Oyebode 2004). Marmot and Wilkinson (2001) posit psychosocial pathways by which structural inequality affects mental health at the community level, including diminished community relationships, such as trust and helpfulness, and increased group distinctions marked by racism and sexism. Similarly, Kawachi describes three pathways by which income inequality may affect mental health: (1) underinvestment in human capital, (2) disruption of the social fabric leading to disinvestment in social capital, and (3) psychological distress resulting from social comparisons (2000).

Gender Inequality

A consistent finding in psychiatric epidemiology is that women report more psychological distress than men regardless of social class (Kessler and McRae 1981; Mirowsky and Ross 2003). This has been attributed to the sex role hypothesis that women find their social roles more stressful and less rewarding than men (Kessler and McRae 1981). Specifically, the occupational status of women tends to be lower than that of men, and at the same time, women earn less while carrying more family responsibilities (Mirowsky and Ross 2003). While some argue that the gender difference in psychological distress is a measurement artifact, others argue that it reflects the reality of the social and economic disadvantage of women compared to men (Mirowsky and Ross 2003). For example, poor women experience more frequent and traumatic life events (including domestic violence) than others, and have less control over protective resources (Belle and Doucet 2003; Miranda and Green 1999).

Gender inequality in wages in the USA has long been documented. The "wage gap" has putatively decreased since the 1970s, from women earning 59 cents to each dollar earned by men, to a 2008 estimate of 78 cents to the dollar (Semega 2009). However, significant inequalities still exist. Data from the U.S. Census Bureau 2006 American Community Survey show that among full-time, year-round workers with earnings, women's median income is 77% of men's ($32,649 compared to $42,210) and women's mean income is 71% of men's ($40,849 compared to $57,726). This is despite the generally higher levels of education of women compared to men. Wage inequality by level of education is even more striking, with women with some college education or more earning only 66% of the median income of men with the same level of education. In addition, although unemployment rates for women and men are similar (5.9% and 5.5%, respectively), far fewer women are in the labor force (71.5% of women versus 83.2% of men), and fewer of them are employed (67.2% of women versus 77.8% of men). Finally, 14.7% of women live below the federal poverty level compared to 11.9% of men. While 15% of all American families with minor children are below the federal poverty level, 36.9% of female-headed households with minor children live in poverty (U.S. Department of Commerce 2006).

This overrepresentation of women in the lower social classes, as measured by income and employment in the USA, is a manifestation of gendered social stratification and structures of power, and has consequences for women's mental health. Although the direct consequences of social class on women's mental health is well established (Belle 1990), few researchers have attempted to assess the indirect effects of gendered social structures. A notable exception is the research conducted by Chen et al. (2005) on a stratified random sample of 7,789 women in all 50 states. They characterized states using composite indices of women's economic autonomy, employment and earnings, and reproductive rights. In multilevel models controlling for individual age, race, education, and income, high scores on these indices were significantly associated with lower depression scores among women. This research demonstrates that in addition to direct deleterious mental health consequences of material disadvantage, gender inequality itself has negative consequences for women's mental health. Further, it suggests that promoting women's social status can improve their mental health by reducing economic insecurity, experiences of discrimination, and unfavorable social comparisons.

Gender and Race Inequality

Black Americans are almost three times as likely as other Americans to be living in severe poverty (Woolf et al. 2006). In 2005, about 27% of African American women were living below the federal poverty line, compared to 14% of all American women (United States Census Bureau 2005). These class and race inequalities among women are not only entrenched, but also appear to be growing (Kawachi 2000). In addition to low social class, experiences of racial discrimination are a significant risk factor for psychological distress among African American women (Williams 2002), and it is difficult to disentangle the effects of race and social class in part because of inadequate sampling of Black Americans in most large-scale psychiatric epidemiologic studies (Williams 1986).

The National Survey of Black Americans (NSBA) and its successor, the National Survey of American Life, are exceptions. In their analysis of women using data from the NSBA, Jackson and Mustillo (2001) found that lower social class and concerns about gender discrimination, but not family roles or racial discrimination, were significantly associated with psychological distress among Black women. Whether the effect of inequality on women's mental health is a direct result of deprivation or an indirect result of negative social comparisons, these findings suggest that class and race, as well as other social contexts such as sexual identity, disability, and age, will continue to be important factors in the diagnosis and treatment of women's mental disorders.

The Community Context of Women's Mental Health

There is a growing body of research that has demonstrated the significant role played by community factors in mental health outcomes. This research is characterized by the use of multilevel analytic models, which allow for the simultaneous statistical assessment of group and individual characteristics. In a review of the literature, Truong and Ma (2006) found overwhelming evidence of neighborhood effects on women's mental health, adjusting for individual characteristics. Factors such as neighborhood poverty (percentage of residents with income below the federal poverty level), neighborhood safety (frequency of crime), and neighborhood built environment (housing quality), were all significantly associated with a variety of measures of mental health symptomatology and mental disorder diagnoses. These neighborhood effects were not as strong as individual level effects, and the neighborhood measures used varied widely. However, the consistency of the findings, despite methodological differences and publication bias, indicate the importance of considering community level as well as individual level risk factors in understanding women's mental health.

Few studies have used multilevel analysis to examine the effect of community characteristics on women's mental health in particular, and those that do also examine social class and race/ethnicity. For example, a study of Detroit residents found that higher levels of psychological distress in Black women were attributable to residence in areas of concentrated poverty, regardless of a woman's individual level of impoverishment (Schulz et al. 2000). In this study, a woman's individual income mediated the negative mental health effect of residence in high-poverty neighborhoods, but did not protect them from the psychological distress associated with neighborhood disorder and racial discrimination (Schulz et al. 2006).

Similarly, in a multilevel analysis of 700 African-American women, Cutrona et al. (2000) found women's perceptions of community disorder to be significantly associated with levels of psychological distress. There also was a cross-level interaction between community and individual factors such that mental health benefit of a positive life outlook was significantly more pronounced for women living in communities characterized by high social cohesion, compared to those with positive outlooks in less cohesive communities. In a more recent study, Cutrona et al. (2005) also found that women living in neighborhoods characterized by economic disadvantage and social disorder had a higher incidence of major depression, adjusting for individual level characteristics. They conclude that neighborhood disadvantage/disorder is a vulnerability factor that increases individual women's susceptibility to onset of major depression.

Although not extensively examined using multilevel methods, it has been shown that the nature of the built environment in poverty areas is also detrimental to women's mental health. Living in high-rise, multiple dwelling units, or in poorly maintained buildings is associated with excess psychological distress among women with children (Evans 2003; Siefert et al. 2007). Poor-quality housing can create physical health problems such as respiratory conditions in women and their children, which can negatively impact women's mental health. In addition, housing has an important psychosocial influence on women's perceptions of security, control, permanence, and continuity (Siefert et al. 2007) and is therefore a vital component of mental health and well-being.

Besides neighborhood, communities can be made of shared common social identity (Campbell and Murray 2004). For example, significant communities for women may include family, friends, and civic, social, and religious organizations. These networks can both directly benefit and harm psychological well-being (Gray and Keith 2003). Family and other social ties can be stressful if they involve chronic problems, internalized discrimination, or challenging role expectations, such as socialization toward motherhood, independence, caregiving, and extended family obligations (Brown 2003). Belle and Doucet (2003) cite evidence that for poor women, social networks are more harmful than beneficial because they are associated with reduced resilience and negative behaviors, such as drinking and drug use, and family conflict. Although, in general, social networks are not as defined by geography as in the past, among poor urban women, isolation continues to limit social connections outside of local neighborhoods (Berkman and Clark 2003).

A Contextual Approach to Women's Mental Health Services Research

Society and social policy must change in order to engage in mental illness prevention at the primary level. Alegria et al. (2003) have described how specific public policies regarding housing, education, and income supports reduce social inequalities in mental health by equalizing social conditions. These policies include Section 8 housing vouchers, the Individuals with Disabilities Education Act, and the

Earned Income Tax Credit. Programs that promote employment, education, and stable housing; enhance community organizations and engagement for collective efficacy; and combat gender inequalities could alleviate the social production of psychological distress among women.

Such programs could be guided by emerging public mental health models oriented toward promoting positive qualities of daily functioning at the individual, family, and community levels (Magyary 2002). In these models, protective factors and processes can be individual or environmental characteristics that decrease the probability of developing mental health problems. Such positive mental health factors would be ecologically embedded in a socioeconomic environmental context as called for by the Basic Behavioral Science Task Force of the National Institute of Mental Health National Advisory Mental Health Council (1996). For women's mental illness prevention, such policies could emphasize career development, quality housing, and flexible childcare programs that enhance women's economic status and social networks.

This approach is responsive to the prevention of mental health problems and the promotion of positive mental health in the context of developmental epidemiologically based prevention research theory that can inform policies (Kellam et al. 1999). In this context, conceptual models are used to identify proximal targets for intervention that are mediators or moderators of the distal outcome, including mental illness or psychological distress. The theory is developmental in the sense that hypotheses focus on antecedent factors in the individual's life that interact with environmental factors to influence the lifecourse leading to poor mental health. Kellam et al. (1999) argue that a strong developmental theory should include risk and protective factors at the individual and environmental levels, including culture and social class specific to women. This research model is also relevant to the Community Science Model of Community Psychology. As described by Wandersman (2003), this model has an explicit emphasis on integrating prevention research and practice, and the active participation of the community (locus of practice) in the research.

Therefore, future public policies and programs based on this model should emphasize a community-strengths approach, promoting mutual learning and empowerment, equalizing power among participants, and integration of research and practice (Bruce et al. 2002; Schulz et al. 2002). This approach could result in development of career skills, development of long-term community capacity and resources for community organizations (Kelley et al. 2005), increased interagency and university ties (Lantz et al. 2001), and community leadership development (Kelly et al. 2004), all of which could benefit the status of women in the community. Thus, development of knowledge regarding community influences on women's mental health could also result in direct benefits to community mental health.

Implications of Contextual Approach

There are implications of the contextual approach to women's mental health in terms of the types of individual level services that should be available. First, the community location and proximity of services are important. Allard et al. (2003) found that among women receiving welfare benefits in the Detroit metropolitan area, those who lived within 1.5 miles of a mental health service provider were 30% more likely to utilize services than those who had to travel further. They suggest that mental health services programs for low-income women could mitigate the negative effect of distance by providing transportation assistance, onsite childcare, improved outreach and marketing, and linkages with community programs and organizations. The importance of outreach and marketing is supported by research showing that for racial/ethnic minority women, access to mental health services is influenced by the economic status of their neighborhood of residence. African American and Hispanic/Latina women living in low-poverty areas are significantly more likely to be referred to mental health services from the criminal justice system than by social services or by self/family/friends (Chow et al. 2003).

The damaging mental health effects of individual and community gender inequality could be mitigated by improving awareness of gender issues among mental health providers and other community health professionals. Interventions that incorporate systems change and combine prevention and treatment goals have shown potential benefits to affective disorder outcomes (Bruce et al. 2002). In addition to targeting mental health service providers, community interventions should include educational campaigns about the effects of gender inequality and community characteristics on women's mental health.

Siefert et al. (2007) found that among low-income women, those who had access to a loan in a crisis and help with childcare were less than half as likely to screen positive for major depression as others, even given significant poverty, food insecurity, and other risk factors for depression. Therefore, preventive mental health services in the community should be resource-intensive, including components such as emergency relief funds and access to childcare. Women's mental health services could also benefit from explicit linkages with community organizations that address social issues for women (e.g, education, employment, housing, and safety), and these organizations should be encouraged to include health and mental health components in their activities. Such synergistic linkages would benefit community organizations by enhancing their internal competencies and building new organizational relationships and external resources (Foster-Fishman et al. 2001; Maton 2008).

The Social Context of Recovery Services

The National Consensus Statement on Mental Health Recovery (USDHHS 2004) defines recovery as, "… a journey of healing and transformation enabling a person with a mental health problem to live a meaningful life in a community of his or her choice while striving to achieve his or her full potential." It further notes that recovery as a process and outcome has implications at individual, family, community, provider, organizational, and systems levels. This multilevel approach to recovery has also been described as an ecological perspective, incorporating the individual, their environment, and the interactions between the two (Onken et al. 2007). These elements and their synergistic interplay can work to facilitate or hinder recovery. In particular, "Recovery relies on an environment that provides opportunities and resources for new or resumed social roles, engagement in relationships with others and meaningful integration in the larger society" (Onken et al. 2007, p. 16).

Research has shown that mental health services that support recovery are influenced by their environment. For example, in a study of supported employment services for people with psychiatric disabilities, Cook et al. (2006) demonstrated that county unemployment rate was significantly associated with employment outcomes across multiple states throughout the country. However, they also found that study participants who received best practice supported employment had significantly better outcomes than those who did not, regardless of local unemployment. The participants who had the best employment outcomes in terms of having competitive jobs and working more hours were those who both received best practice supported employment services and lived in an area of relatively low unemployment. Other environment factors can also interact with recovery services, such as employment or housing discrimination based on age, race/ethnicity, gender, or the stigma of mental disorder (Burke-Miller et al. 2006; Cook and Burke 2002).

It is important to consider the social context of recovery especially because the environments of women living with mental illness are often socially marginalized, economically dire, legally unfair, and emotionally isolated (Cook and Burke 2002). The onus for the change required for successful recovery can not only lie on the individual, but on social change as well. Services that emphasize self-determination, such as consumer-operated services and self-directed care, can empower women to be in charge of their own recovery and facilitate recovery at the individual and community levels (Cook 2005).

Implications for Women's Mental Health

Social determinants of women's mental health include social class and race. Further, mediating factors are specific to social context on multiple levels, including community resources, group support, and individual identity. Response to socially determined stressors is specific to women, both as individuals and as members of communities and social networks.

Prior research has identified a number of both individual and community-level factors associated with poor women's mental health and psychological distress. Growing levels of already debilitating poverty in the USA (Woolf et al. 2006) suggest that psychological distress is likely to be an ongoing public health problem among poor women living in urban communities. Community mental health services and practice should focus on community-level prevention as well as on individual-level therapy and recovery services that emphasize self-determination for women with mental illness.

References

Alegria, M., Perez, D. J., & Williams, S. (2003). The role of public policies in reducing mental health status disparities for people of color. *Health Affairs, 22,* 51–64.

Allard, S. W., Tolman, R. M., & Rosen, D. (2003). Proximity to service providers and service utilization among welfare recipients: The interaction of place and race. *Journal of Policy Analysis and Management, 22*(4), 599–613.

Basic Behavioral Science Task Force of the National Advisory Mental Health Council. (1996). Basic behavioral science research for mental health: Sociocultural and environmental processes. *American Psychologist, 51,* 722–731.

Belle, D. (1990). Poverty and women's mental health. *American Psychologist, 45*(3), 385–389.

Belle, D., & Doucet, J. (2003). Poverty, inequality, and discrimination as sources of depression among U.S. women. *Psychology of Women Quarterly, 27,* 101–113.

Berkman, L. F., & Clark, C. (2003). Neighborhoods and networks: The construction of safe places and bridges. In I. Kawachi, & L. F. Berkman (Eds.), *Neighborhoods and health.* New York, NY: Oxford University Press.

Brown, D. R. (2003). A conceptual model of mental well-being for African American women. In D. R. Brown & V. M. Keith (Eds.), *In and out of our right minds: The mental health of african american women* (pp. 1–22). New York, NY: Columbia University Press.

Bruce, M. L., Smith, W., Miranda, J., Hoagwood, K., & Wells, K. (2002). Community-based interventions. [special issue]. *Journal of Mental Health Services Research, 4,* 205–214.

Burke-Miller, J. K., Cook, J. A., Grey, D. G., Razzano, L. A., Blyler, C. R., Leff, H. S., et al. (2006). Demographic characteristics and employment among people with severe mental illness in a multisite study. *Community Mental Health Journal, 42*(2), 143–159.

Campbell, C., & Murray, M. (2004). Community health psychology: Promoting analysis and action for social change. *Journal of Health Psychology, 9*(2), 187–196.

Chen, Y. Y., Subramanian, S. V., Acevedo-Garcia, D., & Kawachi, I. (2005). Women's status and depressive symptoms: A multilevel analysis. *Social Science and Medicine, 60,* 49–60.

Chow, J. C., Jaffee, K., & Snowden, L. (2003). Racial/ethnic disparities in the use of mental health services in poverty areas. *American Journal of Public Health, 93*(5), 792–797.

Cook, J. A. (2005). "Patient-Centered" and "Consumer-Directed" Mental Health Services. Prepared for the Institute of Medicine, Committee on Crossing the Quality Chasm – Adaptation to Mental Health and Addictive Disorders.

Cook, J. A., & Burke, J. (2002). Public policy and employment of people with disabilities: Exploring new paradigms. *Journal of Behavioral Science & the Law, 20,* 541–557.

Cook, J. A., Mulkern, V., Grey, D. D., Burke-Miller, J., Blyler, C., Razzano, L. A., et al. (2006). Effects of unemployment rate on vocational outcomes in a randomized trial of supported employment for individuals with psychiatric disabilities. *Journal of Vocational Rehabilitation, 25*(2), 71–84.

Current Population Survey, Annual Demographic Survey March Supplement, United States Census Bureau, 2005.

Cutrona, C. E., Russell, D. W., Brown, P. A., Clark, L. A., Hessling, R. M., & Gardner, K. A. (2005). Neighborhood context, personality, and stressful life events as predictors of depression among African American women. *Journal of Abnormal Psychology, 114*(1), 3–15.

Cutrona, C. E., Russell, D. W., Hessling, R. M., Brown, P. A., & Murry, V. (2000). Direct and moderating effects of community context on the psychological well-being of African American women. *Journal of Personality and Social Psychology, 79,* 1088–1101.

Eaton, W. W. (2001). *The sociology of mental disorders.* Westport, CT: Praeger Publishers.

Evans, G. W. (2003). The built environment and mental health. *Journal of Urban Health, 80*(4), 536–555.

Foster-Fishman, P. G., Berkowitz, S. L., Lounsbury, D. W., Jacobson, S., & Allen, N. A. (2001). Building collaborative capacity in community coalitions: A review and integrative framework. *American Journal of Community Psychology, 29*(2), 241–261.

Gray, B. A., & Keith, V. M. (2003). The benefits and costs of social support for African American women. In D. R. Brown & V. M. Keith (Eds.), *In and out of our right minds: The mental health of African American women* (pp. 242–257). New York, NY: Columbia University Press.

Jackson, P. B., & Mustillo, S. (2001). I am woman: The impact of social identities on African American women's mental health. *Women and Health, 32,* 33–59.

Kawachi, I. (2000). Income inequality and health. In L. F. Berkman & I. Kawachi (Eds.), *Social epidemiology* (pp. 76–94). New York, NY: Oxford University Press.

Kawachi, I., & Berkman, L. F. (2003). Introduction. In I. Kawachi & L. F. Berkman (Eds.), *Neighborhoods and health* (pp. 1–19). New York, NY: Oxford University Press.

Kellam, S. G., Koretz, D., & Moscicki, E. K. (1999). Core elements of developmental epidemiologically based prevention research. *American Journal of Community Psychology, 27,* 463–482.

Kelley, M. A., Baldyga, W., Baraja, F., & Rodriquez-Sanchez, M. (2005). Capturing change in a community-university partnership: The Si Se Puede Project. *Preventing Chronic Disease, 2*(2), A22.

Kelly, J. G., Azelton, L. S., Lardon, C., Mock, L. O., Tandon, S. D., & Thomas, M. (2004). On community leadership: Stories about collaboration in action research. *American Journal of Community Psychology, 33,* 205–216.

Kessler, R. C. (2003). Epidemiology of women and depression. *Journal of Affective Disorders, 74,* 5–13.

Kessler, R. C., & McRae, J. A. (1981). Trends in the relationship between sex and psychological distress: 1957–1976. *American Sociological Review, 46,* 443–452.

Krieger, N. (2002). A glossary for social epidemiology. *Epidemiological Bulletin, 23*(1), 7–11.

Krieger, N. (Ed.). (2004). *Embodying inequality: Epidemiologic perspectives.* Amityville, NY: Baywood Publishing Company.

Lantz, P. M., Viruell-Funetes, E., Israel, B. A., Softley, D., & Guzman, R. (2001). Can communities and academia work together on public health research? Evaluation results from a community-based participatory research partnership in Detroit. *Journal of Urban Health, 78,* 495–507.

Lynch, J. W., & Kaplan, G. A. (2000). Socioeconomic position. In L. F. Berkman & I. Kawachi (Eds.), *Social epidemiology* (pp. 13–35). New York, NY: Oxford University Press.

Magyary, D. (2002). Positive mental health: A turn of the century perspective. *Issues in Mental Health Nursing, 23,* 331–335.

Marmot, M., & Wilkinson, R. G. (2001). Psychosocial and material pathways in the relation between income and health: A response to Lynch et al. *British Medical Journal, 322,* 1233–1236.

Maton, K. I. (2008). Empowering community settings: Agents of individual development, community betterment, and positive social change. *American Journal of Community Psychology, 41,* 4–21.

Mays, V. M., Cochran, S. D., & Barnes, N. W. (2007). Race, race-based discrimination, and health outcomes among African Americans. *Annual Review of Psychology, 58,* 201–225.

McKinlay, J. B., & Marceau, L. D. (2000). To boldly go… *American Journal of Public Health, 90,* 25–33.

McLeod, J. D., & Kessler, R. C. (1990). Socioeconomic status differences in vulnerability to undesirable life events. *Journal of Health and Social Behavior, 31,* 162–172.

Miranda, J., & Green, B. L. (1999). The need for mental health services research focusing on poor young women. *Journal of Mental Health Policy and Economics, 2,* 73–80.

Mirowsky, J., & Ross, C. E. (2003). *Social causes of psychological distress.* New York, NY: Walter de Gruyter, Inc.

Murali, V., & Oyebode, F. (2004). Poverty, social inequality, and mental health. *Advances in Psychiatric Treatment, 10,* 216–224.

Onken, S. J., Craig, C. M., Ridgway, P., Ralph, R. O., & Cook, J. A. (2007). An analysis of the definitions of and elements of recovery: A review of the literature. *Psychiatric Rehabilitation Journal, 31*(1), 9–22.

Schulz, A. J., Israel, B. A., Zenk, S. N., Parker, E. A., Lichtenstein, R., Shellman-Weir, S., et al. (2006). Psychosocial stress and social support as mediators of relationships between income, length of residence and depressive symptoms among African American women on Detroit's eastside. *Social Science & Medicine, 62,* 510–522.

Schulz, A., Krieger, J., & Galea, S. (2002). Addressing social determinants of health: Community-based participatory approaches to research and practice. *Health Education and Behavior, 29,* 287–295.

Schulz, A. J., Williams, D. R., Israel, B. A., Becker, A, Parker, E., James, S. A., et al. (2000). Unfair treatment, neighborhood effects, and mental health in the Detroit metropolitan area. *Journal of Health and Social Behavior, 41*(3), 314–332.

Semega, J. (2009). Men's and women's earnings by state: 2008 American Community Surveys. American Community Survey Reports, U.S. Bureau of the Census, Washington, DC.

Siefert, K., Finlayson, T. L., Williams, D. R., Delva, J., & Ismail, A. I. (2007). Modifiable risk and protective factors for depressive symptoms in low-income African American mothers. *American Journal of Orthopsychiatry, 77*(1), 113–123.

Truong, K., & Ma, S. (2006). A systematic review of relations between neighborhoods and mental health. *Journal of Mental Health Policy and Economics, 9,* 137–154.

United States Department of Commerce. Bureau of the Census, 2008-12-15, American Community Survey (ACS): Public Use Microdata Sample (PUMS), 2006.

United States Department of Health and Human Services. (1999). *Mental health: A report of the surgeon general.* Rockville, MD: U.S. Department of Health and Human Services, Substance Abuse and Mental Health Services Administration, Center for Mental Health Services, National Institutes of Health, National Institute of Mental Health.

United States Department of Health and Human Services. (2004). *National concensus statement on mental health recovery.* Rockville, MD: U.S. Department of Health and Human Services, Substance Abuse and Mental Health Services Administration, Center for Mental Health Services.

Wandersman, A. (2003). Community science: Bridging the gap between science and practice with community-centered models. *American Journal of Community Psychology, 31,* 227–242.

Williams, D. R. (1986). The epidemiology of mental illness in Afro-Americans. *Hospital and Community Psychiatry, 37,* 42–49.

Williams, D. R. (2002). Racial/ethnic variations in women's health: The social embeddedness of health. *American Journal of Public Health, 92*(4), 588–597.

Woolf, S. H., Johnson, R. E., & Geiger, H. J. (2006). The rising prevalence of severe poverty in America: A growing threat to public health. *American Journal of Preventive Medicine, 31*(4), 332–341.

Chapter 18
Racial and Ethnic Disparities

Yuri Jang, David A. Chiriboga and Marion Ann Becker

Introduction

The primary objective of this chapter is to provide information on economic, psychiatric, and cultural factors that influence service access by racial/ethnic minority women. A secondary objective is to discuss the policy implications of existing research for mental health services that are provided to this population. These objectives draw from the extent and nature of the problems faced by minority women. According to the recent estimates, of the nearly 153 million women living in the USA, more than 31 million (20%) are members of racial/ethnic minorities (U.S. Census Bureau 2007). Their health, therefore, both physical and mental, assumes significance in terms of health services provision and overall social policy.

The disadvantages faced by men and women from racial/ethnic groups are well documented and include lower socioeconomic status, poorer health conditions, lower utilization of services, and higher rates of premature death, disease, and disability (Smedley et al. 2003). Despite a decade-long effort to close the gap in health status and socioeconomic status between majority and minority populations, disparities continue to exist (Satcher 2007; Smedley et al. 2003; U.S. Department of Health and Human Services (DHHS) 2001). The disparities are particularly problematic and entrenched for racial/ethnic women, because these women are often faced with multiple economic and social disadvantages and are more likely to be subjected to racism, sexism, and classism (Brown and Keith 2003). The devalued social status of minority women, in turn, has important implications not only for their physical health, but also for the topic on which this chapter focuses— their mental health.

Y. Jang (✉)
Department of Aging & Mental Health Disparities, Florida Mental Health Institute,
University of South Florida, Tampa, FL 33612, USA

B. L. Levin, M. A. Becker (eds.), *A Public Health Perspective of Women's Mental Health*,
DOI 10.1007/978-1-4419-1526-9_18, © Springer Science+Business Media LLC 2010

Minority Women's Mental Health

One of the most widely replicated findings in the mental health literature is the greater prevalence of depression among women compared to men. Most studies have reported that women are up to twice as likely as men to suffer from depression (Blazer et al. 1994; Kessler 2003). Regardless of whether the method of assessment is based on self-report or diagnostic interview, women manifest more signs and symptoms of depression (Blazer et al. 1998; Kessler 2003; Nolen-Hoeksema et al. 1999). The finding holds true not only for non-Hispanic Whites but also for racial/ethnic minority groups (Cochran et al. 1999; Myers and Rodriguez 2002; Rosen et al. 2003). Factors such as low income and education, unemployment or employment in low-status and high-stress jobs, large family size, marital dissolution, family conflicts, trauma exposure, single parenthood, racism, and discrimination, which are often observed in the lives of minority women, put these women at a higher risk for depression (McGrath et al. 1990).

The confluence of all of these contributing factors varies from group to group. Historical and contextual circumstances that are specific to each racial/ethnic group should also be considered when assessing the mental health of minority women. For example, the fact that many Native American women are victims of incest, rape, and other forms of sexual assault may contribute to their particularly high levels of mental health problems and substance abuse (McGrath et al. 1990; Walters and Simoni 2002).

Immigration, especially in the context of refugee status, has a pervasive influence on mental health. Women who are immigrants must deal with the need to adapt to the host culture. It is well documented that lack of acculturation limits opportunities for social participation and socioeconomic advancement and causes various forms of mental distress (Berry 2002; Chiriboga et al. 2002; Myers and Rodriguez 2002).

In addition to the challenges associated with acculturation, a host of traumatic experiences may precede arrival in the USA. This is especially true for refugees. In the case of Southeast Asian refugee women, the prevalence of posttraumatic stress disorder is high due to their unique history (McGrath et al. 1990; Yee and Chiriboga 2007). Appreciation of the historical and contextual background facilitates a more effective assessment and treatment of mental health problems in minority women.

Minority women are more likely to be exposed to stressful life circumstances due to their multiple roles, including employment, housekeeping, childrearing, and family caregiving (Brown and Keith 2003). Coincident with their traditional gender role as a "kin keeper" and the strong emphasis on family in minority cultures, minority women are more likely to be positioned as caregivers of young children, aging parents, and ill and/or disabled relatives. Particularly when their resources are limited, minority women are likely to experience role overload, which may lead to mental distress.

It is interesting that a line of research has shown the unique strengths and resilience of racial/ethnic minorities in coping with adversities in life. African-American women fare better than White women when faced with stressful life situations such as caregiving (Roth et al. 2001) and bereavement (Balaswamy and Richardson 2001). There is a wide range of variation in the way individuals appraise and respond to life stresses, and cultural values and beliefs play a significant role in this process. It has been suggested that African-American women may be hardier in response to life stresses because they are better socialized to cope with uncertainty or adversity in life (Gibson 1986). Studies have found that religious beliefs and values are important resources for African-American women in coping with crises and challenges (Jang et al. 2005). The beneficial role of a strong family and community support has also been documented in studies of minority populations (Dilworth-Anderson and Burton 1999; Noh and Kaspar 2003). In addition, cultural identity is a protective factor against life stress among various groups of minority women (Jones et al. 2007; Walters and Simoni 2002).

Culture and Mental Health

Although personal history plays an important role in mental health and response to treatment across all groups, the experience and manifestation of mental disorders is often mediated by cultural factors (Kleinman 2004). For example, although somatization (the physical expression of mental distress such as pains and aches in the absence of physiological causes) is a common idiom of mental distress (Simon et al. 1999), it is especially prevalent among racial/ethnic minorities and women (Lin and Cheung 1999; Lu et al. 1995; U.S. DHHS 2001). Myers et al. (2002) reported that African-American and Hispanic women express more somatic complaints than White women even after the effects of socioeconomic status are controlled.

Researchers have identified a number of mental disorders that are specific to certain cultural groups, and the *Diagnostic and Statistical Manual of Mental Disorders* (4th ed.) classifies these as culture-bound syndromes (U.S. DHHS 2001). Examples of recognized culture-bound syndromes include (a) *ataque de nervios* among Hispanics ("uncontrollable shouting, crying, trembling, and aggression typically triggered by a stressful event involving family"); (b) *taijin kyofusho* among the Japanese ("intense fear that one's body displeases, embarrasses, or is offensive to other people in appearance, odor, facial expressions, or movement"); and (c) *hwa-byung* among Koreans ("chest discomfort, burning up, feelings of suffocation, and heat sensation caused by the suppression of anger"; American Psychiatric Association 1994). In the assessment of cultural groups, studies have shown that women and those with low acculturation are more vulnerable to culture-bound syndromes (Pang 1998). However, it is likely that many such syndromes are as yet unidentified in the literature.

Gender and culture influence not only prevalence and symptom presentation but also response to treatment (Kornstein 2002). Increasing attention is being paid to differential responses to treatments across racial/ethnic and gender groups (Kornstein 2002; Ward 2007). Due to racial/ethnic differences in drug metabolism and pharmacodynamics, treatment responses to psychiatric medications vary across groups (Lin and Cheung 1999; Strickland et al. 1997), a fact that has important implications for medication dosages and potential side effects. The health beliefs of different racial/ethnic groups, because they include views about causality and cure, may also affect how interventions are viewed and how effective they are (Alvidrez 1999). This line of study suggests the need for a group-specific approach to the assessment and treatment of mental disorders.

Studying variation by specific groups brings up the question of what is meant when culture is posited as a source of variation. Health professionals often use the term *culture* to refer to values and beliefs, including health beliefs associated with clients from differing backgrounds. Used in this way, culture may help providers to understand that a particular client may be responding and understanding in ways that are atypical—or, at least, may have a greater potential for responding in atypical ways than might be the norm. *Acculturation* is another useful term. It is generally defined in terms of an individual's knowledge about the host culture (Berry 2002). This concerns not only the ability to speak the language of the host culture, but also knowledge about appropriate behavior, attire, use of public and private transportation, and the healthcare system.

Proficiency in English is a central dimension of both acculturation and assimilation. Generally, those who are more educated and hold higher paying jobs experience fewer problems with acculturation and assimilation (Moyerman and Forman 1992). Controlling for socioeconomic status, however, does not eliminate the differences. Among older Mexican-Americans, for example, those lower on acculturation report more symptoms of depression, even if they are second-generation Mexican-Americans (Chiriboga et al. 2002; Gonzalez et al. 2001).

As noted, the ability to use, and the actual use of, English is a central component of most conceptual frameworks and instruments related to acculturation in the USA. Part of the reason for this may be that in the absence of linguistic proficiency, an individual is likely to encounter many barriers to service access and utilization. The social context, however, is a critical factor. For example, a Chinese-American living in San Francisco's Chinatown, a Mexican-American in a *barrio* along the border with Mexico, or a Cuban-American living in Miami may not encounter problems accessing the healthcare system. A deciding factor concerning the efficacy of the social support network may be whether there is anyone who can facilitate interactions with the more formal systems of care (Doty 2003). Chiriboga et al. (2002) reported that among older Mexican-Americans, the more often Spanish was used in family gatherings, the greater was the probable depression of the participants. This finding supports the hypothesis that when an extended family as a whole lacks English proficiency, it is less able to support individual family members in need of mental health treatment because of problems accessing the healthcare system.

There is evidence that individuals who are less acculturated are less likely to seek help for their mental health problems. Generation and immigration status also make a difference. There is evidence that first-generation Mexican-American children have less access to health care and lower rates of utilization than White and Black children, but this disadvantage is reduced for successive generations (Burgos et al. 2005; Tienda and Mitchell 2006).

These findings concerning the relationship of acculturation to service utilization have a direct bearing on women's health. By and large, immigrant women operate at lower levels of acculturation than men. The reasons behind this difference are unclear. To explore one of the possible reasons, we present results obtained from a study modeled after the four Established Populations for Epidemiologic Studies of the Elderly (Cornoni-Huntley et al. 1990). One of the largest epidemiological studies of Mexican-Americans, the study included face-to-face interviews with a multistage probability sample of 3,030 Mexican-American men and women aged 65 and older (Chiriboga et al. 2007; Markides et al. 1999). The sampling frame drew from a five-state region: Texas, New Mexico, Arizona, Colorado, and California. An acculturation score was derived from 16 questions that dealt with facility with English; whether friends, neighbors, and work associates were primarily Anglos or Hispanics; and settings in which either English or Spanish was used (Chiriboga et al. 2002). A median split was used to classify participants as higher or lower in acculturation. In analyses conducted for this chapter, and as expected on the basis of the existing literature, men were more acculturated than women: 54.8% of the men and only 46.4% of the 1,757 women were classified as highly acculturated ($\chi^2 = 20.59$, $p = .000$).

The basic gender difference, however, is only part of the story. It was hypothesized that one source of the gender difference might lie in differential exposure to non-Hispanics, and that a proxy variable for this differential exposure might be work history. To explore this possibility, we divided all participants (men and women) into those who had never worked versus those who had. Very few men had no work history, compared to 81% of the women. The results for the women indicated that among those reporting a work history, 49.5% were categorized among the more highly acculturated; among those without a work history, only 33.5% were so categorized. Another way of looking at this is that slightly more than 50% of women who had worked were listed as lower in acculturation, but the same was true of two-thirds of women who had never worked. These differences were significant ($\chi^2 = 28.13$, $p = .000$) and suggest that Mexican-American men and women with a shared history of prior work exposure may not differ in any meaningful way in level of acculturation. As pointed out by Sue and Sue (2008), as more and more immigrant and minority women enter the labor force, they are likely to break free from traditional roles and become more independent.

We also looked at the relationship between acculturation and both depressive symptomatology (as measured by the Center for Epidemiological Studies—Depression scale (CES-D); Radloff 1977) and service utilization (as measured by whether the participant had seen a dentist within the past 2 years). In both cases, the results suggest that high acculturation and a work history act as protective factors. For men and women with a work history, there was a significant difference in the proportion of the highly acculturated who scored at the probable depression level of 16 or above on the CES-D: 20% of those who had worked scored as probably depressed compared to 36% of those who had not worked ($\chi^2 = 15.20$, $p = .000$). The differences were not significant for those lower in acculturation, who on average were more likely to be judged as probably depressed. Among women only, the highly acculturated with a work history were again significantly less likely to have scores of 16 or greater on the CES-D: 24.5% compared to 36% for those without a work history ($\chi^2 = 5.87, p = .015$; one-sided Fisher's exact test $p = .01$). The associations for women lower on acculturation were not significant.

To explore utilization, we looked at a question that dealt with how long ago the participant had visited a dentist. The more acculturated, whether male or female, were more likely to report having visited a dentist within 2 years. The differences were not marked, but they were still significant. For example, 44% of the more acculturated women had visited the dentist within 2 years compared with 36% of those who were lower in acculturation ($\chi^2 = 10.94$, $p = .001$). Moreover, highly acculturated women with a work history (45%) were more likely than acculturated women without a work history (35%) to have visited the dentist within the past 2 years. This latter difference was significant (one-sided Fisher's exact test $p = .02$), whereas among women low in acculturation, work history had no effect.

Overall, the results confirm that acculturation is associated with mental health and with service utilization and that, for women, work history also plays an important role. At the same time, a number of studies suggest that although Mexican-American women who immigrated to the USA have higher rates of affective disorders than immigrant men, their rates are actually lower than those of their US-born counterparts (Grant et al. 2004; Vega et al. 2004).

Mental Health Services Utilization

Gender role, culture, acculturation, and other factors discussed in this chapter are not simply esoteric academic issues but ones that affect access to care and service utilization. Underutilization of mental health services among minorities is well documented (Cook et al. 2007; Snowden and Yamada 2005; U.S. DHHS 2001). Despite evidence that women are more sensitive to personal emotions and more willing to talk about their emotional distress (Burns and Rapee 2006; Fischer and Turner 1970), mental health service utilization rates are low among minority women. Instead of seeking help from mental health professionals, minority women prefer to get guidance for their emotional problems from informal sources such as family, friends, and religious communities (U.S. DHHS 2001).

The lowest rates of utilization for minority women tend to be most evident among recent immigrants, who often have more mental health problems (Katz and Gagnon 2002). In one study, clinicians were asked about their experiences providing care to immigrant women suffering from postpartum depression. Teng et al. (2007) identified two barriers to care. The first barrier involved practical issues, such as the women not knowing that services were available, not knowing where the services could be obtained, and having limited proficiency with English. The second barrier involved cultural issues, such as the perceived stigma associated with mental health problems. Providers also mentioned that they themselves experienced barriers to adequate provision of care, including the lack of appropriate assessment tools and language problems.

Whether immigrants or not, minority women face still other barriers to mental health service utilization. These barriers include limited or no insurance coverage, inability to pay for services, and lack of transportation and child care. All are impediments to mental health service use, and all are more likely to be encountered among women from minority populations (U.S. DHHS 2001). Of particular concern is that minority women represent a substantial portion of the uninsured population. Compared to White women, African-American women are twice as likely and Hispanic women are three times as likely to lack insurance coverage (Agency for Healthcare Research and Quality 2007).

In addition to access, cultural beliefs and the stigma attached to mental disorders have served as key barriers to service use among minority women (U.S. DHHS 2001). A stigma on mental illness is common throughout the world (World Health Organization 2001); however, it is particularly embedded in minority cultures (Leong and Lau 2001). Minorities tend to lack general knowledge about mental health (U.S. DHHS 2001) and disbelieve the medical model of depression that portrays depression as a disease requiring professional treatment (Karasz 2005). Minorities often view depression as a sign of weakness or lack of discipline and willpower (Leong and Lau 2001; Mills et al. 2004). Particularly in Asian cultures, in which endurance and internalization of emotional troubles is considered a woman's virtue, outward help-seeking for personal emotion is discouraged (Leong and Lau 2001). Such cultural characteristics mean Asian-Americans seek mental health services long after the onset of symptoms, resulting in the need for more intensive and extended treatment (Lin and Cheung 1999; Snowden and Cheung 1990).

Even if minorities access mental health services, the quality of services that they receive is often inadequate. According to the *National Healthcare Disparities Report* (Agency for Healthcare Research and Quality 2005), minority mental health service users receive lower quality care than do Whites. Also, adherence to treatment regimes among minority service users is lower than among Whites. Dropout rates from counseling and nonadherence to psychiatric medication are consistently higher among minority groups than Whites (Sue and Sue 2008). Some studies have reported that engagement in counseling and treatment adherence is improved when the race/ethnicity of client and therapist is matched, elucidating the benefits of cultural competence in mental health services (Smith et al. 2008). Exemplary factors that facilitate minority clients' compliance and satisfaction with services may include language competence, appreciation of cultural beliefs and values, respect, trust, and responsiveness to clients' need.

Implications for Women's Mental Health

In the U.S. Surgeon General report *Mental Health, Culture, Race, and Ethnicity* (U.S. DHHS 2001), eliminating racial disparities in the utilization of mental health services was identified as a top priority. Despite increased attention to mental health disparities during the ensuing years, it is evident that racial/ethnic minority women with psychiatric disorders still rarely use mental health services. Recent research indicated that utilization disparities among Hispanics and African-Americans compared to Non-Hispanic Whites actually worsened from 2000 to 2004 (Cook et al. 2007; Dobalian and Rivers 2008). Such disparities increase the likelihood that a major depressive disorder will become a chronic illness resulting in decreased daily functioning (Breslau et al. 2005; Williams et al. 2007).

These findings underline the urgent need for policy initiatives and service delivery strategies to improve mental health services for minority women. There is a critical need for additional research to explore specific risk and protective factors among these at-risk populations, along with barriers to, and facilitators of, service utilization. Culturally sensitive, gender-specific intervention programs should be developed and implemented to increase service use and improve community-wide well-being. Understanding sociocultural characteristics related to healthcare, including service access issues, is necessary to better serve minority populations. Designing programs specifically targeted to promote mental health literacy, increase awareness of available services, foster navigation of health and mental health systems, and reduce the stigma associated with mental disorders is a vital component of rendering mental health disparities a thing of the past.

References

Agency for Healthcare Research and Quality. (2005). *National healthcare disparities report.* Rockville, MD: U.S. Department of Health and Human Services.

Agency for Healthcare Research and Quality. (2007). *Health care for minority women.* Rockville, MD: U.S. Department of Health and Human Services.

Alvidrez, J. (1999). Ethnic variations in mental health attitudes and service use among low-income African American, Latina, and European American young women. *Community Mental Health Journal, 35,* 515–530.

American Psychiatric Association. (1994). *Diagnostic and statistical manual of mental disorders* (4th ed.). Washington, DC: Author.

Balaswamy, S., & Richardson, V. (2001). The cumulative effects of life event, personal and social resources on subjective well-being of elderly widowers. *International Journal of Aging and Human Development, 53,* 311–327.

Berry, J. (2002). Conceptual approaches to acculturation. In K. Chun, P. Organista, & G. Marin (Eds.), *Acculturation: Advances in theory, measurement, and applied research* (pp. 17–37). Washington, DC: American Psychological Association.

Blazer, D., Kessler, R., McGonagle, K., & Swartz, M. (1994). The prevalence and distribution of major depression in a national community sample: The national comorbidity survey. *American Journal of Psychiatry, 151,* 979–986.

Blazer, D., Landerman, L., Hays, J., Simonsick, E., & Saunders, W. (1998). Symptoms of depression among community-dwelling elderly African American and white older adults. *Psychological Medicine, 28,* 1311–1320.

Breslau, J., Kendler, K. S., Su, M., Gaxiola-Aguilar, S., & Kessler, R. C. (2005). Life-time risk and persistence of psychiatric disorders across ethnic groups in the United States. *Psychological Medicine, 35,* 317–325.

Brown, D., & Keith, V. (2003). *In and out of our right minds: The mental health of African American women.* New York, NY: Columbia University Press.

Burgos, A. E., Schetzina, K. E., Dixon, L. B., & Mendoza, F. S. (2005). Importance of generational status in examining access to and utilization of health care services by Mexican American children. *Pediatrics, 115,* e322–e330.

Burns, J., & Rapee, R. (2006). Adolescent mental health literacy: Young people's knowledge of depression and help seeking. *Journal of Adolescence, 29,* 225–239.

Chiriboga, D., Black, S., Aranda, M., & Markides, K. (2002). Stress and depressive symptoms among Mexican American elders. *Journal of Gerontology: Psychological Sciences, 57B,* P559–P568.

Chiriboga, D. A., Jang, Y., Banks, S. M., & Kim, G. (2007). Acculturation and its effects on symptom structure in a sample of Mexican American elders. *Hispanic Journal of Behavioral Sciences, 29*(1), 83–100.

Cochran, D., Brown, D., & McGregor, K. (1999). Racial differences in the multiple social roles of older women: Implications for depressive symptoms. *The Gerontologist, 39,* 465–472.

Cook, B. L., McGuire, T., & Miranda, J. (2007). Measuring trends in mental health care disparities, 2000–2004. *Psychiatric Services, 58,* 1533–1540.

Cornoni-Huntley, J., Blazer, D. G., Lafferty, M. E., Everett, D. F., Brock, D. B., & Farmer, M. E. (Eds.). (1990). *Established populations for epidemiologic studies of the elderly: Vol. 2. Resource data book* (National Institutes of Health Publication No. 90–495). Washington, DC: National Institute on Aging.

Dilworth-Anderson, P., & Burton, L. (1999). Critical issues in understanding family support and older minorities. In T. P. Miles (Ed.), *Full color aging: Facts, goals, and recommendations for America's diverse elders* (pp. 93–105). Washington, DC: The Gerontological Society of America.

Dobalian, A., & Rivers, P. A. (2008). Racial and ethnic disparities in the use of mental health services. *Journal of Behavioral Health Services Research, 32*(2), 128–143.

Doty, M. (2003, February). *Hispanic patients' double burden: Lack of health insurance and limited English* (Publication No. 592). New York, NY: Commonwealth Fund.

Fischer, E., & Turner, J. (1970). Orientations to seeking professional help: Development and research utility of an attitude scale. *Journal of Consulting and Clinical Psychology, 35,* 79–90.

Gibson, R. (1986). Older black Americans. *Generations, 10,* 35–39.

Gonzalez, H. M., Haan, M. N., & Hinton, L. (2001). Acculturation and the prevalence of depression in older Mexican Americans: Baseline results of the Sacramento area Latino study on aging. *Journal of the American Geriatrics Society, 49,* 948–953.

Grant, B. F., Stinson, F. S., Hasin, D. S., Dawson, D. A., Chou, S. P., & Anderson, K. (2004). Immigration and lifetime prevalence of *DSM-IV* psychiatric disorders among Mexican Americans and non-Hispanic whites in the United States: Results from the national epidemiologic survey on alcohol and related conditions. *Archives of General Psychiatry, 61,* 1226–1233.

Jang, Y., Borenstein, A., Chiriboga, D., & Mortimer, D. (2005). Depressive symptoms among African American and white older adults. *Journal of Gerontology: Psychological Sciences, 60B,* P313–P319.

Jones, H., Cross, W., & DeFour, D. (2007). Race-related stress, racial identity attitudes, and mental health among black women. *Journal of Black Psychology, 33,* 208–231.

Karasz, A. (2005). Cultural differences in conceptual models of depression. *Social Science & Medicine, 60,* 1625–1635.

Katz, D., & Gagnon, A. (2002). Evidence of adequacy of postpartum care for immigrant women. *Canadian Journal of Nursing Research, 34,* 71–81.

Kessler, R. C. (2003). Epidemiology of women and depression. *Journal of Affective Disorders, 74,* 5–13.

Kleinman, A. (2004). Culture and depression. *New England Journal of Medicine, 351,* 951–953.

Kornstein, S. (2002). Gender-based difference in the treatment of depression. In K. Pearson, S. Sonawalla, & J. Rosenbaum (Eds.), *Women's health and psychiatry.* Philadelphia, PA: Lippincott, Williams & Wilkins.

Leong, F., & Lau, A. (2001). Barriers to providing effective mental health services to Asian Americans. *Mental Health Services Research, 3,* 201–214.

Lin, K., & Cheung, F. (1999). Mental health issues for Asian Americans. *Psychiatric Services, 50,* 774–780.

Lu, F., Lim, R., & Mezzich, J. (1995). Issues in the assessment and diagnosis of culturally diverse individuals. In J. Oldham & M. Riba (Eds.), *Review of psychiatry* (pp. 477–510). Washington, DC: American Psychiatric Press.

Markides, K. S., Stroup-Benham, C. A., Black, S. A., Satish, S., Perkowski, L. C., & Ostir, G. (1999). The health of Mexican American elderly: Selected findings from the Hispanic EPESE. In M. Wykle & A. Ford (Eds.), *Planning services for minority elderly in the 21st century* (pp. 72–90). New York, NY: Springer.

McGrath, E., Keita, G. P., Strickland, B. R., & Russo, N. F. (1990). *Women and depression: Risk factors and treatment issues.* Washington, DC: American Psychological Association.

Mills, T., Alea, N., & Cheong, J. (2004). Differences in the indicators of depressive symptoms among a community sample of African-American and Caucasian older adults. *Community Mental Health Journal, 40,* 309–331.

Moyerman, D. R., & Forman, B. D. (1992). Acculturation and adjustment: A meta-analytic study. *Hispanic Journal of Behavioral Sciences, 14,* 163–200.

Myers, H., Lesser, I., Rodriguez, N., Mira, C., Hwang, W., Camp, C., et al. (2002). Ethnic differences in clinical presentation of depression in adult women. *Cultural Diversity and Ethnic Minority Psychology, 8,* 138–156.

Myers, H., & Rodriguez, N. (2002). Acculturation and physical health in racial and ethnic minorities. In K. M. Chun, P. B. Organista, & G. Marin (Eds.), *Acculturation: Advances in theory, measurement, and applied research* (pp. 163–185). Washington, DC: American Psychological Association.

Noh, S., & Kaspar, V. (2003). Perceived discrimination and depression: Moderating effects of coping, acculturation, and ethnic support. *American Journal of Public Health, 93,* 232–238.

Nolen-Hoeksema, S., Larson, J., & Grayson, C. (1999). Explaining the gender difference in depressive symptoms. *Journal of Personality and Social Psychology, 77,* 1061–1072.

Pang, K. (1998). Symptoms of depression in elderly Korean immigrants: Narration and the healing process. *Culture, Medicine and Psychiatry, 22,* 93–122.

Radloff, L. S. (1977). The CES-D scale: A self-report depression scale for research in the general population. *Applied Psychological Measurement, 1,* 385–401.

Rosen, D., Spencer, M., Tolman, R., Williams, D., & Jackson, J. (2003). Psychiatric disorders and substance abuse dependence among unmarried low-income mothers. *Health and Social Work, 28,* 157–165.

Roth, D., Haley, W., Owen, J., Clay, O., & Goode, K. (2001). Latent growth models of the longitudinal effects of dementia caregiving: A comparison of African American and white family caregivers. *Psychology and Aging, 16,* 427–436.

Satcher, G. (2007, August). *Culture, race, ethnicity, and mental health: A dialogue.* Plenary address at the 115th Annual Convention of the American Psychological Association, San Francisco, CA.

Simon, G., VonKorff, M., Piccinelli, M., Fullerton, C., & Ormel, J. (1999). An international study of the relation between somatic symptoms and depression. *New England Journal of Medicine, 341,* 1329–1355.

Smedley, B., Stith, A., & Nelson, A. (2003). *Unequal treatment: Confronting racial and ethnic disparities in health care.* Washington, DC: National Academies Press.

Smith, L., Constantine, M. G., & Dize, C. B. (2008). The territory ahead for multicultural competence: The "spinning" of racism. *Professional Psychology: Research and Practice, 39,* 337–345.

Snowden, L., & Cheung, F. (1990). Use of inpatient mental health services by members of ethnic minority groups. *American Psychologist, 45,* 347–355.

Snowden, L., & Yamada, A. (2005). Cultural differences in access to care. *Annual Review of Clinical Psychology, 1,* 143–146.

Strickland, T., Stein, R., Lin, K. M., Risby, E., & Fong, R. (1997). The pharmacologic treatment of anxiety and depression in African Americans: Considerations for the general practitioner. *Archives of Family Medicine, 6,* 371–375.

Sue, D. W., & Sue, D. (2008). *Counseling the culturally diverse: Theory and practice* (5th ed.). Hoboken, NJ: Wiley.

Teng, L., Blackmore, E. R., & Stewart, D. E. (2007). Healthcare worker's perceptions of barriers to care by immigrant women with postpartum depression: An exploratory qualitative study. *Archives of Women's Mental Health, 10*, 93–101.

Tienda, M., & Mitchell, F. (2006). *Multiple origins, uncertain destinies: Hispanics and the American future.* Washington, DC: National Academies Press.

U.S. Census Bureau. (2007, July 1). *Annual estimates of the population by sex, race, and Hispanic origin for the United States.* Washington, DC: U.S. Department of Commerce.

U.S. Department of Health and Human Services. (2001). *Mental health: Culture, race, and ethnicity—A supplement to* Mental health: A report of the Surgeon General. Rockville, MD: U.S. Department of Health and Human Services, Substance Abuse and Mental Health Services Administration, Center for Mental Health Services, National Institutes of Health, National Institute of Mental Health.

Vega, W., Sribney, W., Aguilar-Gaxiola, S., & Kolody, B. (2004). 12-month prevalence of *DSM-III-R* psychiatric disorders among Mexican Americans: Nativity, social assimilation, and age determinants. *Journal of Nervous and Mental Disease, 192,* 532–541.

Walters, K., & Simoni, J. (2002). Reconceptualizing native women's health: An "indigenist" stress-coping model. *American Journal of Public Health, 92*, 520–524.

Ward, E. (2007). Examining differential treatment effects for depression in racial and ethnic minority women: A qualitative systematic review. *Journal of the National Medical Association, 99,* 265–274.

Williams, D. R., González, H. M., Neighbors, H., Nesse, R., Abelson, J. M., Sweetman, J., et al. (2007). Prevalence and distribution of major depressive disorder in African Americans, Caribbean blacks, and non-Hispanic whites: Results from the National Survey of American life. *Archives of General Psychiatry, 64,* 305–315.

World Health Organization. (2001). *World health report 2001. Mental health: New understanding, new hope.* Geneva, Switzerland: Author.

Yee, W. B. K., & Chiriboga, D. A. (2007). Issues of diversity in health psychology and aging. In C. M. Aldwin, C. L. Park, & A. Spiro, III (Eds.), *Handbook of health psychology and aging* (pp. 286–312). New York, NY: Guilford Press.

Chapter 19
Parenting and Recovery for Mothers with Mental Disorders

Joanne Nicholson

Introduction

Parenting is a significant role for many mothers with mental disorders, offering both opportunities to facilitate as well as impede recovery. The purpose of this chapter is to provide an ecological approach to motherhood and recovery, acknowledging the complex nature of the relationships between mothers and children, and considering the context in which these relationships grow and develop. National prevalence data are used to describe mothers with mental disorders and the background and experiential characteristics that shape their life contexts. Key components for interventions are described, drawing from relevant literature and previous studies, and implications for mental health policy and services delivery are discussed.

Parenting is a significant life role for the majority of American women, including those with mental disorders (Mowbray et al. 1995; Nicholson et al. 2004). Not only is success in this role a normal life goal for many, but functioning as well as possible as parents, particularly for mothers with mental disorders and related disabilities, would seem to be intimately related to the recovery process and successful functioning in other major life domains (e.g., employment, community living, and personal health and well-being). The achievement of maximum community participation for women with mental disorders may hinge on addressing the disabilities conveyed by these disorders for women in their functioning as mothers.

The relationship between motherhood and other aspects of the lives of women with mental disorders is complex. For example, a woman's status and functioning as a parent may influence the goals she sets for employment and her capacity to achieve them. The relationships between a woman's mental health, her mothering status and responsibilities, and her ability to obtain and sustain employment warrant increased attention, particularly given the impact of welfare reform in the

J. Nicholson (✉)
Department of Psychiatry, Center for Mental Health Services Research, University of Massachusetts Medical School, 55 Lake Avenue North, Worcester, MA 01655, USA

B. L. Levin, M. A. Becker (eds.), *A Public Health Perspective of Women's Mental Health*, DOI 10.1007/978-1-4419-1526-9_19, © Springer Science+Business Media LLC 2010

USA and expectations regarding women and work (see, for example, the work of Lennon et al. 2001). Parenting may contribute positively to women's lives in the community by providing opportunities for meaningful activity that is valued by society in relationships with others, including family, friends, and neighbors. Community integration may, in turn, provide access to resources and opportunities for support in the parenting role, including the informal assistance of grandparents, parent–peer activities, or routine contact with pediatricians and other helping professionals (Nicholson et al. 1998b). Mothers' personal health and well-being are deeply intertwined with that of their children. Demonstrating the complex interaction of maternal and child well-being, researchers have documented that successful treatment of mothers' depression is associated with a reduction in their children's diagnoses and symptoms (Weissman et al. 2006). Mothers with mental disorders whose resources are limited may choose, out of necessity, to prioritize meeting their children's needs at the expense of meeting their own (Nicholson et al. 1998a). For example, mothers may feel compelled to purchase sneakers for their children rather than psychiatric medication for themselves.

The complexity of the relationships among these variables suggests the value of an ecological model of parenting and recovery for mothers with mental disorders. While parenting has been seen as a set of interactions and transactions between parent, child, and familial and social contexts (Belsky 1984; Patterson and Fisher 2002), the links between parenting and mental health recovery have only recently been suggested (Nicholson et al. 2006; Nicholson and Henry 2003).

The objectives of this chapter are (1) to present an ecological perspective on parenting and recovery for mothers with mental disorders, (2) to describe these mothers, their experiences, and needs, (3) to extrapolate from the existing literature key components and processes of relevant interventions, and (4) to discuss the implications for mental health policy and services delivery.

An Ecological Perspective on Parenting and Recovery

An ecological model of recovery provides the framework for exploring the relationships between individual adult characteristics, including illness characteristics, characteristics of the parent–child environment, and the interactions and transactions between the two (Onken et al. 2007). In this most recent analysis of the literature, recovery is conceptualized as more than alleviating symptoms or recovering from an illness per se. An ecological model of recovery emphasizes participation in meaningful life roles, community inclusion, and social integration (Onken et al. 2007). The individual is placed in life context, and recovery is seen as a process that evolves over time.

The person-level elements of recovery that involve interaction with others in the immediate life context are of particular interest in considering mothers with mental disorders and their families. According to Onken et al. (2007), these elements include hope, agency, self-determination, meaning/purpose, and awareness/potentiality. Hope, the notion that change and a better future are possible, is essential to mustering the energy and resources to overcome the disabling impact of mental disorders. Agency, or goal-directed determination, is based on a sense of competence that can be supported by an environment, or fostered, as an individual overcomes environmental obstacles to recovery. Recovery rests upon self-determination; the individual must chose his or her own goals, life path, and the steps along that path. A sense of meaning or purpose in life is derived from the individual's interactions with an environment that provides opportunities for success in meaningful, relevant activities. Awareness and potentiality imply an individual's understanding that change is possible, that recovery is a process that requires opportunities to build strengths, and that relapse and setbacks may be a part of the process (Onken et al. 2007). Functioning is not necessarily disorder-driven, and the concept of recovery transcends diagnostic categories.

Parenting is a meaningful life role, relevant to many women, that provides a set of interactions and transactions that are quite likely related to the expression of mental disorders and the recovery process. Therefore, the functioning, well-being, and recovery process of mothers with mental disorders are likely to be influenced by the characteristics and actions of their children, their interactions with them, and their familial and social context, as well as by the disabling aspects of their disorders. Motherhood may present opportunities for, or obstacles to, recovery for women with mental disorders. Success in parenting may promote feelings of agency and self-determination; mothers may take pride in contributing to the health and well-being of children, and setting and achieving goals for managing a home. On the other hand, if the impairments conveyed by mental disorders impede successful functioning, the experience of failure in the parenting role can have profound repercussions for mothers. In addition, barriers to or deficits in the resource environment may contribute to disparities in parenting capacity by undermining the efforts of mothers with mental disorders to care for their children, and may serve as obstacles to the recovery process. Examples of the potential for parenting experiences to promote or hinder recovery are provided in Table 19.1[1] through the use of quotes from mothers with serious mental disorders who participated in a series of studies over the past decade (Nicholson and Henry 2003; Nicholson et al. 1998a, b, 2001b).

Given that recovery is a process, with anticipated times of growth and progress, and times of relapse and setback, the functioning of women with mental disorders may vary at any one point in time as well as over time across the roles they play. For example, a mother with a mental disorder may function well in the home, but may not have the energy or organizational skills to balance motherhood and employment outside the home. Or, a mother may function well and meet role expectations quite capably until a relapse or setback occurs. Then her need for resources and supports may increase for a time until her functioning improves again.

[1] Quotes from mothers with serious mental health disorders are taken from previous studies (Nicholson and Henry 2003; Nicholson et al. 1998a, b)

Table 19.1 Parenting provides a context for recovery

Elements of recovery[a]	Promote recovery	Hinder recovery
Hope: The expectation of better things in the future	"My children give me strength, they give me hope, they give me the will to survive…"	"They think once you've been abused you are going to abuse your own kids."
Sense of agency: The assumption of individual competency to overcome challenges	"I think in my circumstances my mental illness has made me stronger. You have to try twice as hard. You have to prove things to people."	"If you can't take care of yourself, you're definitely not going to be able to take care of somebody else…"
Self-determination: The opportunity to set goals, make choices, and determine a life path	"…I gotta' do it for me and my kids, to show them a better way…"	"…You know, some people think you shouldn't have a baby because you have a mental illness and because you're on medication."
Meaning and purpose: The ability to pursue and undertake productive activities of interest	"…In reality I don't want to go [to the hospital]. I want to be home. I want to be the mother. I want to be in charge of the house…cooking, cleaning, taking care of everybody, changing diapers."	"…speaking for myself as a mother who doesn't have her children…My heart is in chains…"
Awareness and potentiality: To believe that change is possible and achievable	"…my daughter doesn't necessarily have to get it [mental illness]. It's how she's going to grow up."	"When you're doing good, nobody's there for you… but when they find out the least little bit wrong, they're there on you, letting you know all the negative…no positive."

[a] Onken et al. (2007)

Mothers with Mental Disorders

The National Comorbidity Survey (NCS) of the USA is the best source of data regarding the prevalence of motherhood among women with mental disorders (Kessler 1994; Kessler et al. 1994, 1997; Nicholson et al. 2004). Analyses of data from the Part II subsample of the original NCS indicate that 68% of women who meet criteria for mental disorders over the course of their lifetime are mothers (i.e., report having natural-born children; Nicholson et al. 2004). Sixty-seven percent of women with comorbid mental disorder and substance use disorders were parents. These percentages were actually higher than the prevalence of parenthood reported by women with no mental disorder or substance use disorder (62%), and did not capture those adults who reported having only adopted or step, foster, or other unrelated children living with them, or who had ever given birth to a child who subsequently died. Among women who met criteria for severe and persistent mental illness, two-thirds were parents. The majority of women who met diagnostic criteria for any disorders falling into the major NCS diagnostic categories were parents (i.e., affective disorders, anxiety disorders, posttraumatic stress disorder (PTSD), and nonaffective psychosis). Among NCS respondents who were parents, 47% of the mothers had a lifetime prevalence of mental disorders (Nicholson et al. 2004). It is important to note that NCS respondents were living in the community, and their responses do not adequately reflect the experiences of those in the military or institutionalized at the time of the study.

Mothers with mental disorders in the NCS had an average of 2.3 children. The average age of illness onset and average age at birth of their first child varied across diagnostic categories (Nicholson et al. 2004). Mothers who met criteria for anxiety disorders and PTSD over the course of their lifetime had illness onsets, on average, about four or more years *prior* to the births of their first children (Nicholson et al. 2004). Those women who met criteria for affective disorders and nonaffective psychosis had illness onsets, on average, about 4 years *after* giving birth to their first children. Women with nonaffective psychosis had their children generally at younger ages than women whose disorders fell into other diagnostic categories.

The timing of illness onset in relation to the birth of children may be significant in terms of outcomes for women as well as for children. In a study of urban mothers receiving services in public sector settings, women who were parents first and then became ill showed the most positive illness trajectories, as did women whose illness onsets occurred well before the birth of any children (Mowbray et al. 2005). In the Mowbray et al. (2005) study, women whose illness onsets occurred close to the time of the birth of a child fared least well.

Three-quarters of mothers in the NCS who met criteria for any mental disorder were Caucasian, with African-American (12%) and Latina (almost 9%) mothers comprising smaller percentages (Nicholson et al. 2004). This is noteworthy, given that many of the studies over the past 15 years have focused on mothers who are African-American or described in studies as from diverse racial and ethnic backgrounds, largely recruited in public settings or agencies (Mowbray et al. 2001; Nicholson et al. 2001a; White et al. 1995). Consequently, the experiences of Caucasian mothers with mental illness and, in particular, those receiving treatment or services in the private sector, are relatively less well understood.

More mothers with psychiatric disorders are living without partners, compared with mothers who do not provide evidence of mental disorders (approximately 28% and 20%, respectively), lending support to the conclusion that mothers with mental illness, and particularly those with serious mental illnesses, may be more isolated and in greater need of social supports (Mowbray et al. 2000). Women with schizophrenia, for example, compared with women without mental illness, are less likely to have a current partner, and more likely to have a higher number of lifetime sexual partners (Miller and Finnerty 1996; Nicholson and Miller 2008). Family disruptions may be more common when parents have mental disorders due to a higher likelihood of divorce and the impermanent nature of partner relationships, or the increased likelihood of out-of-home placements of children (Nicholson and Miller 2008; Park et al. 2006). In addition, a significantly higher percentage of mothers with mental disorders in the NCS were living below the poverty level, again confirming the likely need for access to basic resources and supports (Mowbray et al. 2001; Nicholson et al. 2004).

Mental disorders often co-occur with other mental disorders (e.g., depression and anxiety), substance use disorders, and other medical conditions (e.g., hypertension, arthritis, etc.; U.S. DHHS 1999). Consequently, mothers may be living with significant physical disorders as well as complex mental health and substance abuse conditions (Larson et al. 2005; Reed and Mowbray 1999). In addition, mothers may have experiences of violence, as victims or as witnesses, during childhood and as adults, and at the hands of caretakers, partners, and strangers (Goodman et al. 1997; McHugo et al. 2005; Nicholson et al. 2006). They may also have a high prevalence of other types of traumatic experiences, such as significant losses, homelessness, and incarceration (McHugo et al. 2005). Women with mental disorders are more likely to be victims of violence than perpetrators; experiences of violence and trauma can contribute to, or exacerbate, mental disorders and substance use disorders (Kendler et al. 2000; U.S. DHHS 1999).

Mothers with mental disorders identify loss of custody or contact with children as a significant concern (Nicholson et al. 1998a, 2001a; Zemencuk et al. 1994). The prevalence of losing custody or contact with children for these women is unknown, though in studies of small-scale, clinic or treatment setting samples, from one-quarter to over three-quarters of mothers with serious mental disorders reported custody loss (Mowbray et al. 2001; Nicholson 2001a). While both maternal mental illness and substance use have been linked to elevated risk of child abuse and neglect, there are no national data on the prevalence with which mothers with mental disorders abuse or neglect their children (Egami et al. 1996; Nicholson et al. 2006). Trauma experiences may play a greater role than mental disorders or substance use disorders alone in precipitating mother–child separations. Mothers with co-occurring mental disorders and substance use disorders who are separated from minor children have significantly greater lifetime and current exposure to stressful events and interpersonal abuse (Nicholson et al. 2006). Mothers may relinquish custody of children involuntarily through a child protective action consequent to abuse and neglect, or voluntarily, perhaps at times of poor functioning or hospitalization, making formal or informal arrangements with family members or friends. Mothers may continue to be involved with their children, visiting with them or providing more active levels of care, even though others bear primary legal or day-to-day responsibility for care giving (Nicholson et al. 1998b; Ritsher et al. 1997).

Given that the children of parents with mental disorders are at a greater risk for developmental and mental health problems (Goodman and Gotlib 1999; Nicholson et al. 2001a; Oyserman et al. 2000), mothers may be challenged to meet their children's needs as well as their own. Their access to family supports for respite or backup may be limited (Nicholson et al. 1998b). Children may have unique educational or emotional needs that would benefit from school or treatment interventions. Mothers' experiences with providers, which may have been positive or negative, may contribute to their willingness and ability to advocate for and access essential services for their children (Henry and Nicholson 2005; Nicholson et al. 1998a).

In addition to the needs common to all parents and families (e.g., safe housing, transportation, stable income, adequate childcare and healthcare, etc.), mothers with mental disorders described illness-specific needs or potential targets of intervention as well (Nicholson and Henry 2003). Mothers may require assistance in balancing the stresses of parenting and family life while living with psychiatric symptoms, managing medications and treatment regimes, and maintaining relationships with providers of services for themselves and for their children. Mothers may request support for and training in strategies for communicating with their children about their mental disorders in age-appropriate ways (Nicholson and Henry 2003).

Depending on the impairments conveyed by particular mental disorders, mothers may have difficulties in interactions with children, reading nonverbal cues or responding to children in appropriately synchronous or contingent ways (Nicholson and Miller 2008). Depression may result in blunted effect; an apathetic or withdrawn mother may not be emotionally available to parent adequately or may not have the energy to provide appropriate levels of stimulation to their children (Nicholson and Henry 2003). Disordered thinking may interfere with a mother's ability to plan and implement strategies to meet basic family needs (e.g., grocery shopping, preparing meals, paying bills), or to recognize patterns in children's behavior, making managing children's behavior quite challenging. Mothers with delusions or hallucinations may misunderstand or misinterpret their children's actions. Depending on their own childhood experiences, mothers may lack a basic knowledge of developmentally appropriate milestones and age-appropriate behavior.

It is important to note that for women with mental disorders, motherhood may provide opportunities for the development and expression of strengths as well. Children and the desire to parent well may provide the motivation for mothers to seek treatment (Nicholson and Henry 2003; Nicholson et al. 1998a). Developing effective strategies for managing a household and meeting children's needs may be very satisfying to mothers, whose successful efforts may lead to feelings of enhanced self-efficacy and pride in fulfilling the maternal role (Nicholson and Miller 2008). Women with mental disorders who set goals, make choices, and determine that their life path includes motherhood, have access to endless opportunities for the development of skills and a sense of competency in a meaningful life role (Onken et al. 2007). Without access to adequate, appropriate supports and resources, however, the opportunities for failure also abound.

Key Intervention Components and Processes

Mothers' and children's functioning, well-being, and experiences are intimately intertwined. Outcomes for each are multiply determined and interrelated. An ecological model of parenting and recovery captures the complexity of these relationships, and suggests that the assessment and treatment or service planning processes must be comprehensive. Intervention supports and solutions must be multimodal and/or targeted to specific, unique needs at different and, potentially, multiple points in time.

Assessment

Mothers' goals, strengths, challenges, resources, and supports must be adequately assessed to develop relevant, meaningful plans for treatment, support, and rehabilitation (Henry and Nicholson 2005; Nicholson and Miller 2008). The assessment must include questions regarding the woman's current parenting status and responsibilities, questions providers often overlook (Henry and Nicholson 2005; Mowbray et al. 2006; Nicholson et al. 1993). Women must be understood in the context of their strengths, hopes, and desires for parenting, and their challenges and concerns. Mothers must be supported in recognizing what they do well and in identifying their individual and interpersonal resources. This information must be placed in the larger context of an understanding of family and community. For example, the strengths and challenges of children, partners, and extended family must be examined. The ultimate focus of an assessment and treatment or service planning is the woman's goals for the future, for herself as a mother, and for her family.

Treatment

Providers can support mothers with mental disorders indirectly by infusing consideration of mothers' parenting choices, demands, and challenges into existing evidence-based practices. Assertive community treatment (ACT), family psychoeducation, supported employment, skills training, symptom self-management, cognitive interventions, and integrated treatment for co-occurring disorders are evidence-based practices for adults that potentially could be applied effectively, with some modifications, to support women with mental disorders as they pursue parenting goals (Mueser et al. 2001; Nicholson and Henry 2003). Optimal pharmacotherapy can support mothers with mental disorders to function as well as possible. The demands and challenges of parenting, including the requirements of the perinatal period, must be considered in making decisions about psychopharmacology. Providers must be aware, not only of the impact of various medications and their side effects on women's general and reproductive health, but of women's goals and desires regarding pregnancy and motherhood.

Providers can directly support women's functioning as mothers via support and rehabilitation strategies specifically targeted to improve parenting. Generic models of parent education, support and skill-building may be applicable, but do not necessarily specifically address the needs of mothers with mental disorders (Nicholson and Henry 2003; Nicholson and Miller 2008). Parenting classes, coaching, and support groups may be useful in providing the basics to parents in general. However, mothers with mental disorders may find traditional parent supports irrelevant, or may perceive barriers to their full participation. They may be uncomfortable engaging in group discussion or revealing information about the challenges they face related to their disorders.

Existing Interventions for Mothers with Mental Disorders

There are no specific interventions for mothers with mental illnesses and their families that have been rigorously independently tested and have achieved the standard of evidence-based practice. However, existing programs or interventions for families living with parental mental disorders share program assumptions or consistent mission statements, theories of change, and program components and processes (Hinden et al. 2002, 2005, 2006; Nicholson et al. 2007). Findings from previous survey and site visit studies suggest the essential ingredients for interventions and provide practice-based guidance for relevant intervention approaches (Nicholson et al. 2007; Shonkoff 2000).

Twenty interventions specifically targeted at parents with mental disorders and their families, identified in a national survey of programs, shared a common commitment to enhancing the functioning of adult family members with mental disorders and supporting the development of their children (Hinden et al. 2006). Shared program assumptions commonly described by program representatives underscored the beliefs that adults with mental disorders deserve the opportunity to parent, have much to offer their children and, with access to appropriate supports, will function well in their role as parents. A further set of common assumptions underscored the ecological perspective, i.e., if parents do better, children do better and vice versa. In addition, prevention and early intervention to improve parenting and support child development can enhance outcomes for both children and parents (Nicholson et al. 2007). These assumptions reflect the underlying beliefs that effective services must be family-centered and strengths-based.

Theories of Change

Providers in programs studied by the researchers recommended what might be described as a pragmatic, eclectic theoretical approach to working with families living with parental mental disorders (Hinden et al. 2006; Nicholson et al. 2007). While programs may have been derived from psychosocial rehabilitation, child attachment/psychodynamic, or psycho-educational approaches, the common theme across providers was the willingness to do "whatever it takes" to enhance parent and family functioning (Hinden et al. 2006; Nicholson et al. 2007). Rather than adherence to a specific theoretical model, providers embraced a comprehensive, practical, nonjudgmental approach to intervention, with a level of intensity that varied over time according to mothers' and families' needs.

Program Components

While programs in a national survey and site visit studies varied in location or setting (e.g., inpatient, community-based, and residential programs), common intervention strategies or program components were found (Hinden et al. 2006; Nicholson et al. 2007). Case management for all family members was considered essential. The family, rather than the individual woman with a mental disorder, was defined as the client unit. Family case management included emotional support and help with problem solving, the coordination of multiple services for family members, and crisis management. Families often required facilitated access to concrete resources and benefits to meet basic family needs, as well as access to formal treatment and social service supports. Parent support, education, and skills training were provided, either center-based or in families' homes. In addition, programs often met family members' needs for advocacy and provided support to mothers in navigating sometimes conflicted relationships with partners, extended family, employers, landlords, school personnel, and other service providers. Programs varied in the provision of more traditional mental health services (e.g., family therapy or dyadic mother–child psychotherapy) and child-focused interventions, such as the evaluation of children's needs, psychotherapy, and early intervention or after-school services.

Key Issues for Policy and Services Delivery

A focus on recovery in the lives of mothers with mental disorders requires a contextualized understanding of women that includes the role of mother and the impact of parenting experiences. Parenting is a meaningful life role. The opportunities provided by parenting and a woman's experiences as a mother cannot be untangled from her mental health, her functioning in other significant life roles, and the supports and challenges conveyed by her family, community, and societal contexts. Mental health services are an essential part of that context. Providers of mental health services have tremendous opportunity to work together with women to support their achievement of maximum community participation if they attend to women's goals, desires, challenges, and successes as mothers.

Implications for Women's Mental Health

Providers and participants in existing programs for mothers with mental disorders recommended that effective services must be *family-centered* (Hinden et al. 2006). Given national prevalence data, it is no longer possible or advisable to deny or avoid the fact that women with mental disorders, including those with serious mental disorders, are becoming mothers and wish to provide care for their children (Biebel et al. 2004, 2006). Women in previous studies pursued motherhood, regardless of whether family members or providers were supportive or advised against it. They faced the same challenges all mothers faced, along with the additional demands of managing a mental disorder. As a mother with a serious mental disorder in one study explained, “You have to go to work. You gotta’ come home. You gotta’ deal with the kids, deal with your own home. Your own problems, you know, really start piling up.” They require treatment, support, and rehabilitation approaches that are effective in addressing their individual needs and also take their goals and roles as mothers into consideration.

Mothers with mental disorders who are separated from their children must be supported in developing alternative ways to nurture as successfully as possible. Whether a separation is temporary (e.g., a short-term hospitalization) or longer-term (e.g., an out-of-home placement and move to adoption), supports must be put in place for mothers as well as children. Mothers can be helped to make visits with children as positive as possible, and to negotiate what may be conflicted relationships with their children’s caregivers, including ex-partners, extended family members, and foster parents. Mothers who have lost contact with their children, either voluntarily or involuntarily, through placement with relatives, guardianship, or adoption, benefit from support in acknowledging their losses and possibly coping with feelings of failure.

Services for mothers with mental disorders must be based on the mother’s strengths. Parents with mental disorders want to be treated with respect and have their strengths acknowledged (Nicholson and Henry 2003). Parent–provider trust, communication, and collaboration are built in the context of relationships in which strengths are emphasized (Hinden et al. 2005).

Mothers with mental disorders often have difficulty identifying their own strengths, and focus on their failures instead. Once mothers come under the scrutiny of the child welfare system via a child protective action, or their involvement with the legal system in a divorce and custody situation, the willingness to trust providers and, therefore, to benefit most from treatment, may be compromised. Mothers with mental disorders may have difficulty identifying strengths in their children as well, and must be encouraged to assist their children in recognizing and accessing the individual and interpersonal resources that promote resilience.

Providers can work together with mothers to reframe their thinking about what may be perceived as deficits into strengths. For example, women may be labeled by providers as “resistant” or “non-compliant” if they “fail” to keep treatment appointments. In fact, mothers’ participation in treatment may be undermined when they do not have adequate childcare and cannot leave children home alone, or if they cannot bring their child along because the clinic does not have a family waiting area.

Symptoms may be reframed as “coping mechanisms” and actually may be the defensive strategies that allow women to survive, particularly in situations in which women have experiences of violent victimization and trauma. A treatment goal might be to replace unhealthy or maladaptive ways of coping with healthier ways. A mother with a serious mental health disorder who is labeled “manipulative” by providers or family members, in fact may have perfected such strategies to survive previous bad, dangerous, or even life-threatening experiences and relationships.

Mothers who are identified as overprotective by providers may, in fact, have real concerns regarding the safety of their children, based on their own unsafe experiences as children. Providers must set aside negative labels to begin to focus on women's strengths, to talk with women about their experiences, their characteristic coping strategies, and the impact of mental disorders on their current functioning and goals as mothers.

Given the prevalence of victimization, the witnessing of violence, serious disruptions and losses, and the potential for impact on the parent–child relationship, services for mothers with mental disorders must be *trauma-informed* (Nicholson et al. 2006). Experiences with their children can serve as reminders to mothers of past events, as well as what their lives were like when they were the ages of their children, providing opportunities to trigger PTSD symptoms. For more information on PTSD, see Chaps. 3 and 5 in this volume.

Relationships with children test boundaries and limits, and raise issues of intimacy, power and control, and loss. Mothers with histories of violence may have difficulty in relationships with other adults, peers, and providers, and may be victimized or reminded of their victimization experiences in these relationships. Perhaps the greatest trauma is prompted by the loss of custody of a child.

Mothers should be asked about their experiences of past trauma and current risk and be encouraged to respond to the extent they are able and at a pace that is comfortable for them. Perhaps even more important are conversations about ways in which anxiety, depression, or PTSD-like responses are triggered in current parenting situations. Mothers may require support to provide a safe home and family environment for their children, particularly if they did not grow up in a safe environment themselves.

References

Belsky, J. (1984). The determinants of parenting: A process model. *Child Development, 55,* 83–96.

Biebel, K., Nicholson, J., Geller, J. L., & Fisher, W. H. (2006). A national survey of state mental health authority programs and policies for clients who are parents: A decade later. *Psychiatric Quarterly, 77,* 119–128.

Biebel, K., Nicholson, J., Williams, V., & Hinden, B. R. (2004). Facilitating systems change: State mental health authorities developing programs and policies for parents with mental illness. *Administration and Policy in Mental Health, 32,* 31–48.

Egami, Y., Ford, E. E., Greenfield, S. F., & Crum, R. M. (1996). Psychiatric profile and sociodemographic characteristics of adults who report physically abusing or neglecting children. *American Journal of Psychiatry, 153*(7), 921–928.

Goodman, L. A., Rosenberg, S. D., Mueser, K. T., & Drake, R. E. (1997). Physical and sexual assault history in women with serious mental illness: prevalence, correlates, treatment, and future research directions. *Schizophrenia Bulletin, 23,* 685–696.

Goodman, S. H., & Gotlib, I. H. (1999). Risk for psychopathology in the children of depressed mothers: A developmental model for understanding mechanisms of transmission. *Psychological Review, 106*(3), 458–490.

Henry, A. D., & Nicholson, J. (2005). Helping mothers with serious mental illness. *Directions in Rehabilitation Counseling, 16,* 19–32.

Hinden, B. R., Biebel, K., Nicholson, J., Henry, A., & Katz-Leavy, J. (2006). A survey of programs for parents with mental illness and their families: Identifying common elements to build an evidence base. *Journal of Behavioral Health Services & Research, 33*(1), 21–38.

Hinden, B. R., Biebel, K., Nicholson, J., Henry, A. D., & Stier, L. (2002). *Steps toward evidence-based practices for parents with mental illness and their families*. Rockville, MD: Substance Abuse and Mental Health Services Administration, Center for Mental Health Services.

Hinden, B. R., Biebel, K., Nicholson, J., & Mehnert, L. (2005). The Invisible Children's Project: Key ingredients of an intervention for parents with mental illness. *Journal of Behavioral Health Services and Research, 32*(4), 393–408.

Kendler, K. S., Bulik, C. M., Silberg, J., Hettema, J. M., Myres, J., & Prescott, C. A. (2000). Childhood sexual abuse and adult psychiatric and substance use disorders in women: An epidemiological and cotwin control analysis. *Archives of General Psychiatry, 57*(10), 953–959.

Kessler, R. C. (1994). The national comorbidity survey of the United States. *International Review of Psychiatry, 6,* 365–376.

Kessler, R. C., Anthony, J. C., Blazer, D. G., Bromet, E., Eaton, W. W., Kendler, K., et al. (1997). The US national comorbidity survey: Overview and future directions. *Epidemiologia e Psichiatria Sociale, 6,* 4–16.

Kessler, R. C., McGonagle, K. A., Zhao, S., Nelson, C. B., Hughes, M., Eshleman, S., et al. (1994). Lifetime and 12-month prevalence of DSM-II-R psychiatric disorders in the United States: Results from the national comorbidity survey. *Archives of General Psychiatry, 51,* 8–19.

Larson, M. J., Miller, L. J., Becker, M., Richardson, E., Kammerer, N., Thom, J., et al. (2005). Physical health burdens of women with trauma histories and co-occurring substance abuse and mental disorders. *Journal of Behavioral Health Services and Research, 32*(2), 128–140.

Lennon, M. C., Blome, J., & English, K. (2001). *Depression and low income women: Challenges for TANF and welfare-to-work policies and programs*. Rockville, MD: Substance Abuse and Mental Health Services Administration, Center for Mental Health Services.

McHugo, G. J., Caspi, Y., Kammerer, N., Mazelis, R., Jackson, E. W., Russell, L., et al. (2005). The assessment of trauma history in women with co-occurring substance abuse and mental disorders and a history of interpersonal violence. *Journal of Behavioral Health Services and Research, 32*(2), 113–127.

Miller, L. J., & Finnerty, M. (1996). Sexuality, pregnancy, and childrearing among women with schizophrenia spectrum disorders. *Psychiatric Services, 47*(5), 502–506.

Mowbray, C. T., Bybee, D., Oyserman, D., & MacFarlane, P. (2005). Timing of mental illness onset and motherhood. *The Journal of Nervous and Mental Disease, 193*(6), 369–378.

Mowbray, C. T., Bybee, D., Oyserman, D., MacFarlane, P., & Bowersox, N. (2006). Psychosocial outcomes for adult children of parents with severe mental illness: Demographic and clinical history predictors. *Health & Social Work, 31*(2), 99–108.

Mowbray, C. T., Oyserman, D., Bybee, D., MacFarlane, P., & Rueda-Riedle, A. (2001). Life circumstances of mothers with serious mental illness. *Psychiatric Rehabilitation Journal, 25*(2), 114–123.

Mowbray, C. T., Oyserman, D., & Ross, S. (1995). Parenting and the significance of children for women with a serious mental illness. *Journal of Mental Health Administration, 22*(2), 189–200.

Mowbray, C. T., Schwartz, S., Bybee, D., Spanj, J., Rueda-Riedle, A., & Oyserman, D. (2000). Mothers with mental illness: Stressors and resources for parenting and living. *Families in Society, 81*(2), 118–129.

Mueser, K. T., Bond, G. R., & Drake, R. E. (2001). Community-based treatment of schizophrenia and other severe mental disorders: Treatment outcomes? *Medscape Mental Health, 6*(1), 1–31.

Nicholson, J., Biebel, K., Hinden, B. R., Henry, A. D., & Stier, L. (2001a). *Critical issues for parents with mental illness and their families*. Rockville, MD: Substance Abuse and Mental Health Services Administration, Center for Mental Health Services.

Nicholson, J., Biebel, K., Williams, V. F., & Katz-Leavy, J. (2004). Prevalence of parenthood in adults with mental illness: Implications for state and federal policy, programs, and providers.

In R. W. Manderscheid & M. J. Henderson (Eds.), *Mental health, United States, 2002* (DHHS Publication No. (SMA) 3938, pp. 120–137). Rockville, MD: Substance Abuse and Mental Health Services Administration, Center for Mental Health Services.

Nicholson, J., Finkelstein, N., Williams, V., Thom, J., Noether, C., & DeVilbiss, M. (2006). A comparison of mothers with co-occurring disorders and histories of violence living with or separated from minor children. *Journal of Behavioral Health Services and Research, 33*(2), 225–243.

Nicholson, J., Geller, J. L., Fisher, W. H., & Dion, G. L. (1993). State policies and programs that address the needs of mentally ill mothers in the public sector. *Hospital and Community Psychiatry, 44,* 484–489.

Nicholson, J., & Henry, A. D. (2003). Achieving the goal of evidence-based psychiatric rehabilitation practices for mothers with mental illness. *Psychiatric Rehabilitation Journal, 27,* 122–130.

Nicholson, J., Henry, A. D., Clayfield, J., & Phillips, S. (2001b). *Parenting well when you're depressed: A complete resource for maintaining a healthy family.* Oakland, CA: New Harbinger Publications.

Nicholson, J., Hinden, B. R., Biebel, K., Henry, A. D., & Katz-Leavy, J. (2007). A qualitative study of programs for parents with serious mental illness and their children: Building practice-based evidence. *Journal of Behavioral Health Services and Research, 34*(4), 395–413.

Nicholson, J., & Miller, L. J. (2008). Parenting. In K. Mueser & D. V. Jeste (Eds.), *The clinical handbook of schizophrenia.* New York, NY: Guilford Press.

Nicholson, J., Sweeney, E. M., & Geller, J. L. (1998a). Mothers with mental illness: I. The competing demands of parenting and living with mental illness. *Psychiatric Services, 49,* 635–642.

Nicholson, J., Sweeney, E. M., & Geller, J. L. (1998b). Mothers with mental illness: II. Family relationships and the context of parenting. *Psychiatric Services, 49,* 643–649.

Onken, S. J., Craig, C. M., Ridgeway, P., Ralph, R. O., & Cook, J. A. (2007). An analysis of the definitions and elements of recovery: A review of the literature. *Psychiatric Rehabilitation Journal, 31*(1), 9–22.

Oyserman, D., Mowbray, C. T., Meares, P. A., & Firminger, K. B. (2000). Parenting among mothers with a serious mental illness. *American Journal of Orthopsychiatry, 70*(3), 296–315.

Park, J. M., Solomon, P., & Mandell, D. S. (2006). Involvement in the child welfare system among mothers with serious mental illness. *Psychiatric Services, 57*(4), 493–497.

Patterson, G. R., & Fisher, P. A. (2002). Recent developments in our understanding of parenting: bidirectional effects, causal models, and the search for parsimony. In M. H. Bornstein (Ed.), *Handbook of parenting: Volume 5. Practical issues in parenting* (pp. 59–88). Mahwah, NJ: Lawrence Erlbaum Associates.

Reed, B. G., & Mowbray, C. T. (1999). Mental illness and substance abuse: Implications for women's health and health care access. *Journal of the American Medical Women's Association, 54,* 71–78.

Ritsher, J. E., Coursey, R. D., & Farrell, E. W. (1997). A survey on issues in the lives of women with severe mental illness. *Psychiatric Services, 48*(10), 1273–1283.

Shonkoff, J. P. (2000). Science, policy, and practice: Three cultures in search of a shared mission. *Child Development, 71,* 181–187.

U.S. DHHS. (1999). *Mental health: A report of the surgeon general.* Rockville, MD: Substance Abuse and Mental Health Services Administration, Center for Mental Health Services.

Weissman, M. M., Pilowsky, D. J., Wickramaratne, P. J., Talati, A., Wisniewski, S. R., Fava, M., et al. (2006). Remissions in maternal depression and child psychopathology. *Journal of the American Medical Association, 295*(12), 1389–1398.

White, C. L., Nicholson, J., Fisher, W. H., & Geller, J. L. (1995). Mothers with severe mental illness caring for children. *The Journal of Nervous and Mental Disease, 183*(6), 398–403.

Zemencuk, J., Rogosch, R. A., & Mowbray, C. T. (1994). The seriously mentally ill woman in the role of parent: characteristics, parenting sensitivity and needs. *Psychosocial Rehabilitation Journal, 18,* 77–92.

Chapter 20
Navigating the Worlds of Information

Ardis R. M. Hanson and Bruce Lubotsky Levin

During the past several decades, major federal reports have repeatedly prioritized two areas of critical importance for improving the health and mental health of Americans: (1) promoting women's mental health services as an essential component of overall health; and (2) the development of a national telecommunication system for surveillance of health and mental health data. Women seek treatment for services across a variety of health and specialized mental healthcare settings, both formal and informal, and each encounter generates data. Although the healthcare field is being encouraged to develop national health information systems, each agency, organization, and delivery system has its own databases, formatting structure, and data collection and reporting requirements, often broken down by gender, age, and ethnicity. Further, each reporting stream may not relate to users and collectors of data across the variety of health and mental healthcare settings.

Not only do a multitude of federal, state, county, and local health and mental health agencies collect and maintain data on women's mental health, academia itself continues to explore women's mental health, providing access through a variety of print and online venues. Therefore, with the vast number and variety of databases and information resources held in countless organizations, where do researchers and policymakers look to access information for use in services research studies and delivery systems, and to develop policy alternatives for improving women's mental health?

This chapter presents how best to navigate the systematized body of knowledge that constitutes women's mental health. The authors integrate the disparate disciplines involved in women's mental health into a working framework focused on information-seeking behaviors. The chapter contents are divided into six sections examining (1) the background of the recurring themes of disparity in mental

A. R. M. Hanson (✉)
Research Library, Louis de la Parte Florida Mental Health Institute,
College of Behavioral & Community Sciences,
University of South Florida, Tampa, FL 33612, USA

B. L. Levin, M. A. Becker (eds.), *A Public Health Perspective of Women's Mental Health*,
DOI 10.1007/978-1-4419-1526-9_20, © Springer Science+Business Media LLC 2010

health services and the importance of developing organized information systems for women's mental health; (2) the intellectual foundation of organizing information; (3) the various types of information available; (4) selected sources of information, including generalist and specialist authors and providers of databases and resources on women's mental health; (5) current and emerging technologies which affect how one finds and retrieves information; and (6) the implications that emerging technologies and information-seeking behaviors have on women's mental health research, services delivery, and policy.

Background

In the seminal publication *Mental Health: A Report of the Surgeon General* (U.S. Department of Health and Human Services, Office of the Surgeon General 1999), mental disorders were reported to be influenced by gender, age, race, and culture. Consequently, the diagnosis and treatment of mental disorders should ideally be tailored to these socioeconomic characteristics. This report also discussed the importance of the confidentiality of health and mental health information systems in light of the movement toward integrated and shared patient information systems. The report influenced a number of subsequent federal agency initiatives urging researchers to expand their studies on gender disparities and their impact on services research within the emerging online health information infrastructure.

Healthy People, 2000 (U.S. Department of Health and Human Services 1991) and *Healthy People, 2010* (U.S. Department of Health and Human Services 2000) also identified the elimination of health disparities by gender as a major goal. These reports also suggested the development of a public health infrastructure by increasing efforts to collect, track, and disseminate national health and mental health data in order to build and maintain national data and surveillance systems containing health and mental health data.

The *President's New Freedom Commission on Mental Health* (2003) noted that stigma, treatment and insurance limitations, and fragmentation of service delivery systems prevented Americans with mental disorders from receiving appropriate and adequate mental healthcare. This complexity in mental health services also reflects the convolution in accessing the multitude of academic databases and catalogs addressing mental health services in America.

While the *President's New Freedom Commission on Mental Health* (2003) identified six overall goals for transforming mental health services delivery in America, two goals were directly relevant to conclusions drawn in *Mental Health: A Report of the Surgeon General* (U.S. Department of Health and Human Services, Office of the Surgeon General 1999), *Healthy People, 2000* (U.S. Department of Health and Human Services 1991), and *Healthy People, 2010* (U.S. Department of Health and Human Services 2000): (1) the elimination of disparities in mental health services and (2) the use of communication and information technology to access mental health services.

The *Surgeon General's Workshop on Women's Mental Health* (U.S. Department of Health and Human Services 2005) developed seven themes pertaining to women's mental health services, including the essential nature of women's mental health services to overall health and the importance of health literacy in sharing information about women's mental health in language that is understandable and information that is of use to all individuals. Health literacy extends beyond lay language. Health literacy also addresses an individual's ability to find, retrieve, understand, and use health information effectively.

From a global perspective, the World Health Organization published the report *Gender in Mental Health Research* (Vikram 2005) which summarized the differences in the prevalence of mental disorders in women and men and encouraged an increased emphasis in public health research on gender issues and their impact on mental health.

Currently, the Obama administration has played an active role in the elimination of health disparities as well as in laying emphasis on the development of health information systems. For example, earlier in his career, State Senator Obama helped pass a mental health parity bill in Illinois. As a US Senator, he supported the bipartisan *Paul Wellstone Mental Health and Addiction Equity Act of 2007*, an updated version of legislation that requires coverage for serious mental illnesses, including substance use disorders, to be provided on the same terms and conditions as are applicable to other physical diseases.

Just as the passage of mental health parity reformed insurance and financing of mental health services, the Obama administration emphasizes the strengthening of health information technology and the elimination of health inequities as a critical part of a continuing strategy to reform health and mental health services in the USA. The Obama administration has pledged nearly $20 billion in the economic stimulus package to build health information technology. In addition, *Health Disparities: A Case for Closing the Gap* (Halle et al. 2009), prepared by the Office for Health Reform, also acknowledged the importance of quality, affordable, and accessible healthcare for women and minority populations as well as for other underserved areas (including rural populations).

Thus, major federal health and mental health reports and legislative initiatives have increasingly prioritized the elimination of mental health disparities as well as encouraged the development of integrated and accessible health and mental health information systems. However, in order to find and access information on women's mental health, one must first understand how information is organized, retrieved, and accessed.

Organizing Information

Instant electronic access to digital information is the single most distinguishing attribute of the information age. However, much as we would like to think that we can type in a couple of words or phrases and magically the exact information we want will appear, the truth is that information-seeking is a much more complicated process. Numerous databases exist within academic, organizational, and governmental institutions, each with its own elaborate retrieval mechanisms.

Within an information-seeking framework, one examines the behaviors and skills of individuals who have a research or clinical question (Weiler 2005; Meho and Tibbo 2003; Solomon 2002). To be able to frame a question, then ask the question using the language of search engines, and finally to successfully retrieve that specific answer amidst thousands or even tens of thousands of possible items can only be accomplished through an understanding of what information exists and, more importantly, how it is organized.

The effectiveness of a system in accessing information is a direct function of the organizing principles upon which it is built (Jordan 2006; Luo et al. 2004; Saade and Alexandre Otrakji 2007). Just as each of the practical fields in mental health rests upon its discipline's knowledge as its underlying base, so does the design of information systems, for organizing those disparate languages, rest upon an intellectual foundation. In order to be an effective (re)searcher, an understanding of how information is organized is essential.

Search engines are not created equal. We search for information in a variety of ways. Generally, we search using an author's name (personal name or organizational name), or a title of a report, or a specific topic. We may restrict the scope of our search by language, year, or type of work (e.g., government report, journal article, or legislation). Where we search also affects how we search and what we will retrieve. Most individuals start with the internet. There are numerous books and websites that address how to be a more effective internet searcher. As one purpose of this chapter is to review targeted, selected resources across a variety of providers, we encourage the readers to investigate the resources listed in the references at the end of this chapter for more information on internet searching (specifically Fink 2005; Friedman 2005; Hock 2007; Notess 2006).

Types of Information

Finding information on women's mental health in today's environment requires us to search across online, print, and media resources. Each resource has specialty content and formats, which may be proprietary, open access, or a combination of open and restricted access. Indexing and/or abstracting services, table of contents (TOC) services, citation databases, and numeric and spatial databases may be in a digital or print format. Each type of resource is different, and understanding these differences can make searching for relevant and pertinent information easier.

Indexing and/or Abstracting Services

Many online indexing and abstracting (I&A) databases started as print resources. *Index Medicus*, which started in 1879, evolved into the free online PubMed database offered by the National Library of Medicine (NLM; National Library of Medicine

2004). *Psychological Abstracts*, also a print resource, slowly morphed into PsycLIT (CD-ROM), then into PsycINFO, its current web-based form. Both databases are indexing and abstracting resources. Skilled indexers read and assign subject headings to all items indexed in PubMed and PsycINFO using the discipline-based vocabularies of the NLM's *Medical Subject Headings* (MeSH) and the American Psychological Association's *Thesaurus of Psychological Index Terms*, respectively (National Library of Medicine 2007; Tuleya 2007). Professional abstractors write abstracts for the indexed item, or the vendor may choose to use author-written abstracts.

The printed *Index Medicus* ceased publication at the end of 2004 and online *PubMed* was recognized as the definitive permanent source of *Index Medicus* (*Index Medicus to cease as print publication* 2004). Unlike *PubMed, PsycINFO* is proprietary, i.e., you must have a current personal or institutional subscription to a vendor, such as *Cambridge Scientific Abstracts*, *OVID*, or *EBSCO*, to have access.

Table of Contents Services

TOC services keep users updated with information about the latest journal publications and Internet-based resources as they become available. Some TOC services are databases, such as *Current Contents Connect*®, which provide access to *complete* tables of contents, with bibliographic information and abstracts from selected scholarly journals across a variety of disciplines. Other TOC services are through journal vendor sites, which are free, or through academic databases, which may be proprietary.

Citation Databases

What we are calling citation databases are the Thomson/ISI citation databases, i.e., *Web of Science*, *Web of Knowledge*, or the Social Science, Science, and Arts and Humanities Citation Indexes, all of which are proprietary resources. Composed of three major content areas, arts and humanities, social sciences, and science, they are multidisciplinary databases of bibliographic information gathered from thousands of scholarly journals. In addition to its basic search features, subject, author, journal, and/or author address, each indexed article also includes the article's cited reference list (i.e., bibliography). This feature allows the user to search the databases for articles that cite a known author or work.

Tracking cited authors or known works has many benefits. As an author, you see who is citing your research and how your research is influencing newer research. You can track the directions in which specific research is progressing based on earlier studies and analyze the impact of published research. It is also an easy way to keep up-to-date with what is happening in a specialized literature and with the works of specific authors in a specific substantive field.

Numeric and Spatial Databases

There are literally thousands of numeric and spatial databases used in mental health and substance abuse services research. These range from open source and proprietary access general statistics databases to demographic and population-based databases. Furthermore, it includes surveillance and epidemiology databases and data available at the micro-, meso-, and macrolevels.

A spatial database is a database optimized to store and query data related to objects in space. A geographic information system (GIS) manipulates numeric and spatial data into a visual display, such as a map, chart, or graph. Since a GIS has the ability to apply spatial operators to data and the ability to link data sets together, it is useful in asking what and where questions pertaining to location and time (Hanson 2001).

When examining the types of data used in women's mental health services research, there are five major types of data. *Demographic and outcomes data* describe the prevalence of conditions such as poverty, household composition, employment, and crime. *Service data* capture what services are currently available to residents. *Resource data* capture the governance and financing systems that control community resources. *Geographic data* map the spatial location of the neighborhood by zip code, census tract, local neighborhood boundaries, or other specific designations. *Infrastructure data* describe transportation systems, storm water and sewage facilities, streets and sidewalks, the age of physical facilities, and other aspects of the physical environment of a neighborhood.

Keeping the five types of data mentioned in the previous paragraph in mind, consider the following questions (Hanson 2001, p. 58):

"What is at X?"
"How do I get from X to Y?"
"Where is this condition true [or not true]?"
"What has changed since …?"
"What are the pattern(s)?"
"What if we change Z?"

The first question asks what exists at a specific location. A GIS can use a variety of data, such as a place name, a postal code, geographical coordinates, or a census block. The second question links two locations and answers what is between points X and Y. The third question, true/not true, asks if that place satisfies certain conditions (e.g., is there a treatment center by bus route #45?). The fourth question looks for the changes at a location at two different moments in time. The fifth question determines patterns, such as surveillance clusters of mental or physical illnesses or the increase of service centers. The last question tries to determine what will happen if something new is added (Hanson 2001).

Tools and Tips: Thesauri, Controlled Vocabulary, and Filters

One of the most important things to remember when searching for information is that the tools that are available for use vary across databases, across disciplines, and across skill levels. It is critical to use the tools that come with online resources to effectively capture the relevant information necessary in women's mental health and substance abuse services research and services delivery. The mantra for searching is simple: A well-constructed search should provide precision and relevance in recall with allowance for serendipity. This simply means that the search results (recall) should be relevant to a specific topic, should have a high degree of precision in terminology and concept, and still allow an individual to capture emergent or novel trends (serendipity).

As in any search, we begin with key concepts, using the language of our everyday workplace. However, our "everyday language" may not be the same "everyday language" articulated by the author or by the specific vocabulary used in a specific database. Specific disciplines each use a specific (controlled) vocabulary found in a specialized thesaurus. A controlled vocabulary encompasses the headings or terms used by indexers within a discipline.

Why don't searches work? There are a number of reasons. *PubMed*, for example, uses an automatic term-mapping feature. That means you can type in your "everyday language" and *PubMed* runs the terms first as a phrase "against" the MeSH headings, then against journal names, and finally against author and investigator names. *PubMed* searches until it finds a match. If no match is found, *PubMed* breaks the phrase down into discrete words and maps each word as an AND with the next word, much like a key concept. If a search does not turn out the way you thought it should, clicking on the DETAILS tab allows you to view the query box and the syntax used to run the search.

For example, if we use the term DUAL DIAGNOSIS AND WOMEN AND TREATMENT, 3,072 items are retrieved; however, the search is not as successful, since *PubMed* is unable to match the phrase "dual diagnosis" and breaks it into separate words. Thus, articles such as "Single-operator double-balloon endoscopy (DBE) is as effective as dual-operator DBE" are retrieved. If we run a search on the terms WOMEN CO-OCCURRING DISORDERS TREATMENT, 456 items that are more relevant appear, such as the article "Women with co-occurring disorders (COD): Treatment settings and service needs," which displays all the terms in the title. However, if we change the display to the *MEDLINE* display, we can see the MeSH terms, which include ADOLESCENT, ADULT, BATTERED WOMEN/* PSYCHOLOGY, CRIME, FEMALE, HUMANS, MENTAL DISORDERS/* THERAPY<MIDDLE-AGED, SUBSTANCE-RELATED DISORDERS/*THERAPY, AND TREATMENT OUTCOME. If we change our search to SUBSTANCE-RELATED DISORDERS/*THERAPY AND FEMALE AND HUMANS, suddenly we have 21,848 articles to review, of which 1,589 are reviews of the literature. Why is this the case? Because CO-OCCURRING DISORDERS is not a MeSH term or phrase. This is one way to start learning which headings will retrieve relevant articles in a specific field.

Filters, or limits, come in many "flavors." They may allow you to restrict the search by author, year, journal, language, full-text/free full-text only, gender, age, type of article, and many more categories, depending on the database used. One of the most useful filters (outside of gender, age, or language) is type of article. Again, using *PubMed*, you can limit your search to clinical trial, practice guideline, or case reports. Two of the best "type of article" filters are meta-analysis and review. Meta-analyses scrutinize methods and methodologies of empirical research. Many evidence-based practice articles focus on meta-analyses to determine best practices for a disorder in an age group and/or of a particular linguistic or cultural group. If we limit our current search by type of ARTICLE = META-ANALYSIS AND AGES = AGED: 65+ YEARS AND LANGUAGES = ENGLISH, there are 13 meta-analyses addressing the efficacy of specific drugs, brief interventions for hazardous drinkers, counseling as intervention for cocaine-abusing methadone-maintenance patients, and effectiveness of brief interventions to reduce alcohol intake in primary healthcare populations: a meta-analysis, among others.

Review articles provide a longitudinal or cross-sectional view of a topic. If we limit our current search by type of ARTICLE = REVIEW AND AGES = AGED: 65+ YEARS AND LANGUAGES = ENGLISH, there are 146 review articles, ranging from psychosocial interventions for cocaine to the global burden of disease from alcohol, illicit drugs, and tobacco. Filters can exclude irrelevance in a search and create relevant and focused searches.

Caveats

Many indexing and abstracting (I&A) resources offer access to full-text; however, access to the resource may be restricted. PsycINFO provides access to selected full-text, based on the institutional holdings. If the institution subscribes to a journal, then online access is available. If not, the user must locate a print copy or request a copy through interlibrary loan. PubMed, for example, provides free access to materials in PubMed Central or through other open-access repositories. However, similar to PsycINFO, not everything in PubMed is available online. However, the strength of article databases is the identification of targeted content. After identification of content, acquiring content can be available on a pay-per-item basis or through libraries.

The same is true of numeric and geospatial data. Whether the data are under the public domain, public sector, or leased proprietary data, issues of intellectual property, data redistribution rights, and derivative rights must be addressed in the use, reuse, or manipulation of geospatial data (Hanson 2008). Although researchers have responsibilities to promulgate their research, retaining rights over how their results are used affects access to primary or derivative data, especially for long-term or multiyear studies (Hanson 2008).

Sources of Information

Let us start with a disclaimer. Information-seeking, finding, and retrieval in women's mental health require complex cognitive and behavioral processes. Numerous entities at all levels create and publish information, including government, academic, professional, consumer, advocacy, and individual, to name just a few. Each entity has its preferred distribution or communication channels, its preferred formats, and its preferred schedules. Limited space does not allow the authors of this chapter to cover all the many authoritative resources available to savvy (re)searchers. The following discussion, by definition, will highlight selected free or academic resources, attempting to address broad content areas as well as to provide a context for future exploration by the reader.

National Library of Medicine (NLM) Gateway

The NLM Gateway provides free "one-stop" shopping for many of the NLM's information databases and catalogs (http://gateway.nlm.nih.gov/gw/Cmd). Within the Gateway, you can search bibliographic, consumer, and other online resources. Bibliographic resources include MEDLINE/PubMed, which contains journal citations from 1950 to the present; the NLM catalog of monographs, serials, and media; and the Bookshelf of full-text biomedical books. Also included in the bibliographic resources are the TOXLINE subset (toxicology), DART (Developmental and Reproductive Toxicology), and Meeting Abstracts. Most of these databases allow you to export your search into citation management software (including ProCite, EndNote, and RefWorks).

Consumer health resources include the Medline Plus suite of resources: Health Topics; Drug Information; Medical Encyclopedia; Current Health News and directories; DIRLINE (Directory of Information Resources Online, organizations, research resources, projects, and database), Genetics Home Reference (genetic conditions), and a Household Products Database.

In the "other information resources," in addition to additional toxicology databases (Hazardous Substances Data Bank), there are HSRProj (Health Services Research Projects in Progress) and ClinicalTrials.gov. HSRProj is an important guide to ongoing grants and contracts in health services research. Searches are by keyword, investigator, and supporting agency. There is also a map feature, where, as of June 2009, there were 145 projects in Florida, with links to a more descriptive record including keywords, abstract, contact information, agency, grant type and number, and status. ClinicalTrials.gov is a registry of federally and privately supported clinical trials conducted in the USA and internationally. Each record includes sponsor, identifier number, purpose, eligibility, contacts, location, topic categories, and MeSH terms. Currently there are 74,322 clinical trials in 167 countries. It also has an excellent FAQ (frequently asked questions) and glossary.

Not only does PubMed provide free access to MEDLINE (16 million references) and indexes and abstracts for approximately 5,000 national and international biomedical journals, there are also two special features of interest to clinicians. On the Clinical Queries page (customized searches on the etiology, diagnosis, prognosis, or treatment of specific diseases), there is another search option for systematic reviews (SRs). This search option allows users to find a variety of resources, including SRs, meta-analyses, and clinical trials reviews. Evidence-based medicine (practice), consensus development conferences, and guidelines are also available. A word about

SRs versus literature reviews. An SR is a more rigorous literature review, as it tries to reduce bias by identifying, appraising, selecting, and synthesizing *all* quality research evidence relevant for that question. Each SR follows a peer-reviewed protocol based on the Cochrane Collaboration protocol for SRs.

The Cochrane Collaboration: Cochrane Reviews

Another source for SRs online is the Cochrane Collaboration Cochrane Reviews (http://www.cochrane.org/reviews/). Unlike PubMed's SRs, which are full-text, the Cochrane Collaboration only makes the abstracts of its reviews available online. Subscriptions to the *Cochrane* suite of databases are often available at universities that have medical schools or schools/colleges of public health. You can search the abstracts (natural language), browse an alphabetical-by-title list, or browse by topic (according to Cochrane Review Groups). For a review of clinical studies, the rigor of an SR cannot be matched. It will not be anecdotal in nature. It will be clear as to the method of analysis and explain why it excludes some research studies while including others.

The PILOTS Database: An Electronic Index to the Traumatic Stress Literature

The PILOTS database (http://www.ncptsd.va.gov/ncmain/publications/pilots/), developed at Dartmouth's Center for Posttraumatic Stress Disorder, covers national and international literature on posttraumatic stress disorder (PTSD) and other mental health consequences of exposure to traumatic events. Each bibliographic record in the PILOTS database contains a bibliographic citation, an abstract or description of the article's content, descriptors or key terms to allow users to construct searches using PILOTS' controlled vocabulary, and the titles of the tests or measures used in the article (if applicable). You can also export your search into citation management software (ProCite, EndNote, and RefWorks). Another benefit is the ability to create a "My Research" online area on PILOTS. There are videos, manuals, and guides for the general public, veterans and their families, and mental health providers.

Centers for Disease Control and Prevention (CDC): WISQARS™, YPLL, NVDRS, ARDI

Within the CDC, there are a number of resources pertinent to women's mental health: WISQARS™; Years of Potential Life Lost (YPLL); the National Violent Death Reporting System (NVDRS); and the Alcohol-Related Disease Impact (ARDI).

WISQARS™ (Web-based Injury Statistics Query and Reporting System; http://www.cdc.gov/ncipc/WISQARS/) is an interactive database system that provides customized reports of injury-related (morbidity and mortality) data. Data are divided into fatal and non-fatal injuries. In addition to injury reports and leading-causes reports on WISQARS™, there are two underutilized data sources: YPLL (http://webappa.cdc.gov/sasweb/ncipc/ypll.html) and the NVDRS (http://www.cdc.gov/ncipc/profiles/nvdrs/). Both datasets allow you to select men or women only or comparison tables of both. The YPLL, which measures the relative impact of lethal forces and diseases on a population, is a useful way to draw attention to the loss of expected years of life as a result of deaths in childhood, adolescence, and early adult life (Gardner and Sanborn 1990). In 2009, there were 2006 data available for YPLL, NVDRS, and WISQARS.

The NVDRS is a state-based surveillance system linking data from law enforcement, offices of vital statistics, crime laboratories, coroners, and medical examiners. It currently covers 17 states (Alaska, California, Colorado, Georgia, Kentucky, Maryland, Massachusetts, New Jersey, New Mexico, North Carolina, Oklahoma, Oregon, Rhode Island, South Carolina, Utah, Virginia, and Wisconsin), with plans to cover all 50 states, the District of Columbia, and the US territories.

Another interactive database, ARDI (http://www.cdc.gov/Alcohol/ardi.htm), generates estimates of alcohol-related deaths and YPLL due to alcohol consumption. Data break outs are by state, age, gender, and cause of death. The ARDI software also allows states to calculate direct healthcare costs, indirect morbidity and morality costs, and nonhealth-sector costs associated with alcohol misuse.

Alcohol and Alcohol Problems Science Database: ETOH

ETOH (http://etoh.niaaa.nih.gov/) is a database of historic national and international alcohol-related research information (1972–2003), produced by the National Institute on Alcohol Abuse and Alcoholism (NIAAA). Highly structured with a controlled vocabulary, there is an AOD Thesaurus basic search to find preferred terms to use in the ETOH search engine. ETOH's bibliographic record contains the citation and information on who funded the project, and if a federal grant, the grant number. After running the search, a list of citations appears. Clicking on the checkbox, then the SUBMIT EDITS button, brings up the abstract. Unfortunately, there are no descriptors attached to the abstract to allow the user to expand or narrow one's search.

Center for the Study and Prevention of Violence (CSPV): VioLit, VioEval

The CSPV (http://www.colorado.edu/cspv/) at the Institute of Behavioral Science at the University of Colorado at Boulder has four databases: VioLit, VioEval, VioPro, and VioSource. VioLit provides bibliographic citations and CSPV-authored abstracts of the violence-related research and literature on juvenile violence. Records contain the article citation, abstract written by CSVP staff, and keywords. Violence Evaluation Instruments Database (VioEval) is a compilation of data collection tools available on violence-related topics and for program evaluation purposes. This is an excellent supplement to Buros Mental Measurements and Test Critiques. As with VioLit, there is a controlled vocabulary available. Choosing VIOLENCE AGAINST WOMEN brings up 30 measures. Records may contain author, title, and publisher information, URL of test publisher website or link to academic journal article, a description of the test, cost information if available, references, and additional keywords, depending on availability of information. VioPro and VioSource carry information about violence prevention programs and violence-related curricula and media, respectively.

FedStats.gov: Topics, MapStats, Statistical Reference Shelf

FedStats.gov provides a one-stop shop for statistics from over 100 agencies covering numerous topics including agriculture (i.e., rural populations), crime, demographics, economics, education, environment, health, income, labor, safety, and more. What is important is the wealth of information available through government agencies. What is also important is the subject structure and description of the resources. It is not an intuitive site. If you look under Topics A–Z, for example, mental health is listed under Hazardous Substances—Cigarettes. However, mental health is also found using a broader population topic, such as children, or hidden in categories covering services, utilization, insurance, and services expenditures. It may be easier for new users to spend time browsing the agency site to become familiar with what products are available.

Quick statistics on states are found using MapStats, which includes a mix of current year minus one (e.g., 2008 statistics in current year 2009) and census data. MapStats provides profiles of a state, a county, a city, or congressional and federal judicial districts. The "Statistics by geography from U.S. agencies" link provides international, national, state, county, and local comparisons across major topic areas and links the topic to the specific agency providing the statistics.

The Statistical Reference Shelf provides full-text access to two seminal reference materials, the *Statistical Abstract of the United States* (1878 to current year minus 1) and *Health, United States* (1975 to current year minus 1). The *Statistical Abstract* is the authoritative and comprehensive summary of social, political, and economic statistics of the USA. Tables are provided in Adobe Acrobat (.pdf) or in Microsoft Excel (.xls). *Health, United States*, provides an annual snapshot of trends on health status and healthcare utilization, resources, and expenditures as well as variation in health, health behaviors, and healthcare in the USA. Race/ethnicity, gender, educational attainment, income level, and geographic location are indicators collected in this volume. Generally, each annual report has a special feature. The 2008 report features young adults, 18–29 years of age. Previous chartbooks featured special sections on access to care, adults 55–64, and urban and rural health.

The National Academies Press (NAP)

The NAP publishes online the 4,000+ reports issued by the National Academy of Sciences, the National Academy of Engineering, the Institute of Medicine, and the National Research Council. An authoritative source for materials addressing critical issues in science and health policy, NAP publications are freely available online for reading, and have executive summaries available for printing or purchase through their website. Unlike Google Books where portions of text may be missing, NAP monographs are full-text and searchable with a simple text search engine. You can start with the simple search feature across all books using a simple construct enclosed within double quotes, e.g., "mental health." The use of double quotations around a phrase results in the words in the phrase adjacent to each other as opposed to the words anywhere in the book. Once the list of books is generated, you can again search within the book using phrases ("within double quotes") or using single words. The search engine does not handle possessives, so you cannot use terms such as "women's mental health". The "show in context" links will take you right to the page where the word or phrase is located, rather than having to skim or read the entire chapter.

In addition, the NAP site provides two research tools, the "Web Search Builder" and the "Reference Finder". The Web Search builder allows you to use the book's keywords to explore within the book, across the NAP collection or across the web. Reference Finder is a "find more like this text" search tool. You can paste up to eight pages of text and ask the Finder to search the NAP reports on the site or to search the web (Google, Yahoo, MSN, and press sites). It extracts a series of keywords from the provided text, puts them into the NAP search engine, then aggregates and displays the NAP texts that seem most appropriate. Both tools allow you to add new terms of your choice to the list that NAP provides.

Current and Emerging Technologies

Web 2.0 is the second generation of web development and web design. O'Reilly (2005, p. 3) describes Web 2.0 as "the business revolution in the computer industry caused by the move to the Internet as a platform, and an attempt to understand the rules for success on that new platform." Web 2.0 has spawned new web-based communities, hosted services, and applications, such as social networking sites, digital media sites (video, audio, and mash-up), wikis, blogs, and social tagging sites (folksonomies, or user-generated taxonomies). These new technologies and applications foster important advances in how we can "pull and push" specific information.

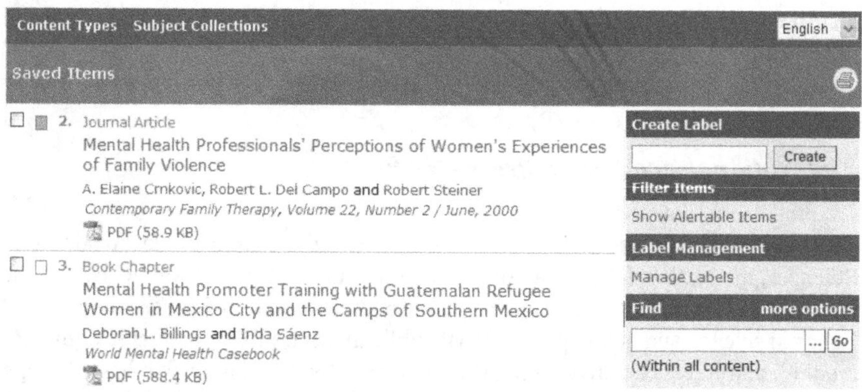

Fig. 20.1 Personal archive for the Journal of Behavioral Health Services & Research. (This image, from springerlink.com, is used with permission of Springer Science+Business Media)

Pull technologies allow the user to request information from a website, such as a database where a query generates a display or exportable information. One example of a pull technology is when you are on a journal article webpage. For example, on Springer's *Journal of Behavioral Health Services & Research* (JBHS&R) website, you have the option for creating a personal archive.

In addition to the citation and abstract, there may be an additional column on the right-hand side of the page. Under Services (see Fig. 20.1), you have the option to find similar articles in the journal or in PubMed. You must be on the webpage to access the service or product.

Push technologies, on the other hand, target services directly to the user. These include RSS (really simple syndication), email alerts (e-alerts), blogs, and wikis to name a few (Fig. 20.2). RSS allows users to subscribe to updates from a website based on subject interest. "Feeds" allows a content provider to syndicate content and "push" content to RSS "readers" located on individual computers. For example, Substance Abuse and Mental Health Services Administration's Health Information Network (SHIN) runs three RSS feeds: new publications, eNetwork archive (e.g., webcasts, etc.), and publications and materials (observances, campaigns, etc.).

- **Email this article**
- **PubMed citations**
- **Find related articles**
- **Find related articles in PubMed**
- **Related subject collections**
- **Alert me to new issues**
- **Alert me when this article is cited**
- **Alert me if corrections are posted**
- **Add to my personal archive**
- **Download to citation manager**

Fig. 20.2 Example of pull and push services for *JBHS&R*. (This image, from springerlink.com, is used with permission of Springer Science+Business Media)

SHIN also provides the option to use an email alert rather than a feeder in those facilities whose HIPAA (Health Insurance Portability and Accountability Act) compliance constraints may not allow the use of syndicated feeds. The National Institute of Mental Health (NIMH) and the Agency for Healthcare Research and Quality (AHRQ) websites, for example, provide RSS feeds whenever the site is updated or changed. As with email, RSS feeds will accumulate on your computer, so it becomes another daily read, store, or delete routine.

For many people, RSS is one more technology to have to monitor and review. E-alerts, which arrive automatically via email, are often the easiest option for users. E-alerts come in a number of "flavors." One type of e-alert is updates from websites. All federal websites provide an option to subscribe to an alert whenever the agency updates a particular page or site. This is a good way to track changes on guidelines or best practices pages, legislative update sites, or new tools, to name just a few. Another e-alert service tracks journal updates. On almost all online journal sites, users can opt to receive e-alerts of the TOC for each new issue (Fig. 20.3).

In addition to the TOC alerts, you can also track when a specific article you like is cited, corrected, or commented upon, when specific authors publish a new paper, or when new articles appear based on keywords chosen. These "Cite Track Alerts" are available in participating journal publishers, such as HighWire Press, Oxford Journals, and Sage Publications.

Blogs and wikis are often downplayed as authoritative sites. A blog, or web log, is a chronologically ordered, periodically updated site, while a wiki is a collaborative authoring software using a web browser. Both applications support hypertext links and RSS, as well as other more complex Web 2.0 applications. Numerous healthcare facilities, providers, and academic/research libraries use blogs and wikis as a way to provide current updates on topics. One example is Massachusetts General's

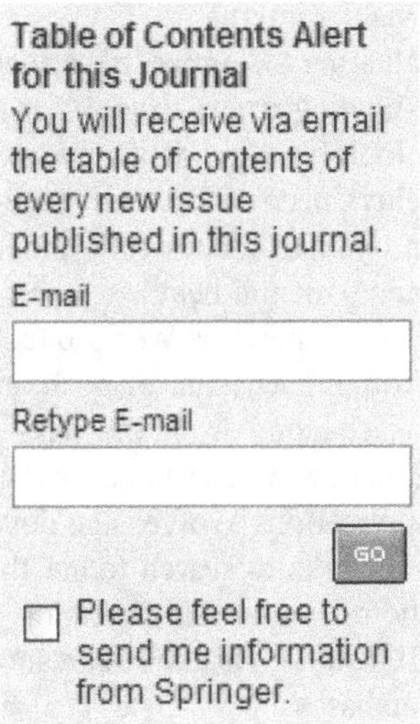

Fig. 20.3 Table of contents alert for the Journal of Behavioral Health Services & Research. (This image, from springer.com, is used with permission of Springer Science+Business Media)

Center for Women's Mental Health, which provides content across the intersection of physical and mental health (http://www.womensmentalhealth.org/blog/). Women and Substance Abuse, a blog about addiction, treatment, and recovery, provides updates on federal and state initiatives, uses both e-alerts and RSS, and lists other blogs and resources. It is run by *Crossroads for Women*, a 30-year-old substance abuse and mental health organization in Maine. The *Loop*, run by the Louis de la Parte Florida Mental Health Institute Research Library at the University of South Florida, provides updates on new resources, grant opportunities, web events, legislation, and trends, and also allows users RSS or to subscribe to its distribution list. Womenshealth.gov, one of many federal agencies, actively advocates linking its site to blogs on women's health and mental health issues. Clearly, depending on one's research, professional, or personal interests, one can push and pull information from a variety of resources, organizations, and formats.

Implications for Women's Mental Health

This chapter briefly examined a number of major national health and mental health reports, all emphasizing the current disparities in health and mental health services in America as well as the urgency and need to develop a national electronic telecommunications system for surveillance of health and mental health data. In order to analyze, evaluate, and propose alternatives to improve women's mental health services delivery through the implementation of policy changes, it is critical to be able to find and access relevant data from national and state sources as well as through the academic literature. Information on women's mental health is published in a variety of formats and locations. The interdisciplinary nature of services research and services delivery together with the proliferation of information results in accessibility issues in obtaining and synthesizing this information directly and free of charge via the internet.

A key to evaluating the impact of services delivery on the implementation of policy change is knowing *where* to look for supporting data, *how* to more effectively and efficiently look for these data, and *what* data sources contain reliable and valid data. (Re)searchers need to become more comfortable with current and emerging technologies in order to successfully navigate the disparate worlds of information regarding women's mental health services. For example, Web 2.0 technologies, as resources, will be old news as Web 3.0 technologies emerge.

As shown in the discussion of push and pull technologies, how we search for information has changed from the days of Web 1.0. Web 3.0 will mean more changes, again, in how we use and access online resources for research as new technologies and applications evolve. The development of a semantic web, which uses *contextual* frameworks to search rather than simply matching words and phrases, will increase the relevance and precision of internet searches. The same semantic technology will also increase the relevance and precision of searches in academic and research databases.

This requires the user to have a more complete understanding of the terminology of his or her field or discipline within the larger framework of women's mental health. Hence, spending the time to understand the conceptual organization of knowledge within disciplines, as evidenced through the many finding tools and databases, is critical for today's researcher.

America faces an unprecedented opportunity to improve women's mental health through both information and technology use and creation. Translating increased knowledge and evidence-based methods into daily practice requires us to ensure effective information-seeking and retrieval behaviors are part of the skill sets provided in established educational curricula within formal education, in continuing professional development, and within the workplace. This integrates the distal and proximal knowledge that practitioners derive from practice and from learning. Such an understanding then becomes another translational tool as we move from research to practice to policy.

References

Index Medicus to cease as print publication. (2004, May–June). *NLM Technical Bulletin, 338*, e2. Retrieved January 12, 2009, from http://www.nlm.nih.gov/pubs/techbull/mj04/mj04_im.html

Fink, A. (2005). *Conducting research literature reviews: From the Internet to paper* (2nd ed.). Thousand Oaks, CA: Sage Publications.

Friedman, B. (2005). *Web search savvy strategies and shortcuts for online research*. Mahwah, NJ: Lawrence Erlbaum.

Gardner, J. W., & Sanborn, J. S. (1990). Years of potential life lost (YPLL) – what does it measure? *Epidemiology, 1*(4), 322–329.

Halle, M., Lewis, C. B., & Seshamani, M. (2009). *Health disparities: A case for closing the gap*. Washington, DC: Office of Health Reform. http://www.healthreform.gov/reports/healthdisparities/disparities_final.pdf

Hanson, A. (2001). Community assessments using map and geographic data. *Behavioral and Social Sciences Librarian, 19*(2), 49–62.

Hanson, A. (2008). Reference services. In J. Abresch, A. Hanson, S. J. Heron, & P. Reehling (Eds.), *Integrating geographic information systems into library services: A guide for academic libraries* (pp. 175–201). Hershey, PA: Information Science Publishing.

Hock, R. (2007). *The extreme searcher's Internet handbook: A guide for the serious searcher* (2nd ed.). Medford, NJ: CyberAge Books.

Jordan, M. (2006). The CARL metadata harvester and search service. *Library Hi Tech, 24*(2), 197–210.

Luo, Y., Liu, X., Wang, X., Wang, W., & Xu, Z. (2004). Design open sharing framework for spatial information in semantic web. In H. Jin, Y. Pan, N. Xiao, & J. Sun (Eds.), *Grid and Cooperative Computing: GCC 2004 Third International Conference, Wuhan, China, October 21–24, 2004, proceedings* (pp. 145–152). Berlin, Germany: Springer-Verlag GmbH.

Meho, L. I., & Tibbo, H. R. (2003). Modeling the information-seeking behavior of social scientists: Ellis's study revisited. *Journal of the American Society for Information Science and Technology, 54*(6), 570–587.

National Library of Medicine. (2004). *Milestones in NLM history.* Retrieved January 6, 2009, from http://www.nlm.nih.gov/about/nlmhistory.html

National Library of Medicine. (2007). *Medical subject headings, use of MeSH in indexing*. Bethesda, MD: U.S. National Library of Medicine, National Institutes of Health, Health & Human Services.

Notess, G. R. (2006). *Teaching Web search skills: Techniques and strategies of top trainers*. Medford, NJ: Information Today, Inc.

O'Reilly, T. (2005). *Web 2.0 compact definition: Trying again*. Sebastopol, CA: O'Reilly Media, Inc. Retrieved May 30, 2009, from http://radar.oreilly.com/archives/2006/12/web_20_compact.html

President's New Freedom Commission on Mental Health (2003). *Achieving the promise: Transforming mental health care in America. Final Report* (DHHS Publication No. SMA-03-3832). Rockville, MD: President's New Freedom Commission on Mental Health. Retrieved May 19, 2009, from http://www.mentalhealthcommission.gov/reports/FinalReport/toc.html

Saade, R. G., & Alexandre Otrakji, C. (2007). First impressions last a lifetime: Effect of interface type on disorientation and cognitive load. *Computers in Human Behavior, 23*(1), 525–535.

Solomon, P. (2002). Discovering information in context. *Annual Review of Information Science and Technology, 36*, 229–264.

Tuleya, L. G. (2007). *Thesaurus of psychological index terms* (11th ed.). Washington, DC: American Psychological Association.

U.S. Department of Health and Human Services. (2005). *Surgeon General's workshop on women's mental health*. Washington, DC: Office of the Surgeon General, U.S. Public Health Service. Retrieved May 19, 2009, from http://www.surgeongeneral.gov/topics/womensmentalhealth/

U.S. Department of Health and Human Services. (1991). *Healthy people 2000: National health promotion and disease prevention objectives*. Washington, DC: U.S. Government Printing Office.

U.S. Department of Health and Human Services. (2000). *Healthy people 2010, With understanding and improving health and objectives for improving health (2 vols.)* (2nd ed.). Washington, DC: U.S. Government Printing Office.

U.S. Department of Health and Human Services, Office of the Surgeon General. (1999). *Mental health: A report of the Surgeon General*. Rockville, MD: Dept. of Health and Human Services, U.S. Public Health Service.

Vikram, P. (2005). *Gender in mental health research*. Geneva, Switzerland: World Health Organization. Available online at http://www.who.int/gender/documents/MentalHealthlast2.pdf. Accessed June 18, 2009.

Weiler, A. (2005). Information-seeking behavior in generation Y students: Motivation, critical thinking, and learning theory. *Journal of Academic Librarianship, 31*(1), 46–53.

Index

E

I

T